MINERAL ABSORPTION IN THE MONOGASTRIC GI TRACT

ADVANCES IN EXPERIMENTAL MEDICINE AND BIOLOGY

Recent Volumes in this Series

Volume 243
EICOSANOIDS, APOLIPOPROTEINS, LIPOPROTEIN PARTICLES,
AND ATHEROSCLEROSIS
Edited by Claude L. Malmendier and Petar Alaupovic

Volume 244
THE EXPANDING ROLE OF FOLATES AND FLUOROPYRIMIDINES
IN CANCER CHEMOTHERAPY
Edited by Youcef Rustum and John J. McGuire

Volume 245
MECHANISMS OF PHYSICAL AND EMOTIONAL STRESS
Edited by George P. Chrousos, D. Lynn Loriaux, and Philip W. Gold

Volume 246
PREDIABETES
Edited by Rafael A. Camerini-Davalos and Harold S. Cole

Volume 247A
KININS V, Part A
Edited by Keishi Abe, Hiroshi Moriya, and Setsuro Fujii

Volume 247B
KININS V, Part B
Edited by Keishi Abe, Hiroshi Moriya, and Setsuro Fujii

Volume 248
OXYGEN TRANSPORT TO TISSUE XI
Edited by Karel Rakusan, George P. Biro, Thomas K. Goldstick, and Zdenek Turek

Volume 249
MINERAL ABSORPTION IN THE MONOGASTRIC GI TRACT:
Chemical, Nutritional, and Physiological Aspects
Edited by Frederick R. Dintzis and Joseph A. Laszlo

Volume 250
PROGRESS IN POLYAMINE RESEARCH:
Novel Biochemical, Pharmacological, and Clinical Aspects
Edited by Vincenzo Zappia and Anthony E. Pegg

A Continuation Order Plan is available for this series. A continuation order will bring delivery of each new volume immediately upon publication. Volumes are billed only upon actual shipment. For further information please contact the publisher.

MINERAL ABSORPTION IN THE MONOGASTRIC GI TRACT

Edited by

Frederick R. Dintzis
and Joseph A. Laszlo

US Department of Agriculture
Agricultural Research Service
Northern Regional Research Center
Peoria, Illinois

SPRINGER SCIENCE+BUSINESS MEDIA, LLC

Library of Congress Cataloging in Publication Data

Mineral absorption in the monogastric GI tract: chemical, nutritional, and physiological aspects / edited by Frederick R. Dintzis and Joseph A. Laszlo.
    p.   cm. — (Advances in experimental medicine and biology; v. 249)
    "Proceedings of an ACS meeting on Mineral Absorption in the Monogastric GI Tract: Chemical, Nutritional, and Physiological Aspects, held June 9–10, 1988, in Toronto, Canada" — T.p. verso.
    Includes bibliographies and index.
    ISBN 978-1-4684-9113-5   ISBN 978-1-4684-9111-1 (eBook)
    DOI 10.1007/978-1-4684-9111-1
    1. Mineral metabolism — Congresses. 2. Intestinal absorption — Congresses. I. Dintzis, Frederick R. II. Laszlo, Joseph A. III. American Chemical Society. Meeting. (195th: 1988: Toronto, Canada) IV. Title. V. Series.
QP165.M63   1989   89-30356
612′.392 — dc19   CIP

Proceedings of an ACS meeting on Mineral Absorption in the
Monogastric GI Tract: Chemical, Nutrional, and Physiological Aspects,
held June 9–10, 1988, in Toronto, Canada

© 1989 Springer Science+Business Media New York
Originally published by Plenum Press, New York in 1989
Softcover reprint of the hardcover 1st edition 1989

Contributors

H. James Armbrecht, Geriatric Research, Education, and Clinical Center, St. Louis Veterans Administration Medical Center, St. Louis, Missouri 63125 and Departments of Medicine and Biochemistry, St. Louis University School of Medicine, St. Louis, Missouri, USA 63104

Frederick L. Baker, U.S. Department of Agriculture, Agricultural Research Service, Northern Regional Research Center, 1815 N. University St., Peoria, Illinois, USA 61604

Marie M. Cassidy, Department of Physiology, The George Washington University Medical Center, Washington, District of Columbia, USA 20037

Elaine T. Champagne, U.S. Department of Agriculture, Agricultural Research Service, Southern Regional Research Center, P.O. Box 19687, New Orleans, Louisiana, USA 70179

James D. Cook, Department of Medicine, University of Kansas Medical Center, Kansas City, Kansas, USA 66103

Robert J. Cousins, Food Science and Human Nutrition Department and Center for Nutritional Sciences, University of Florida, Gainesville, Florida, USA 32611

Sandra A. Dassenko, Department of Medicine, University of Kansas Medical Center, Kansas City, Kansas, USA 66103

Frederick R. Dintzis, U.S. Department of Agriculture, Agricultural Research Service, Northern Regional Research Center, 1815 N. University St., Peoria, Illinois, USA 61604

John W. Erdman, Jr., Division of Food Science, University of Illinois at Urbana-Champaign, 580 Bevier Hall, 905 S. Goodwin Ave., Urbana, Illinois, USA 61801

Peter R. Flanagan, Departments of Medicine and Biochemistry, The University of Western Ontario, London, Ontario, Canada N6A 5A5

Curtis S. Fullmer, Department of Physiology, New York State College of
    Veterinary Medicine, Cornell University, Ithaca, New York, USA 14853

Wesley R. Harris, Department of Chemistry, University of Missouri-St. Louis,
    St. Louis, Missouri, USA 63121

Richard F. Hurrell, Nestle Research Center, Nestec Ltd., Vers-chez-les-Blanc,
    CH-1000, Lausanne 26, Switzerland

Joseph A. Laszlo, U.S. Department of Agriculture, Agricultural Research Service,
    Northern Regional Research Center, 1815 N. University St., Peoria,
    Illinois, USA 61604

Sean R. Lynch, Medical Service, Veterans Administration Medical Center,
    Hampton, Virginia, USA 23667

Timothy J. Peters, Division of Clinical Cell Biology, Clinical Research Centre,
    Watford Road, Harrow, Middlesex, UK HA1 3UJ

Angela Poneros-Schneier, Division of Food Science, University of Illinois at
    Urbana-Champaign, 580 Bevier Hall, 905 S. Goodwin Ave., Urbana,
    Illinois, USA 61801

Kishor B. Raja, Division of Clinical Cell Biology, Clinical Research Centre,
    Watford Road, Harrow, Middlesex, UK HA1 3UJ

Robert J. Simpson, Division of Clinical Cell Biology, Clinical Research Centre,
    Watford Road, Harrow, Middlesex, UK HA1 3UJ

Tim S. Stahly, University of Kentucky, Agricultural Experiment Station,
    Department of Animal Science, Lexington, Kentucky, USA 40546-0215

Raul A. Wapnir, North Shore University Hospital and Cornell University Medical
    College, Department of Pediatrics, Manhasset, New York, USA 11030

Robert H. Wasserman, Department of Physiology, New York State College of
    Veterinary Medicine, Cornell University, Ithaca, New York, USA 14853

Meryl E. Wastney, Department of Pediatrics, Georgetown University, 3800
    Reservoir Road, N. W., Washington, District of Columbia, USA 20007

Don W. Watkins, Department of Physiology, The George Washington University
    Medical Center, Washington, District of Columbia, USA 20037

Preface

The explosion of information published these days in the primary research literature represents in some ways a substantial barrier to the new investigator or researcher crossing over traditional boundaries between fields. Commonly held beliefs and practices of the field's cognoscente often are poorly understood or appreciated by researchers even in closely related areas. Although review articles offer some relief from this situation, a more complete overview of a subject can often only be had through the forum of a book.

The desire to better understand factors influencing mineral absorption in the intestines provided the impetus for us to organize the symposium *Mineral Absorption in the Monogastric GI Tract: Chemical, Nutritional and Physiological Aspects*, held June 9-10, 1988 in Toronto, Canada, as part of the 195th National Meeting of the American Chemical Society and the Third North American Chemical Congress. The criteria for inviting participants was that they be currently active in research pertinent to mineral absorption, be publishing results of their investigations and willing to participate in a forum designed to present diverse considerations of mineral absorption to a multidisciplinary audience.

The individual chapters are mixtures of reviews and original research. Conceptually, the material has been divided into two sections. The first focuses primarily on the mechanisms involved in the transport and uptake of cations such as iron, zinc and calcium from the intestinal lumen, through the epithelial cells, into the blood stream (absorption), and final dispersement to body tissues. The second section provides a amalgam of subjects that impact mineral absorption, mostly dietary components, but other considerations such as age and health related effects are covered as well. The editors realize that the subjects presented here are an incomplete representation of some important aspects of mineral absorption. Nevertheless, they will be pleased if this volume provides the reader an updated view and a deeper appreciation of the field.

The editors thank the authors of these chapters for their contribution of time and knowledge to the original symposium and to this volume. The financial contributions of the Agricultural & Food Division of the American Chemical Society, the Pillsbury Company, and The Gerber Foods Company to the symposium which produced these proceedings are gratefully acknowledged. The support and encouragement of our colleagues within the Agricultural Research Service, United States Department of Agriculture is greatly appreciated. Finally, we thank Plenum Press for providing the opportunity to present this material to a wider audience.

Frederick R. Dintzis   Joseph A. Laszlo

Contents

Section I. Mechanisms of Mineral Absorption

1. Theoretical and Practical Aspects of Zinc Uptake and Absorption 3

    Robert J. Cousins

2. Zinc Absorption in Humans Determined Using In Vivo Tracer
    Studies and Kinetic Analysis 13

    Meryl E. Wastney

3. Mechanisms of Intestinal Brush Border Iron Transport 27

    Robert J. Simpson, Kishor B. Raja and Timothy J. Peters

4. Trace Metal Interactions Involving the Intestinal Absorption

    Mechanisms of Iron and Zinc 35

    Peter R. Flanagan

5. On the Molecular Mechanisms of Intestinal Calcium Transport 45

    Robert H. Wasserman and C. S. Fullmer

6. Equilibration Constants for the Complexation of Metal Ions
    by Serum Transferrin 67

    Wesley R. Harris

Section II. Dietary Influences on Mineral Uptake

7. Protein Digestion and the Absorption of Mineral Elements 95

    Raul A. Wapnir

8.   The Effect of Dietary Proteins on Iron Bioavailability in Man 117

        Sean R. Lynch, R. F. Hurrell, S. A. Dassenko and J. D. Cook

9.   Effect of Gastrointestinal Conditions on the Mineral-Binding
        Properties of Dietary Fibers 133

        Joseph A. Laszlo

10.   In Vivo Mineral Contents of Dietary Fiber Determined by
        EDX Analysis 147

        Frederick R. Dintzis, Frederick L. Baker and Tim S. Stahly

11.   Phytic Acid Interactions with Divalent Cations in Foods
        and in the Gastrointestinal Tract 161

        John W. Erdman, Jr. and Angela Poneros-Schneier

12.   Low Gastric Hydrochloric Acid Secretion and Mineral
        Bioavailability 173

        Elaine T. Champagne

13.   Effect of Age and the Milk Sugar Lactose on Calcium Absorption
        by the Small Intestine 185

        H. James Armbrecht

14.   Dietary Fiber or Bile-Sequestrant Ingestion and Divalent
        Cation Metabolism 193

        Marie M. Cassidy and Don W. Watkins

    Index 209

Section I

Mechanisms of Mineral Absorption

1

Theoretical and Practical Aspects of Zinc Uptake and Absorption

Robert J. Cousins

Considerable effort has been directed toward improving our understanding of the mechanism of zinc absorption. These studies have provided some basic concepts, but they have also underscored the complexity of the process involved. A useful strategy in these experiments is to partition the overall absorption processes into various steps or phases (Cousins, 1982). Nevertheless, it is necessary to retain the ability to integrate findings with isolated systems into a unified model.

A variety of research techniques have been applied to questions related to zinc absorption. In experiments with animals, intestinal segments, everted sacs, isolated membrane vesicles and perfused intestines are among the methods that have been used. In humans, the balance technique in one of many forms, using radioactive or stable isotopes, and responses to oral zinc loading have been used. These approaches with their attendant strengths and weaknesses have been reviewed (Solomons & Cousins, 1984). The phases of zinc absorption that have been studied in animal experiments are intraluminal factors, cellular entry, intracellular metabolism, cellular release, portal transport and perhaps paracellular transport. This brief review will concentrate on, from both a theoretical and practical perspective, some of the more recent literature on each of these phases of zinc absorption.

Intraluminal Factors

Actually very little is known regarding the molecular associations between zinc and binding ligands in dietary components. These ligands include zinc metalloproteins and zinc bound to nucleic acids of both plant and animal origin. These associations are extremely important determinants of zinc availability for uptake, transcellular movement and absorption (Figure 1).

If the zinc binding ligands in the intestinal contents are species that will be absorbed it is likely that association with zinc will result in enhanced zinc absorption. Conversely, if binding is to a nonabsorbable species absorption will be reduced. A variety of dietary constituents and formulations affect zinc absorption (see Cousins, 1985). For example, a diet high in fiber, which may have beneficial

3

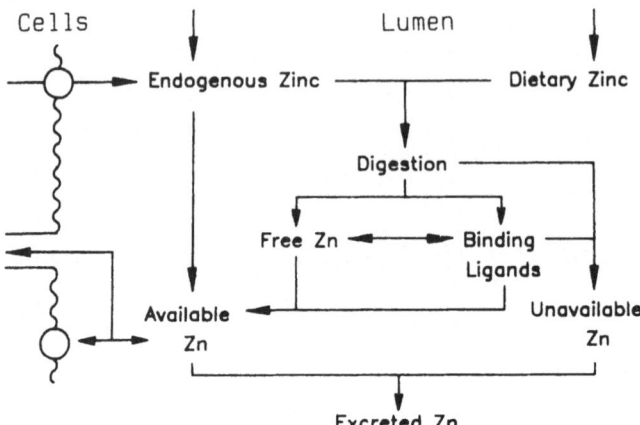

Figure 1. Intraluminal processing of endogenous and dietary zinc. Digestive enzymes generate a variety of products with varying affinities for zinc. Zinc is distributed among these ligands and at intestinal pH exists as free zinc only during transfer between ligands. A portion of luminal zinc is available for uptake by intestinal uptake mechanisms. Zinc not absorbed enters the unavailable pool and is excreted.

effects on digestion and intestinal function, may provide binding sites which limit the supply of available zinc. Furthermore, it is likely that extent of digestion is directly related to availability of zinc (Solomons & Cousins, 1984). Digestive processes influence both endogenous zinc as well as zinc of dietary origins. A decrease in absorption might be expected in malabsorption syndromes where food components are digested to a lesser extent, thus limiting interaction with receptors at the membrane surface.

At the neutral pH of the intestine, zinc does not remain free in solution. The "Free Zn" shown in the diagram is to indicate that Zn atoms may interact with a variety of ligands prior to eventual absorption. The binding affinity of the various ligands then collectively determine availability. This process should be viewed as an equilibrium, however, as shown in Figure 1. Imidazole groups and cysteine are the ligands preferred by zinc. Since metal ions exhibit a marked degree of reactivity (Williams, 1984), considerable interaction among metals may occur at this stage of absorption. The net result of digestion is to present a given quantity of available zinc for interaction with uptake mechanisms. Recent experiments by Roth & Kirchgessner (1985) illustrate the effect of individual dietary proteins on zinc bioavailability.

Uptake Mechanisms

The first step of transepithelial movement of zinc is uptake from the intestinal lumen. This may involve either transport across the brush border membrane (cellular entry) and/or paracellular transport between epithelial cells.

The exact mechanism(s) involved in cellular entry is unknown. Presumably, zinc traverses the unstirred H_2O layer in an exchangeable or diffusable form. A variety of dietary factors may enhance uptake (see Solomons & Cousins, 1984). Individual components do not appear to always have the same documented effects (e.g., EDTA has been shown to both improve and limit absorption). Species differences and methods of measuring the uptake/absorption process may account for these differences.

Zinc transport across the brush border may occur by one or more processes. These are presented diagrammatically in Figure 2. Both bidirectional and unidirectional transport of zinc ion is shown. Presumably this would require interaction with ligands (perhaps macromolecules) that would transfer zinc from the lumen to a carrier protein in the membrane. Membrane receptors for specific proteins or classes of proteins could participate in absorption at this point. Transcellular zinc movement is bidirectional, based on evidence from *in vitro* and *in vivo* techniques (Kowarski et al., 1974; Steel & Cousins, 1985; Hoadley et al., 1987). This may not involve the same transporter molecule(s). Zinc transported as an intact low molecular weight chelate (LMWC) or deposited at the membrane surface with luminal return of the LMWC are also shown as possible mechanisms. There is evidence from the poultry nutrition literature that a chelator added to a feed must have a higher affinity for zinc than ligands in the feed to be effective in promoting absorption (see Kratzer & Vohra, 1986). If this is so, the zinc-LMWC must be absorbed intact or the complex must be degraded within cells and the zinc transferred to a higher affinity ligand. Alternatively as shown, a portion of apparent transepithelial movement could actually follow a paracellular route wherein zinc would move between epithelial cells.

There is an increasing body of kinetic evidence which suggests that cellular entry is concentration dependent. Therefore, the greater the abundance of available zinc from the dietary supply, the greater is the likelihood of cellular uptake. Experiments with isolated brush border membranes of rat intestine have provided evidence for both saturable and nonsaturable processes (Menard & Cousins, 1983). Membrane binding is a factor in vesicle experiments and when binding is accounted for the Km for transport is considerably reduced (Hoadley & Cousins, 1987). When binding to lysed membrane vesicles from zinc adequate rats was used as a correction factor, transport characteristics include a Km (concentration at half maximal velocity) of 100 μM, Jmax (maximum transport velocity) of 2.1 nmol•mg protein^{-1}•min^{-1} and a Kd (diffusion constant) of 1.5 ml•mg protein^{-1}•min^{-1}. The latter represents the first order term and thus represents passive uptake. In contrast, membrane vesicles from zinc depleted rats produced a similar Km and Kd, 130 μM and 1.5 ml•mg protein^{-1}•min^{-1}, respectively, while the Jmax was increased to 5.5 nmol•mg protein^{-1}•min^{-1}. Therefore, when correction factors are similarly applied the transport rate appeared to more than double in vesicles from nutritionally zinc depleted rats.

A perfusion technique where the intestinal lumen is perfused with solutions of various concentrations of zinc and the vascular supply is also isolated and perfused

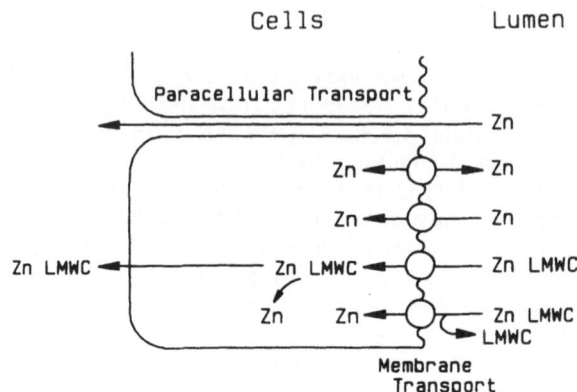

Figure 2. Potential modes of zinc entry across brush border membrane. Bidirectional and unidirectional transport is illustrated. Zinc transport as an intact low molecular weight complex (LMWC) or after donation to a receptor is also illustrated. A significant portion of uptake is saturable. Transport rates via this mode increase with low dietary zinc intake. Nonsaturable paracellular zinc transport is also shown as an entry mechanism.

provides a useful tool for the measurement of zinc uptake and transport kinetics (Smith & Cousins, 1980; Hoadley et al., 1987). Perfusion with intestines from zinc adequate and zinc deficient rats showed that the Km of saturable uptake under these conditions was identical. This series of experiments will be discussed in the later section dealing with an integrated model of uptake and transport. It should be emphasized, however, that a feature shown by the data from experiments with isolated membrane vesicles and perfusion experiments with intact intestine is that transport and uptake, respectively, appear to be increased two to three fold in response to zinc deficiency. This suggests that a reduction in zinc content of the diet can be partially offset by a homeostatic increase in zinc transport mechanisms at the brush border membrane.

A portion of transepithelial zinc movement appears to be nonsaturable. As has been reasoned for calcium movement in the intestine, nonsaturability may be accounted for by movement between cells (Bronner, 1987). A comparable paracellular transport process for zinc is shown in Figure 2. However, since transport of zinc by membrane vesicles also appears to have a nonsaturable phase, the nonsaturable mechanism may be a component of membrane transport rather than paracellular zinc transport.

Intracellular Mechanisms

Since the early 1970s considerable attention has focused on intracellular steps in the regulation of zinc absorption. This area and the rationale involved has been reviewed (see Cousins, 1985). Briefly, it was demonstrated that induction of the synthesis of metallothionein, a low molecular weight zinc and copper binding

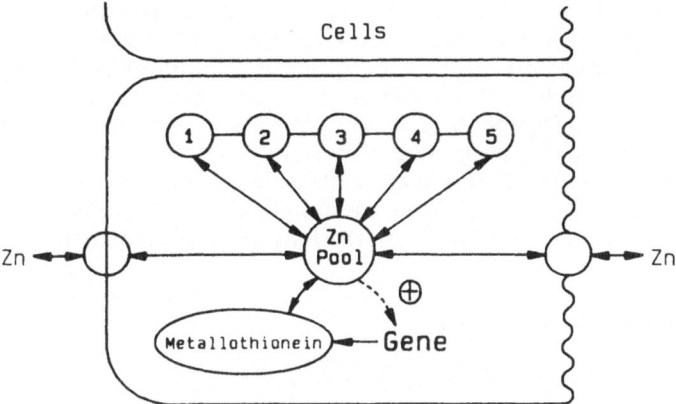

Figure 3. Zinc within intestinal cells interacts with a variety of binding ligands. At least six ligands are identified by high performance liquid chromatography. One of these is metallothionein, an inducible ligand responsive to dietary zinc, that binds a significant portion of zinc entering mucosal cells from the lumen.

protein, resulted in a decrease in copper and/or zinc absorption (Figure 3). It is clear from recent experiments that dietary zinc intake has a much greater control of expression of the metallothionein gene than does copper (Blalock et al., 1988). However, with regard to the intestine, regulation by the dietary zinc supply is only significant when the copper intake is low. When the dietary intake of zinc is constant, metallothionein synthesis is constant. In contrast, intestinal metallothionein synthesis is increased when zinc status is acutely increased, even if copper intake is adequate (Menard et al., 1981). Zinc is subsequently bound to these polypeptides with a shift in kinetics of transepithelial zinc movement. A basic concept involved in intracellular interaction during absorption is that metallothionein, as an inducible intracellular ligand, can influence the cellular concentration of zinc and thus control its metabolism (see Cousins, 1985). A important property of metallothionein is that bound zinc is exchangeable and not irreversibly bound. This adds to the physiological importance of this protein as a possible damping agent for metal transport in this tissue.

An important aspect of metallothionein's role as an intracellular regulator is its higher binding affinity for copper than zinc (Dunn et al., 1987). When induced by zinc, which activates the promoter more effectively at lower cellular concentrations than does copper, the protein preferentially binds copper. This reduces the cellular level of copper available for transport out of the cell. Our experience has been that fairly divergent levels of dietary copper and zinc are necessary to show this effect (Oestreicher & Cousins, 1985). Nevertheless, Brewer & associates (1983) have effectively used this zinc induction/copper binding relationship to create negative copper balance in Wilson's Disease patients. This therapeutic intervention appears to limit copper accumulation which is a major factor in the pathogenesis of this disease. More dramatic increases in intestinal metallothionein occur with fasting (Hoadley et al., 1988).

It has been shown repeatedly that high molecular weight species bind a substantial portion of [65]Zn after oral administration (Smith & Cousins, 1980; Norton & Heaton, 1980). Recently, using high resolution liquid chromatography, we have shown that zinc binds to at least five proteins that have higher molecular weights than metallothionein (Hempe & Cousins, 1988). Distribution of zinc among these proteins differs with time, suggesting a variety of binding constituents are involved in intracellular transport. Experiments with isolated cells showed that a number of these intracellular proteins increase in abundance upon dietary zinc restriction (Hoadley & Cousins, 1985). These interactions are represented in Figure 3.

Basolateral Membrane Transport

Information on the transport of zinc from intestinal cells is limited. The most direct data have been obtained from experiments with perfused intestines and isolated membrane vesicles. The perfusion experiments will be described in the following section.

A generalized scheme for basolateral transport of zinc is shown in Figure 4. Basolateral membrane vesicles for zinc transport studies were prepared by a Percoll density gradient method (Oestreicher & Cousins, 1984). Na^+-K^+ ATPase was used to measure purity of the membrane preparation. Considerable binding of zinc to these membranes was observed. Nevertheless, uptake could be separated into saturable and nonsaturable components. Kinetic analysis of initial rates define a Km of 24 μM and a Jmax of 17 nmol•mg protein^{-1}•min^{-1}. Values from vesicles of zinc depleted rats were 33 μM and 14 nmol•mg protein^{-1}•min^{-1}, respectively, and were comparable to those for control vesicles. Zinc transport at the basolateral membrane should be energy dependent, by analogy to the calcium transport system (Bronner, 1987). However, a problem is encountered in attempting to demonstrate ATP-dependent zinc transport. Specifically, ATP binds zinc tenaciously under in vitro conditions. Therefore, when ATP is added to these incubations the effective zinc concentration is lowered to a point where little free zinc is available for transport by the vesicles. Using calculations based on simultaneous equations, it is possible to adjust the zinc concentrations of incubations to compensate for this chelation effect. When this adjustment is made, ATP produces a four- to six-fold stimulation of zinc transport. Therefore, energy dependency is possible at this point in transcellular zinc movement.

Transfer of zinc from the intestine to the plasma compartment exhibits nonsaturable kinetics *in vivo* (Hoadley et al., 1987). Transport data from in vitro experiments suggest saturable kinetics. Our interpretation of this apparent discrepancy is that within intestinal cells the concentration of free zinc is extremely low. Presumably zinc transfer from the basolateral surface is regulated in such a way that a low concentration of zinc for transport is maintained. Therefore, *in vitro* kinetic experiments where the zinc concentration is varied over a considerable range may not closely approximate the *in situ* situation. These kinetics show a saturable system but the actual zinc concentration *in situ* is so narrowly maintained that *in vivo* measurements suggest a first order transmembrane process.

Albumin appears to be the principal transport molecule in plasma (Smith et al., 1979; Smith & Cousins, 1980). This suggests that other zinc binding proteins in plasma arise through secretion from the liver and other tissues. The limited

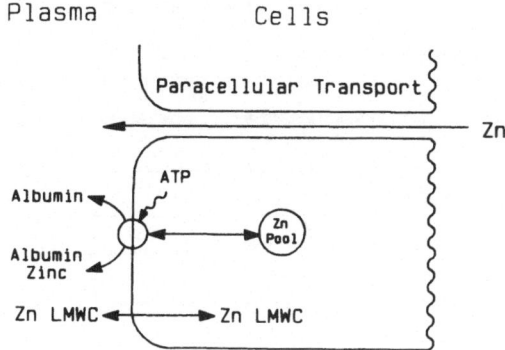

Figure 4. Zinc transport from the basolateral membrane of mucosal cells may be controlled by an ATP-driven mechanism. At normal intracellular zinc concentrations, zinc movement from mucosal cells is probably nonsaturable. Albumin is the plasma carrier for zinc.

amount of data available suggest that the albumin content of plasma has an influence on the extent of absorption (Smith et al., 1979). There is also a limited amount of data which suggests that some zinc chelates are transported across the basolateral membrane intact. However, data with a variety of LMWC molecules do not provide evidence for zinc transport with plasma as LMWC (Hempe & Cousins, 1988).

Integrated Model of Zinc Absorption

The theoretical aspects of the zinc absorption process described above can be used to develop a conceptual mode of how zinc absorption occurs (Figure 5). The dietary zinc content appears to regulate the zinc acquisition and retention system. This may have evolved from a primitive mechanism of single cell organisms. The mechanism may have some characteristics of the vitamin D controlled calcium absorption system (Bronner, 1987). However, the latter probably evolved later, with the need for extra calcium to maintain the skeletal system of vertebrates.

A two period perfusion system for rat intestine was used to simultaneously evaluate uptake and cellular release of zinc under comparable *in vivo* conditions (Hoadley et al., 1987). Both the lumen and vascular supply are perfused. Uptake was monitored as the disappearance of ^{65}Zn from intestines perfused with various concentrations of zinc (5-200 μM). Uptake data were fitted by nonlinear regression to accommodate saturable and nonsaturable components. A Km of 32 μM was obtained for perfusions using intestines from either zinc adequate or zinc depleted rats. The apparent maximum rate of uptake was 57 nmol Zn$\bullet$g$^{-1}\bullet$30 min^{-1} in the zinc adequate group. In the zinc depleted group this apparent rate was three-fold greater (183 nmol Zn$\bullet$g$^{-1}\bullet$30 min^{-1}). Fasting also increased zinc uptake, but to a lesser extent than zinc depletion (Hoadley et al., 1988). When these findings are integrated into a conceptual model of absorption the data suggest that a saturable mechanism for zinc acquisition is activated when the dietary

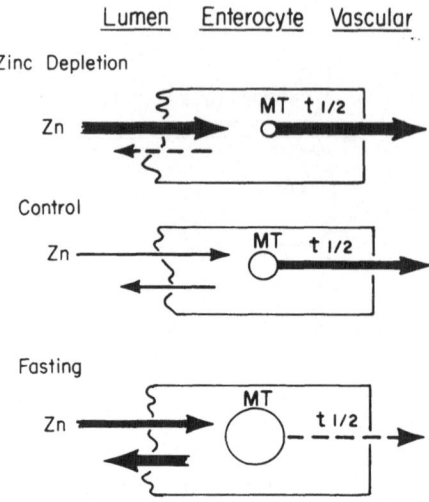

Figure 5. Effects of dietary zinc depletion and fasting on relative transcellular zinc movement. Dietary zinc depletion increases uptake and absorption but decreases cellular metallothionein and cell to lumen transfer. Fasting increases uptake, cellular metallothionein and cell to lumen transfer but decreases absorption. (Reproduced with permission from Hoadley et al., *J. Nutr.* 118, 497-502, 1988.)

zinc supply is low. In keeping with this observation is the finding that the diffusion constant (Kd) for the first-order term (including paracellular transport) is unaffected by dietary zinc. The Kd is about 1.9 ml$\cdot$g$^{-1}\cdot$30 min^{-1} under both dietary conditions. It is reasonable to assume that when dietary zinc is limited, a carrier(s) or receptor(s) is activated or produced. Saturable uptake kinetics would be expected as would a stimulation of uptake rate.

The second part of the two period perfusion model follows efflux of zinc from the vascularly perfused intestine. Specifically, ^{65}Zn taken up during Period I was subsequently monitored within intestinal cells, the lumen and the vascular compartment over a 40 min period (Hoadley et al., 1987). Secretion into the lumen was greater in intestines from the zinc adequate group. Conversely, absorption was less in this group. Rates of mucosal ^{65}Zn transferred to the vascular perfusate were approximately two-fold greater in the zinc depleted group. However, in both groups the luminal zinc during Period I was proportional to the actual transfer rate. Furthermore, linear regression showed that transfer rates from intestine to the vascular compartment was a linear function of the intracellular ^{65}Zn pool. This rate changed with time with the greatest change found in the zinc depleted group. The net result was that the ^{65}Zn half-life was shorter in the zinc deficient group. Collectively, these results show that portal transfer of mucosal ^{65}Zn was nonsaturable, and may involve a rapidly exchanging zinc compartment that was stimulated in zinc depleted rat intestine.

The results of these various studies with the rat model agree fairly closely with data obtained from human subjects (Babcock et al., 1982; Wastney et al., 1986). Specifically, absorption kinetics for zinc are consistent with a saturable transport mechanism. In addition, secretion from the intestinal mucosa into the lumen may provide a homeostatic function as has been shown in Figure 5 derived from experiments with rats.

Fasting had the opposite effect on the rate of mucosal ^{65}Zn transfer to the vascular compartment compared to zinc depletion (Hoadley et al., 1988). Specifically, transfer of ^{65}Zn was less than found in the control group. The half-life of the ^{65}Zn pool within mucosal cells was shorter (15.7 min) in the zinc depleted group compared to that found with the control (25.7 min) or fasted (71.3 min) groups. The half-life of this rapid transport pool was directly proportional to the mucosal metallothionein content (Figure 5). It was proposed that intracellular metallothionein levels contribute to the greater rate of ^{65}Zn transfer to the vascular compartment in zinc depletion and lower rate in fasting. However, metallothionein could act as a facilitator of zinc absorption under some conditions as the proportion of mucosal zinc in the transport pool is directly correlated with cellular metallothionein levels.

Summary

The purpose of this review is to describe our present understanding of the theoretical aspects of zinc uptake and absorption. An attempt has been made to include a selected amount of older literature to illustrate specific points. The zinc acquisition system appears to respond to the dietary zinc supply and the extent of digestive capacity. Up regulation of the uptake process with limited zinc intake seems to increase the pool of zinc that is subsequently exported from mucosal cells to the vascular compartment. Intracellular factors such as metallothionein influence the rate and/or extent of zinc acquisition and are regulated by dietary zinc availability and physiological factors.

References

Babcock, A. K., Henkin, R. I., Aamodt, R. L., Foster, D. M., & Berman, M. (1982) *Metabolism* 31, 335-347.

Blalock, T. L., Dunn, M. A., & Cousins, R. J. (1988) *J. Nutr.* 118, 222-228.

Brewer, G. J., Hill, G. M., Prasad, A. S., Cossack, Z. T., & Rabbani, P. (1983) *Ann. Intern. Med.* 99, 314-320.

Bronner, F. (1987) *J. Nutr.* 117, 1347-1352.

Cousins, R. J. (1982) in *Clinical, Biochemical and Nutritional Aspects of Trace Elements* (Prasad, A.S., Ed.) pp. 117-128, Alan R. Liss, New York.

Cousins, R. J. (1985) *Physiol. Rev.* 65, 238-309.

Dunn, M. A., Blalock, T. L., & Cousins, R. J. (1987) *Proc. Soc. Exp. Biol. Med.* 185, 107-119.

Hempe, J. M., & Cousins, R. J. (1988) *FASEB J.* 2, A865.

Hoadley, J. E., & Cousins, R. J. (1985) *Fed. Proc.* 44, 3413A.

Hoadley, J. E., & Cousins, R. J. (1987) *Fed. Proc.* 46, 1644A.

Hoadley, J. E., Leinart, A. S., & Cousins, R. J. (1987) *Am. J. Physiol.* 252, G825-G831.

Hoadley, J. E., Leinart, A. S., & Cousins, R. J. (1988) *J. Nutr.* 118, 497-502.

Kowarski, S., Blair-Stanek, C. S., & Schachter, D. (1974) *Am. J. Physiol.* 226, 401-407.

Kratzer, F. H., & Vohra, P. (1986) in *Chelates in Nutrition*, CRC Press, Inc., Boca Raton, FL.

Menard, M. P., & Cousins, R. J. (1983) *J. Nutr.* 113, 1434-1442.

Menard, M. P., McCormick, C. C., & Cousins, R. J. (1981) *J. Nutr.* 111, 1353-1361.

Norton, D. S., & Heaton, F. W. (1980) *J. Inorg. Biochem.* 13, 1-9.

Oestreicher, P., & Cousins, R. J. (1984) *Fed. Proc.* 43, 4646A.

Oestreicher, P., & Cousins, R. J. (1985) *J. Nutr.* 115, 159-166.

Roth, H. P., & Kirchgessner, M. (1985) *J. Nutr.* 115, 1641-1649.

Smith, K. T., & Cousins, R. J. (1980) *J. Nutr.* 110, 316-323.

Smith, K. T., Failla, M. L., & Cousins, R. J. (1979) *Biochem. J.* 184, 627-633.

Solomons, N. W., & Cousins, R. J. (1984) in *Absorption and Malabsorption of Mineral Nutrients* (Solomons, N. W., & Rosenberg, I. H., Eds.) pp 125-197, Alan R. Liss, New York.

Steel, L., & Cousins, R. J. (1985) *Am. J. Physiol.* 248, G46-G53.

Wastney, M. E., Aamodt, R. L., Rumble, W. F., & Henkin, R. I. (1986) *Am. J. Physiol.* 251, R398-R408.

Williams, R. J. P. (1984) *Endeavor* 8, 65-70.

2

Zinc Absorption in Humans Determined Using In Vivo Tracer Studies and Kinetic Analysis[1]

Meryl E. Wastney

Absorption of zinc from the gut is the first in a series of processes in which zinc is taken up by the body, utilized in the tissues and then excreted. The absorption and metabolism of adequate quantities of zinc are important in humans since zinc deficiency is associated with symptoms of impaired growth, delayed maturity, skin lesions and taste and smell dysfunction (Prasad, 1979).

Absorption refers to the rate that zinc is taken up from the gut and to the mechanism by which zinc is transported into the body and studies have been undertaken *in vivo* and *in vitro* to examine both aspects (Solomons & Cousins, 1984). Kinetic studies undertaken with radioisotopes in humans have examined the rate of zinc absorption and also aspects of the mechanism of absorption by kinetic analysis of the data through modeling (Foster et al., 1979; Babcock et al., 1980; Wastney et al., 1986).

A model is a mathematical description of a system that represents a hypothesis of how the system functions (Berman, 1982). A model simulates the behavior of a system in that the model solution fits observed data obtained from the system. Modeling can be used to propose and test mechanisms by which a system functions and to determine dynamic properties of a system. Since data are limited (by sampling sites, times and conditions), a model consistent with the data represents a hypothesis of how the system functions and once data are obtained that are not fitted by the model the hypothesis must be revised and a new model proposed (Phair, 1982).

Modeling is a powerful tool for investigating metabolism since it allows processess that occur simultaneously (e.g., transport and metabolism) to be evaluated separately. The philosophy behind development of a model of metabolism is that the model must be consistent with known physiology and with available data from the system (Berman, 1982). A model may be used as a research tool to explore the

---

1   This work was supported by NIH Grant AG06840.

detailed metabolism of a compound or on a less complex level to determine a specific parameter, and the former approach was chosen for the investigation of zinc metabolism in humans (Foster et al., 1979).

A model for zinc metabolism in humans was developed from data, obtained following administration of zinc radiotracers, from plasma, red blood cells, (RBC), urine, feces and by external counting, over whole body, liver and thigh regions (Foster et al., 1979; Babcock et al., 1982; Wastney et al., 1986). The model has been used to explore the mechanisms by which zinc is metabolized, to determine parameters of zinc metabolism (including absorption, tissue uptake, secretion and excretion of zinc), and to study sites of regulation of zinc metabolism (Foster et al., 1979; Babcock et al., 1982; Wastney et al., 1986). The purpose of this paper is to 1) describe some aspects of the process of zinc absorption in humans, 2) describe how absorption has been calculated from *in vivo* kinetic data using the model and 3) discuss the significance of absorption as one parameter of zinc metabolism.

Experimental Procedures

Kinetic studies of zinc metabolism. This model for zinc metabolism in humans was developed from kinetic data obtained from a series of three studies. In each study tracer, (^{69m}Zn, $t_{1/2} = 13.6$ hr or ^{65}Zn, $t_{1/2} = 245$ d), was administered to subjects in the fasting state and activity was measured in seven tissues, (plasma, RBC, urine, feces and by external counting, over liver and thigh regions and whole body) by gamma-ray spectroscopy (Aamodt et al., 1979; Aamodt et al., 1982). Serum zinc concentration and urinary zinc excretion were determined in each study by flame aspiration atomic absorption spectrophotometry (Meret & Henkin, 1971).

The first studies were undertaken in patients with taste and smell dysfunction (Foster et al., 1979) since zinc is considered to have a role in taste and smell function (Henkin, 1984). Patients (n=17) were initially given ^{69m}Zn orally and activity measured for 5 d in the tissues described above, excluding whole body (Aamodt et al., 1979; Foster et al., 1979). One to three months later ^{69m}Zn was administered intravenously and activity was measured in the same six tissues for a further 5 d (Aamodt et al., 1979; Foster et al., 1979).

The second series of studies were undertaken using ^{65}Zn (Aamodt et al., 1982; Babcock et al., 1982). Tracer was administered orally to patients with taste and smell dysfunction (n=10) and activity was measured in feces for 7 d and the other six tissues, described above, for 9 mo while the patients were on their normal diets (basal intake of 10 mg Zn/d) and (except for feces and urine) for a further 9 mo while patients took an additional 100 mg Zn/d (zinc loading), (Aamodt et al., 1982; Babcock et al., 1982).

The third series of studies were undertaken in normal subjects using ^{65}Zn (Wastney et al., 1986). Tracer was administered orally (n=25) or intravenously (n=7) and activity was measured in feces for 7 d and the other six tissues, described above, for 270 d while subjects were on their normal diets (containing approximately 10 mg Zn/d) and (except for feces) for a further 270 d while the subjects took an additional 100 mg exogenous Zn/d (zinc loading), (Wastney et al., 1986).

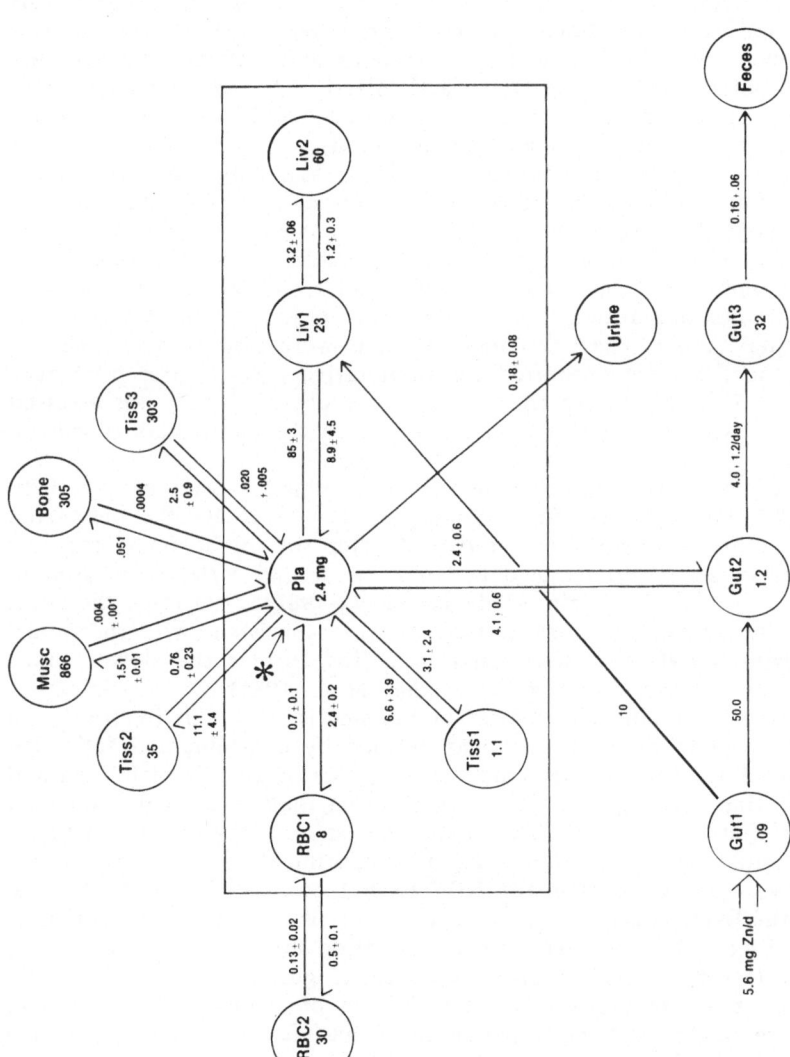

Figure 1. A model for zinc metabolism in humans (Wastney et al., 1986). The asterisk indicates the site of tracer entry (intravenous administration). The double arrow indicates the site of entry of tracee, or unlabelled zinc, (orally in the diet). Compartments representing gut (Gut1, Gut2 and Gut3), plasma (Pla), RBC (RBC1, RBC2), tissues (Tiss1, Tiss2 and Tiss3), liver (Liv1, Liv2), muscle (Musc) and bone are shown with the zinc mass (mg) of each compartment. Fractional rate constants (mean±SD, fraction/d) are given for normal subjects (n=7), (Wastney et al., 1986). The box encloses compartments that turnover rapidly (in less than 2 d).

Data analysis and model development. Data were analysed by compartmental analysis using SAAM/CONSAM (Simulation, Analysis and Modeling and the Conversational version of SAAM, Berman et al., 1983; Berman & Weiss, 1978).

SAAM/CONSAM is a general equation-solving program that can be applied to both linear and non-linear systems. A model may be entered directly, by writing the equations, or indirectly by entering parameters in which case the program sets up a compartmental model defined by the parameters. The program was specifically developed for analysing biological systems and has an interface that allows biological problems to be easily set up and solved. Changes in experimental conditions can be readily simulated by allowing initial conditions and parameter values to change during solution (Berman & Weiss, 1978).

Data were analysed by compartmental analysis by assuming that zinc in the body is located in compartments that turnover at different rates. The data of each individual were analysed using SAAM/CONSAM by entering parameters of the model, their initial values, initial conditions, (describing how the tracer was administered), and the data (consisting of tracer data from the tissues and zinc concentration of plasma and urine). The program set up and solved the equations of the compartmental model. The calculated solutions were displayed by printing and plotting and the fits were optimized by an iterative least-squares procedure (Berman & Weiss, 1978). The fit of the model to the observed data was assessed by the plots, the statistics of the fits and the errors on the parameters (Foster & Boston, 1983).

Development of the model has been described in detail (Foster et al., 1979, Babcock et al., 1982; Foster et al., 1984; Wastney et al., 1986). Briefly, data from the first series of studies over 5 d were used to develop the initial model for zinc metabolism (Foster et al., 1979) while data from the second series were used to define the longer-term kinetics of zinc (Babcock et al., 1982). Data from the latest series describing zinc kinetics in normal subjects were consistent with the model developed from patient data and were used to define further the slower tissue compartments of zinc, in muscle and bone (Wastney et al., 1986).

The current model for zinc metabolism in humans is shown in Figure 1. In the model, zinc absorption from the gut was defined by data obtained following oral administration of tracer, and the rapid tissue uptake of zinc from plasma and the secretion of zinc into gut were defined from data obtained following intravenous administration of tracer. The model consists of three compartments in the gut, (Gut1, Gut2 and Gut3, Figure 1), a compartment representing plasma (Pla, Figure 1), two compartments in the RBC (RBC1 and RBC2, Figure 1), two compartments in the liver, (Liv1, Liv2, Figure1), three tissue compartments (Tiss1, Tiss2, and Tiss3, Figure 1), compartments representing muscle (Musc, Figure 1) and bone, and two loss pathways, via urine and feces (Figure 1).

The pattern of zinc kinetics in tissues following oral tracer administration, generated using the model and mean parameter values for a normal population (Figure 1), are shown in Figure 2. Since activity was measured in liver before it was detected in plasma following oral tracer administration (Figure 2a) a rapid pathway was required for zinc uptake from the gut into liver (Gut1 to Liv1, Figure 1). This pathway probably represents uptake of zinc from the portal circulation (Foster et al., 1979). A compartment lower in the gut (Gut2, Figure 1) represented the major site of zinc absorption. Compartment Gut3 (Figure 1) was required to account for the delay that occurred before administered tracer

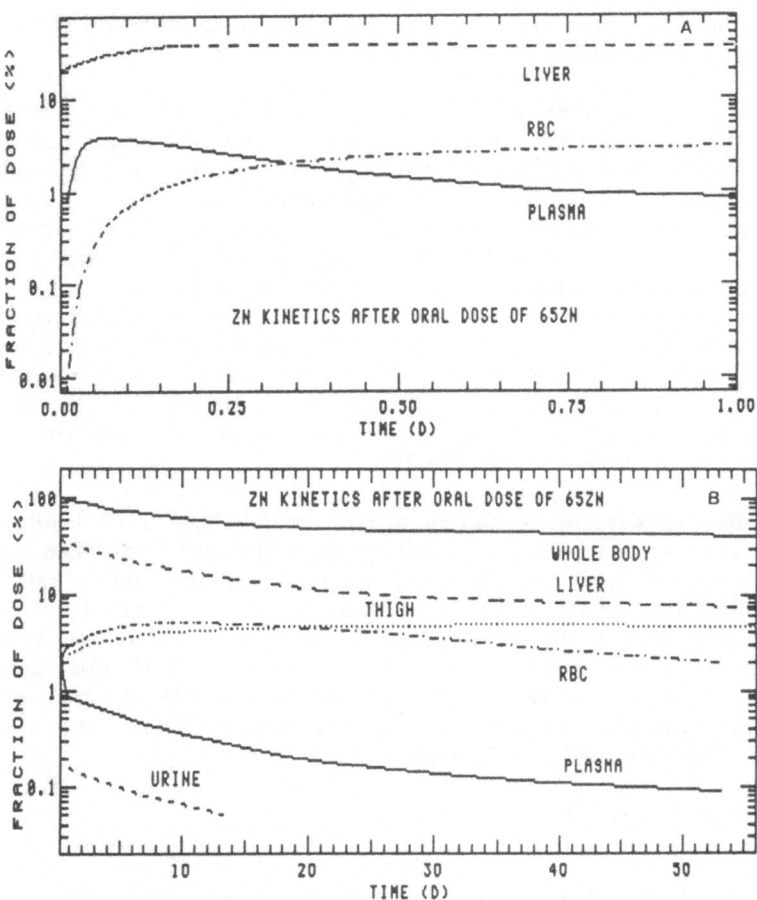

Figure 2. Tissue activity calculated using the model and parameter values for a normal population (Figure 1) in a) liver, red blood cells (RBC) and plasma for 1 d following oral tracer administration and b) whole body, liver, thigh, RBC, and plasma for 56 d and urine for 14 d following oral tracer administration.

appeared in feces. This compartment may represent zinc that enters gut cells and is released back into gut without being absorbed or pools of zinc lower in the gut.

RBC data were fitted by two compartments (RBC1 and RBC2, Figure 1) representing a rapid and slow phase of zinc uptake from blood (Figure 2a). The kinetics of liver zinc (Figure 2a) were fitted by two compartments (Liv1 and Liv2, Figure 1) representing rapid and slow zinc exchange plus fractions of blood (21%), and one of the tissue compartments (9% of Tiss3, Figure 1). Zinc kinetics associated with the thigh (Figure 2b) were fitted by a combination of tissue compartments (2% of Tiss1, 13% of Tiss2 and 7% of Tiss3), blood (5% of RBC1, RBC2 and Pla), muscle (17% of Musc) and bone (21%), (Figure 1). The zinc kinetics of bone have not been described and the parameters were based on calcium kinetic data (Wastney et al., 1986).

   Calculation of absorption. Absorption was defined as the transport of zinc from gut into blood or liver. Zinc which passed through the gut without entering the gut cells or which entered gut cells and was released back into gut without entering plasma was considered to be unabsorbed since this fraction of dietary zinc did not enter plasma and become available for use in tissues. Absorption was calculated by the model as the fraction of tracer entering liver (Gut1 to Liv1, Figure 1) plus the fraction entering plasma (Gut2 to Pla, Figure 1).
   The pattern of appearance of tracer in plasma for the first time (absorption function) was calculated using the model and normal population parameter values (Figure 1), (Figure 3a). The total tracer absorbed was separated into the fraction absorbed via liver (Gut1 to Liv1) and directly via plasma (Gut2 to Pla), (Figure 3a). The absorptive function (Figure 3a) was integrated over time to provide the cumulative absorption of zinc (Figure 3b).

   Definition of sites of regulation of zinc metabolism. Zinc loading invoked regulation of zinc metabolism at specific sites within the body. The locations of these sites were defined through modeling by fitting the kinetic data from the basal and zinc loading states (i.e., zinc intake of 10 vs 110 mg/d) simultaneously by the model (Figure 1). Parameter values in the model were allowed to differ systematically until the model fitted both sets of data. With this approach the minimum number of differences necessary to fit the data obtained during zinc loading were identified and these parameters represented sites of regulation of zinc metabolism (Babcock et al., 1982; Wastney et al., 1986).

Results

   Zinc absorption. Mean parameter values determined for a normal population (n=7) are included on Figure 1. In normal subjects 59% of tracer administered orally in the fasting state was absorbed, calculated (Wastney et al., 1986);

Absorption from the first site via liver, (Gut1 to Liv1, Figure 1)

$$= \frac{10}{(10 + 50)} \qquad (1)$$

$$= 0.167$$

Absorption from the second site directly into plasma, (Gut2 to Pla, Figure 1)

$$= \frac{4.1}{(4.1 + 4.0)} \qquad (2)$$

$$= 0.506$$

$$\text{Total absorbed} = 0.167 + (1 - 0.167) * 0.506 \qquad (3)$$

$$= 0.167 + 0.421$$

$$= 0.588$$

For normal subjects most zinc (42%) entered plasma directly and only 17% was absorbed via liver (Equation 3). Absorption peaked at 0.04 d (1 hr) and continued over 0.25 d (6 hr), (Figure 3a). After 0.25 d (6 hr) 47% of the zinc dose had been absorbed from the gut representing 80% of the total (59%, Equation 3) absorbed (Figure 3b).

Sites of regulation of zinc metabolism. The change in whole body zinc kinetics with zinc loading following an oral dose is shown in Figure 4. The model (Figure 1) was solved with mean parameter values from the basal state (with dietary zinc intake of 10 mg/d) and during zinc loading (when zinc intake increased by 100 mg/d of exogenous zinc), (Wastney et al., 1986). Tracer was lost from the body more rapidly with the higher zinc intake (Figure 4).

Two sites of regulation of zinc metabolism, absorption and excretion in urine, were defined from the studies in patients with taste and smell dysfunction (Babcock et al., 1982). In addition to these two sites, three additional sites of regulation, (secretion into gut, exchange of zinc with RBC and release of zinc by muscle), were defined using more extensive data obtained from normal subjects (Wastney et al., 1986). In normal subjects, when zinc intake increased by ten-fold fractional changes were; absorption decreased from 59±10% to 7±2%, secretion into gut decreased by 37%, uptake of zinc by RBC decreased by 60%, release of zinc by muscle increased by 117% and excretion into urine increased by 128% (Wastney et al., 1986). In terms of mass, plasma zinc concentration increased two-fold and the amount of zinc excreted in urine increased five-fold while the calculated mass of zinc in RBC, liver and thigh did not change (Wastney et al., 1986).

Discussion

Modeling has been used used to examine the the mechanism of zinc absorption in humans, to calculate the amount of zinc absorbed and to evaluate absorption as a site of regulation of zinc metabolism.

Mechanism of absorption. The mechanism of zinc absorption is complex, since it possibly occurs from different sites in the gut, involves transport ligands in the gut, binding proteins within the gut cells and a transport mechanism from the gut cell to plasma (Cousins, 1985). In the model (Figure 1) absorption is simplified. It is represented by two pathways from the gut (Figure 1) as these were sufficient to fit the data obtained from plasma, RBC, liver, thigh, whole body, urine and feces (Babcock et al., 1982; Wastney et al., 1986).

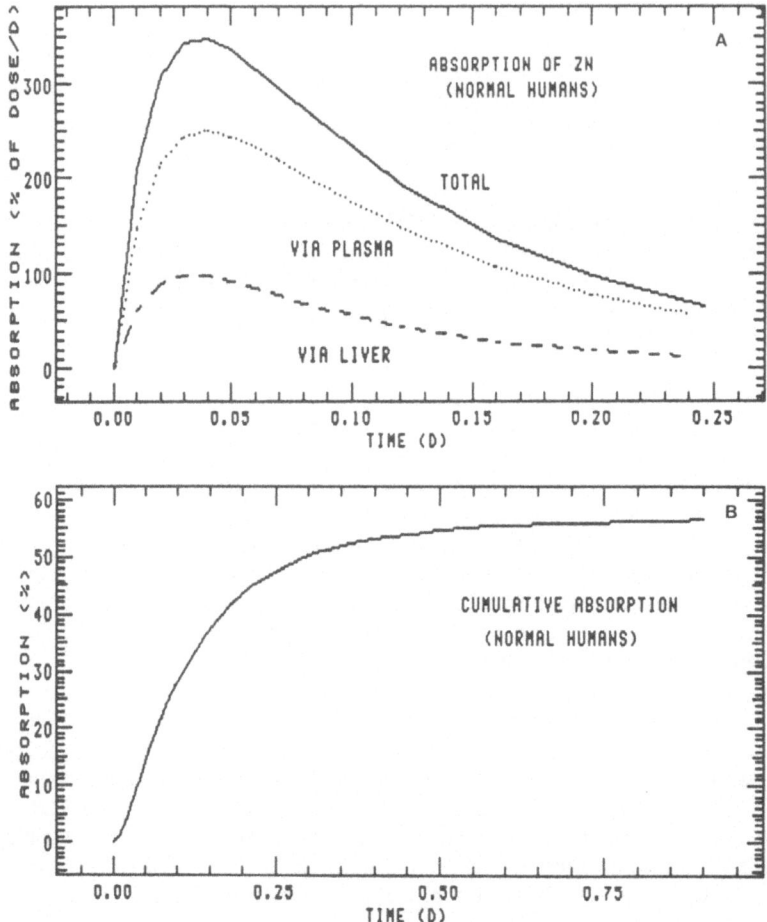

Figure 3. Absorption of zinc tracer into plasma following oral administration determined for normal subjects using the model (Figure 1) and parameter values for normal subjects (Wastney et al., 1986) a) the total appearance of tracer (solid line), tracer absorbed directly into plasma (dotted line) and tracer absorbed via liver (dashed line) and b) cumulative absorption (% of dose) occurring over 1 d.

Deconvolution of plasma data obtained following oral and intravenous tracer administration described an absorption function that enabled a more complex model for absorption to be developed (Foster et al., 1979). (The function determined for normal subjects is shown in Figure 3a.) The absorption model consisted of absorption pathways from a series of compartments in the gut that were considered to represent different sites of absorption. Zinc absorption occurred after 14 min and since passage through the stomach is about an hour it was suggested

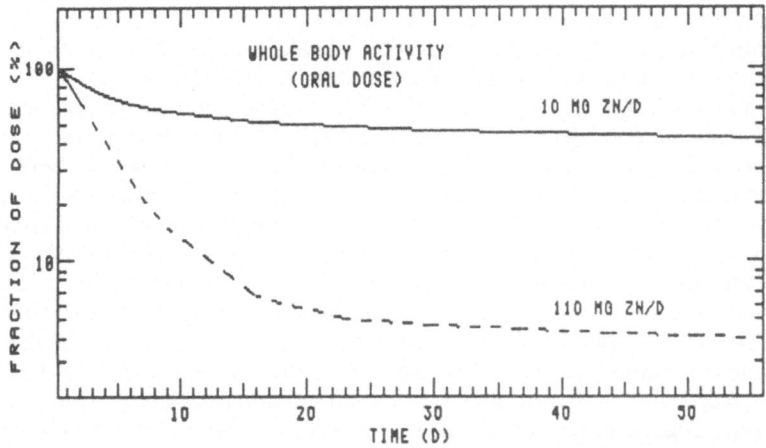

Figure 4. Whole body activity following oral administration of tracer to normal subjects determined using the model and parameter values for a normal population (Figure 1) while on a basal zinc intake of 10 mg/d (solid line) and on an additional 100 mg exogenous Zn/d (dashed line), (Wastney et al., 1986).

that some absorption must occur in the stomach (Foster et al., 1979). Passage through the small intestine is about 4 hr and it was considered that the rest of the zinc was absorbed from the duodenum (Foster et al., 1979). By comparison with calcium data it was determined that zinc and calcium were predominantly absorbed from the duodenum but zinc, unlike calcium, was also absorbed at a site lower than the duodenum, from the jejunum and/or ileum (Foster et al., 1979). In support of this prediction, data obtained from rats (Methfessel & Spencer, 1973) and dogs (Naveh et al., 1988) suggest that the duodenum has the greatest capacity to absorb zinc and studies in humans have shown that zinc absorption from the colon is small (Sandstrom et al., 1986). Further details of the absorptive mechanism of zinc can be incorporated into the model as data become available.

Calculation of absorption. Absorption of zinc has been determined by a number of methods including balance studies (Hartley et al., 1974), zinc tolerance tests (Andersson et al., 1976; Sullivan et al., 1979) and techniques using tracers, such as fecal monitoring (Janghorbani & Young, 1980), regression analysis of fecal excretion of tracer (Janghorbani et al., 1985) whole body counting (Arvidsson et al., 1978; Payton et al., 1982) and by comparing whole body retention after oral versus intravenous tracer administration (Aamodt et al., 1981; Molokhia et al., 1980). Although it is not always explicitly stated, each technique assumes a model of absorption and has underlying assumptions about the process that affect the value determined for absorption. An advantage of representing the physiological system by a compartmental model, as described in this manuscript, is that assumptions of the model can be recognized from the configuration of the model. Another advantage of using compartmental modeling to determine absorption is that data from a number of tissues can be analysed simultaneously. This 1) ensures that a consistent solution is obtained, 2) allows parameter values for other process of metabolism (e.g., secretion and excretion in addition to absorption) to be determined and 3) allows the error on each parameter to be calculated.

The model (Figure 1) was used to analyze data from an independent study, using data from one subject in the literature (Furchner & Richmond, 1962). Data were reported following oral administration of ^{65}Zn for the whole body (for 650 d) and feces (for 4 d) while the subject was on their normal diet (~12 mg Zn/d) and whole body (for 14 d) and feces (for 3 d) when zinc intake was increased by an additional 10 mg Zn/d (Furchner & Richmond, 1962), (Figure 5). A good fit was obtained to the data while the subject was on 12 mg Zn/d using average population parameter values and allowing only absorption to vary (Figure 5). Although the model was developed from data obtained over only 270 d a good fit was obtained to whole body data obtained from this subject over 650 d (Figure 5a) suggesting that kinetics determined for the slow compartments of the model (muscle and bone, Figure 1) can be applied over a longer-term. In this subject absorption of tracer was high (over 90%) and most (79%) occurred from the first site in the gut (Gut1, Figure 1). The remaining tracer (21% of the dose) and secreted tracer were absorbed from the second site lower in the gut (Gut2, Figure 1) at the population value of 50% (Equation 2). Details of the subject were not provided to assist in interpretation of this result (Furchner & Richmond, 1962).

When zinc intake increased to ~22 mg/d for 30 d prior to tracer administration, data from whole body and feces were fitted by the model (Figure 1) by decreasing absorption from 90% to 46% (Figure 5b and c). These results agree with Payton et al. (1982) who also calculated a progressive decrease in fractional absorption when subjects were given increasing amounts of zinc, and the later studies of Wastney et al. (1986) where absorption decreased from 59% to 7% when zinc intake increased from 10 to 110 mg/d. These studies illustrate how absorption functions as a site of regulation of zinc metabolism in humans.

Absorption as one site of regulation of zinc metabolism. What is the relationship of absorption to zinc metabolism and is this parameter a good indicator of zinc status? Since all zinc enters the body from the gut, absorption is often considered to be an index of zinc status. If this were the only parameter regulating zinc metabolism absorption would be a useful indicator of zinc status. However, regulation of long-term human zinc metabolism involves four, or more, sites in addition to absorption, (RBC exchange, secretion into gut, excretion into urine and release from a slowly turning over compartment, considered to be muscle, Wastney

Figure 5. Data (symbols) from one subject (Furchner & Richmond, 1962) following an oral dose of ^{65}Zn and values calculated by the model (lines) using parameter values from a normal population (Figure 1), while the subject was on ~12 mg Zn/d (squares and solid line) and ~22 mg Zn/d (diamonds and dashed line), a) whole body activity over 650 d while on 12 mg Zn/d, b) whole body activity over 14 d, while the subject was on 12 mg Zn/d and 22 mg Zn/d, c) and fecal data over 4 d while the subject was on 12 mg Zn/d and over 3 d while the subject was on ~22 mg Zn/d.

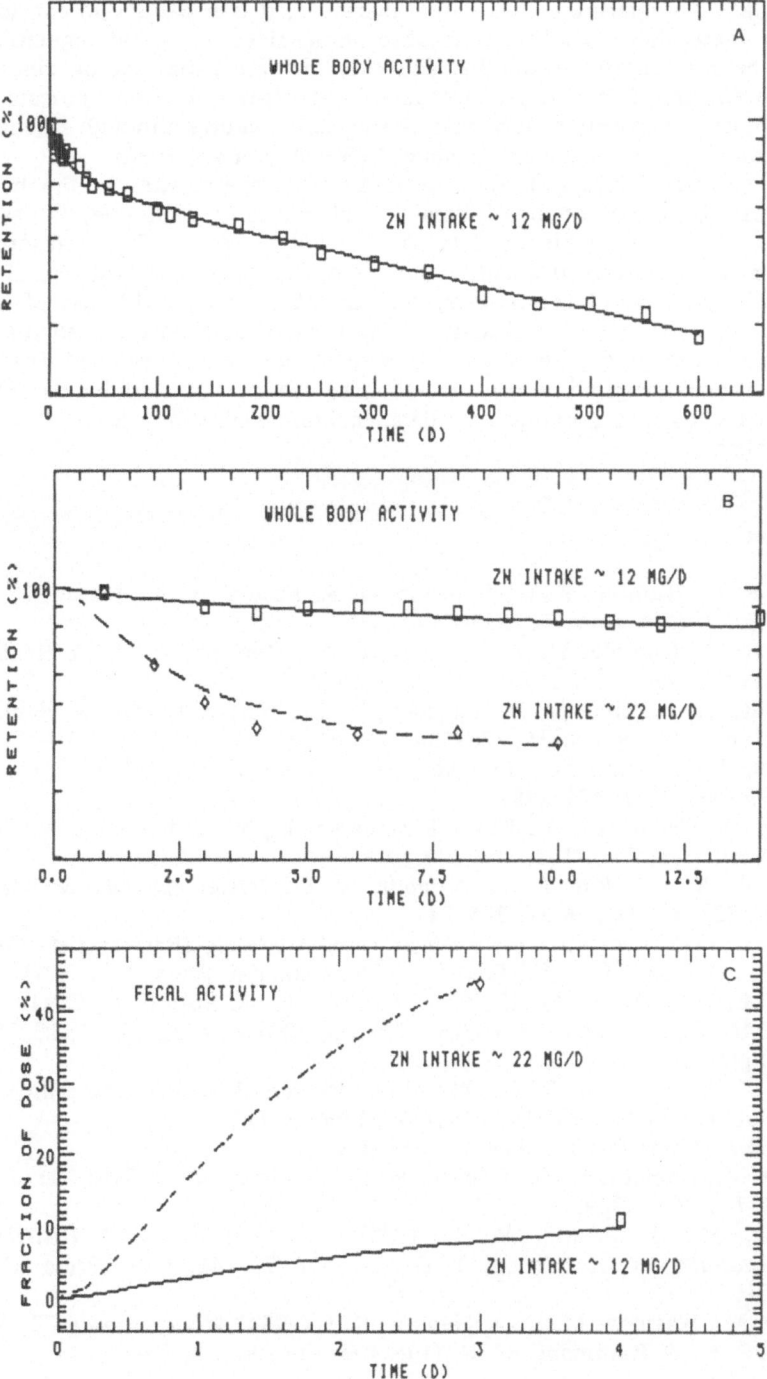

et al., 1986). To determine zinc status, therefore, it is necessary to consider metabolism at these sites, in addition to absorption, since abnormal regulation at one site may be compensated at another site with the result that overall zinc metabolism is not affected. For example, a change in absorption may not indicate a change in zinc status as absorption decreased during zinc loading although calculated zinc levels in some tissues remained unchanged (Wastney et al., 1986).

One method of assessing zinc metabolism at several sites in the body is by kinetic analysis of data obtained from several tissues by modeling, as described in these studies. Modeling kinetic data has enabled processes of zinc absorption and metabolism to be described quantitatively. With the greater availability of computing facilities and modeling software, such as SAAM/CONSAM, use of models as biological research tools should assist in the further quantitative evaluation of zinc metabolism. The model described in these studies was developed from *in vivo* data. Additional insight into zinc metabolism can be obtained by developing the model further by incorporating new data, including *in vitro* data, on specific areas of metabolism.

References

Aamodt, R. L., Rumble, W. F., Johnston, G. S., Foster, D., & Henkin, R. I. (1979) *Am. J. Clin. Nutr.* 32, 559-569.

Aamodt, R. L., Rumble, W. F., Johnston, G. S., Markley, E. J., & Henkin, R. I. (1981) *Am. J. Clin. Nutr.* 34, 2648-2652.

Aamodt, R. L., Rumble, W. F., Babcock, A. K., Foster, D. M. & Henkin, R. I. (1982) *Metabolism* 31, 326-334.

Andersson, K-E., Bratt, L., Dencker, H. & Lanner, E. (1976) *Europ. J. Clin. Pharmacol.* 9, 423-428.

Arvidsson, B., Cederblad, A., Bjorn-Rasmussen, E., & Sandstrom, B. (1978) *Int. J. Nucl. Med. Biol.* 105, 104-109.

Babcock, A. K., Henkin, R. I., Aamodt, R. L., Foster, D. M., & Berman, M. (1982) *Metabolism* 31, 335-347.

Berman, M. (1982) in *Lipoprotein Kinetics and Modeling* (Berman, M., Grundy, S. M., & Howard, B. V., Eds) pp 3-36, Academic Press, New York.

Berman, M., Beltz, W. F., Greif., P. C., Chabay, R., & Boston, R. C. (1983) *CONSAM User's Guide.* US Govt. Printing Office, 1983-421-132:3279, Washington DC.

Berman, M. & Weiss, M. F. (1978) *SAAM Manual.* U.S. Printing Office, [DHEW Publication No (NIH) 78-180], Washington DC.

Cousins, R.J. (1985) *Physiol. Rev.* 65, 238-309.

Foster, D. M., Aamodt, R. L., Henkin, R. I., & Berman, M. (1979) *Am. J. Physiol.* 237, R340-R349.

Foster, D. M., & Boston, R. C. (1983) in *Compartmental Distribution of Radiotracers* (Robertson, J. D., Ed.) pp 73-142, CRC Press, Cleveland, OH.

Foster, D. M., Wastney, M. E., & Henkin, R. I. (1984) *Math. Biosci.* 72, 359-372.

Furchner, J. E., & Richmond, C. R. (1962) *Health Phys.* 8, 35-40.

Hartley, T.F., Dawson, J.B., & Hodgkinson, A. (1974) *Clin. Chim. Acta* 52, 321-333.

Henkin, R. I. (1984) *Biol. Trace Elem. Res.* 6, 263-280.

Janghorbani, M., & Young, V.R. (1980) *Am. J. Clin. Nutr.* 33, 2021-2030.

Janghorbani, M., Young, V. R., & Ehrenkranz, R. A. (1985) in *Trace Elements in Nutrition of Children* (Chandra, R. K., Ed.) pp 63-85, Vevey/Raven Press, New York.

Methfessel, A. H., & Spencer, H. (1973) *J. Appl. Physiol.* 34, 58-62.

Meret, S., & Henkin, R. I. (1971) *Clin. Chem.* 17, 369-373.

Molokhia, M., Sturniolo, G., Shields, R., & Turnberg, L. A. (1980) *Am. J. Clin. Nutr.* 33, 881-886.

Naveh, Y., Bentur L., & Diamond, E. (1988) *J. Nutr.* 118, 61-64.

Payton, K. B., Flanagan, P. R., Stinson, E. A., Chodirker, D. P., Chamberlain, M. J., & Valberg, L. S. (1982) *Gastroent.* 83, 1264-1270.

Phair, R. D. (1982) in *Lipoprotein Kinetics and Modeling* (Berman, M., Grundy, S. M., & Howard, B. V., Eds.) pp 37-40, Academic Press, New York.

Prasad, A. S. (1979) *Ann. Rev. Pharmacol. Toxicol.* 20, 393-426.

Sandstrom, B., Cederblad, A., Kivisto, B., Stenquist, B., & Andersson, H. (1986) *Am. J. Clin. Nutr.* 44, 501-504.

Solomons, N. W., & Cousins, R. J. (1984) in *Absorption and Malabsorption of Mineral Nutrients* (Solomons, N. W., & Rosenberg, I. H., Eds.) pp 125-197, Alan R. Liss, N.Y.

Sullivan, J. F., Jetton, M. M., & Burch, R. E. (1979) *J. Lab. Clin. Med.* 93, 485-492.

Wastney, M. E., Aamodt, R. L., Rumble, W. F., & Henkin, R. I. (1986) *Am. J. Physiol.* 251, R398-R408.

3

Mechanisms of Intestinal Brush Border Iron Transport[1]

Robert J. Simpson[2], Kiskor B. Raja and Timothy J. Peters

Mucosal uptake represents the first cellular step in iron absorption and is the point at which the cell biochemistry of iron absorption and the nutritional chemistry of dietary iron interact. Mucosal uptake was identified as a distinct step in the iron absorption process about 30 years ago (Manis & Schachter, 1962) and several groups of workers have since investigated the kinetics and mechanism of mucosal uptake in experimental animals *in vivo* and with various *in vitro* preparations. Different viewpoints regarding mucosal uptake emerged from these studies and key experimental findings were not always in agreement. For example, studies with *in vitro* incubated tissue failed to agree on whether the initial uptake step is regulable, saturable or regional (Sheehan, 1976; Acheson & Schultz, 1972; Cox & O'Donnell, 1982). *In vivo* studies also conflict as to whether uptake shows saturation kinetics (Wheby et al., 1964; Thompson & Valberg, 1971; Moore et al., 1964).

Studies on isolated brush border membrane Fe transport, which we equate with mucosal uptake, disagree as to the involvement of specific protein carriers in brush border membrane iron transport (Marx & Aisen, 1981; O'Donnell & Cox, 1982; Muir & Hopfer, 1985). We therefore previously set out to conduct a wide ranging and comprehensive study of the mechanism of mucosal iron uptake using mouse intestine both *in vivo* and *in vitro* and using both normal mice and mice with adaptive enhancement of iron absorption.. Hypoxia was selected as a rapid method of evoking enhanced intestinal iron uptake by adult mice, simply placing mice in a hypobaric chamber (0.5 atmospheres—equivalent to an altitude of approximately 5000 m) for 3 days produces a 3-5 fold stimulation in iron absorption. Initial studies were performed with two forms of bioavailable iron;

1 This work was supported by the U.K. Medical Research Council.
2 Author to whom correspondence should be addressed.

27

Fe/ascorbate and Fe/nitrilotriacetate (NTA). The former complex is more physio-logical but is less stable and less well defined. The latter is better defined, more stable but probably unphysiological. These two solutions displayed some distinct properties of ^{59}Fe uptake, raising the question of whether these differences arise solely from differences in chemistry of Fe between the solutions, or from the pres-ence of more than one distinct mechanism for mucosal Fe uptake.

In this paper we will therefore describe kinetic results obtained using each model solution and provide a model for intestinal Fe uptake incorporating these observations.

Experimental Procedures

Measurements of mucosal Fe uptake *in vivo* were performed with tied-off seg-ments of proximal mouse intestine as previously described (Simpson & Peters, 1986; Simpson et al., 1986; Raja et al., 1987a). Incubation media were prepared fresh and contained 0.1 M mannitol, 0.1 M NaCl, 20 mM Hepes-NaOH buffer, pH 7.4. *In vitro* mucosal Fe uptake was determined with pieces of duodenum (2-6 mg wet weight) (Raja et al., 1987a,b).

Male, 6-8 week old, mice (strain To) were used throughout. Hypoxia was induced by placing mice in a hypobaric chamber (0.5 atmospheres) for 3 days (Raja et al., 1987b). Food and water was supplied *ad lib*. The enhanced absorp-tion observed in hypobaric-treated mice was similar to that seen in normobaric mice exposed for 3 days to 10% O_2 (Raja et al., 1988). Fe/ascorbate (1:20) solu-tions for *in vitro* incubations were prepared by mixing 10 mM $FeCl_3$ in 10 mM HCl with a freshly prepared 0.1 M solution of Na ascorbate. The mixture was then added to a stock buffer giving final concentrations 16 mM Hepes (pH 7.4), 125 mM NaCl, 3.5 mM KCl, 1 mM $CaCl_2$, 10 mM $MgSO_4$, 10 mM D-glucose, 5 nM [^{57}Co]-cyanocobalamin (specific activity 0.5-1.0 kBq pmol^{-1}), Fe in the range 45-450 μM and ascorbate in the range 0.9-9 mM. The mixture was bubbled with 95% O_2/5% CO_2 at 37°C for at least 30 min to ensure pH, temperature and O_2 equilibration of the medium before the pieces of duodenum were added to com-mence an uptake determination. Fe/NTA solutions were prepared as above except that 90-900 μM NTA was substituted for the ascorbate. In some experiments, $CaCl_2$ and $MgSO_4$ were omitted from the mixture. Brush border membrane vesicle Fe uptake was determined with ^{59}Fe/ascorbate in 0.1 M mannitol, 0.1 M NaCl, 20 mM Hepes (pH 7.4) (Simpson & Peters, 1984, 1985). Uptake measurements were performed after 5 min preincubation at 37°C.

In some experiments 100 μM ^{51}CrEDTA (1:4) was substituted for Fe/chelate. ^{51}CrEDTA is a stable metal complex which is excluded from cells and therefore is an excellent marker for extracellular fluid and paracellular (i.e., between cells) absorption pathways (Garnett et al., 1967; Bjarnason & Peters, 1984).

Statistical methods. Where data were normally distributed (Royston, 1983), differences were tested by students' *t*-test. Where data were not normally distri-buted, Wilcoxons' rank sum test was employed (Wetherill, 1967).

Results

Uptake of iron by mouse proximal intestine *in vitro*, from various solutions, is shown in Figure 1. The uptake from FeEDTA (1:2) can be seen to be similar to that of the extra-cellular fluid marker ^{51}CrEDTA. Both metal complexes show little uptake after correction for extracellular fluid space with ^{57}Co-cyanocobalamin. Similar uptake was obtained with Fe NTA when a very large excess of NTA (100:1, NTA:Fe) was present. *In vivo* experiments also show similar results (Simpson & Peters, 1986). The uptake of Fe from Fe/ascorbate is similar to uptake from Fe(NTA)$_2$, both being greater than the extracellular fluid markers.

Table I shows the effect of metabolic inhibitors, dinitrophenol and NaF on *in vitro* mucosal Fe uptake. Uptake from both Fe(NTA)$_2$ and Fe/ascorbate was significantly inhibited, especially when both inhibitors were present.

Table II shows the effect of hypoxia on mucosal uptake of Fe *in vivo* and *in vitro*. These data show that uptake from freshly prepared Fe/ascorbate by tied-off segments does not respond to hypoxia while uptake from Fe(NTA)$_2$ is greatly increased. Isolated brush border vesicle Fe uptake shows little increase in response to hypoxia, irrespective of the Fe solution. With *in vitro* incubated tissue, mucosal uptake is strikingly enhanced from both Fe/ascorbate and Fe(NTA)$_2$ solutions but the increase in uptake from Fe(NTA)$_2$ is muted by the presence of divalent cations, MgSO$_4$ and CaCl$_2$.

Figure 2 shows the availability of Fe to the chelator ferrozine in O$_2$ bubbled Fe/ascorbate solutions. When ferrozine is added to Fe/ascorbate solutions, different forms of Fe can be distinguished, viz rapidly available Fe ($t_{1/2}$ for complex formation < 1 s), slowly available Fe ($t_{1/2}$ 1-1000 s), non-available Fe ($t_{1/2}$ >> 1000 s) (Dorey et al., 1987). Rapidly available Fe appears to represent ferrous and weakly chelated ferric species. Figure 2 shows that the rapidly available form of Fe disappears quickly from O$_2$ bubbled Fe ascorbate solutions as used for the *in vitro* studies above. We have previously shown that freshly prepared, air equilibrated, Fe/ascorbate contains substantial rapidly-available Fe on the timescale of the uptake measurements made with brush border vesicles and from *in vivo* tied loops (Simpson & Peters, 1987).

Discussion

Paracellular mechanism of mucosal Fe uptake. Our results show that mucosal Fe uptake from suitably stable Fe solutions (Fe EDTA (1:2), Fe NTA (1:100)) of low molecular weight (< 1000 dalton) can be explained by paracellular (i.e., between cell) uptake (Bjarnason & Peters, 1984) mechanisms, as observed with the stable extracellular fluid marker ^{51}CrEDTA. This mechanism may be expected to be non-saturable and non-regulated and may form a small but significant basal uptake from any solution containing low molecular weight Fe. The presence of such a mucosal uptake mechanism may explain the well known incomplete suppression of Fe absorption in Fe overload (Crosby, 1966).

Cellular mechanisms of mucosal uptake. The data presented for Fe uptake both *in vivo* and *in vitro*, show additional uptake, presumably attributable to cellu-

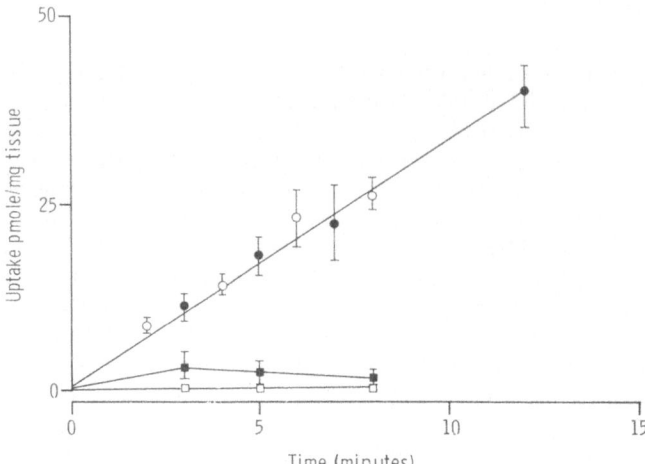

Figure 1. *In vitro* mucosal uptake of ^{59}Fe from various chelates. Mucosal uptake from ^{59}Fe labelled chelates, Fe NTA (1:2) (●); Fe EDTA (1:2) (□) and Fe/ascorbate (1:20) (○), was measured as in the text. Also shown is uptake of ^{51}CrEDTA (■). All metals present at 90 μM. Uptakes were corrected for uptake of the extracellular fluid marker ^{57}Co-cyanocobalamin.

Table I. Effect of metabolic inhibitors on *in vitro* mucosal Fe uptake[a]

Experiment	Inhibition of ^{59}Fe uptake (%)[b]	
	250 μM ^{59}Fe(NTA)$_2$	250 μM ^{59}Fe/ascorbate (1:20)
0.1 mM dinitrophenol	22.6 ± 3.1 (4)	18.9 ± 2.9 (5)
10 mM NaF	26.8 ± 3.5 (6)	35.8 ± 3.8 (4)
Both inhibitors	43.4 ± 2.9 (4)[c]	55.4 ± 3.4 (3)[d]

[a] Incubation time 5 min, see text for details. Data are mean ± SEM for (n) determinations.
[b] Inhibition of uptake performed in parallel with control tissue from same animal.
[c] P < 0.02 compared to other inhibitors above.
[d] P < 0.01 compared to dinitrophenol above.

lar processes. The responses of this uptake to hypoxia depend on the chemistry of the Fe solution and the preparation used.

We previously showed that the uptake of Fe from Fe(NTA)$_2$, in particular, the effects of hypoxia and divalent cations (particularly Ca^{2+}) on uptake could be explained by a two mechanism hypothesis (Raja et al., 1987c). One mechanism relates to uptake of 'weakly chelated' Fe the other to 'strongly chelated' Fe. This second pathway depends on metabolic energy and is greatly enhanced in response

Table II. Effect of hypoxia on Mucosal Fe uptake

Experiment[a]	State	Mucosal ^{59}Fe Uptake			
		^{59}Fe(NTA)$_2$		^{59}Fe/ascobate (1:20)	
In vivo tied-off segment[b]	Normal	60 ± 2.0 (3)		45.4 ± 2.0 (8)	
	Hypoxic	377 ± 36 (8)[f]		55.7 ± 5.9 (11)	
Brush border membrane vesicles[d]	Normal	0.89 ± 0.24 (16)		8.5 range 5.9-17 (17)	
	Hypoxic	1.38 ± 0.26 (17)[e]		9.9 range 7.4-19.5 (15)	
In vitro incubated tissue[c]		Vmax	Km	Vmax	Km
With MgSO$_4$ and CaCl$_2$	Normal	10.5 ± 0.9	103 ± 20 (9)	10.2 ± 1.3	111 ± 31 (6)
	Hypoxic	22.7 ± 2.5[f]	103 ± 17 (8)	33.4 ± 6.0[e]	99 ± 28 (7)
Without MgSO$_4$ or CaCl$_2$	Normal	9.4 ± 1.0	66 ± 9 (5)	ND[g]	ND
	Hypoxic	35.6 ± 6.1[e]	90 ± 21 (5)	ND	ND

[a] For further details see text.
  Given values are means ± SEM for (n) determinations.
[b] pmol/10 min/mg tissue.
[c] Vmax (pmol/min/mg tissue), Km (μM).
[d] nmol/min/mg protein (Fe/ascorbate),
  nmol/5 min/mg protein (Fe(NTA)$_2$).
[e] $P < 0.01$.
[f] $P < 0.001$.
[g] Not determined.

to hypoxia. This hypothesis explains the effect of divalent cations on the hypoxic response (Table II) by suggesting that divalent cations affect the stability of Fe(NTA)$_2$ by competing with Fe for NTA and stimulating uptake by one mechanism but inhibiting uptake by the other (see Figure 3 for diagram).

The data presented above further suggest that the same, two mechanism hypothesis may be used to explain the uptake of Fe from Fe/ascorbate solutions. We have previously shown that brush border vesicle membrane Fe transport can explain *in vivo* mucosal uptake if freshly prepared Fe/ascorbate solutions are used (Simpson et al., 1986). Furthermore, we have suggested that Fe transport from Fe(NTA)$_2$ by isolated brush border membrane vesicles can explain a minor portion of Fe uptake, seen with intact mucosa, which is stimulable by divalent cations (especially Ca^{2+}) (Raja et al., 1987c) but only slightly by hypoxia. Recent investigation of the mechanism of this brush border membrane transport process has revealed that it can be explained by non-esterified fatty acid-mediated Fe transport and that this transport can be from fresh Fe/ascorbate or (more slowly) from Fe(NTA)$_2$ (Simpson et al., 1988). The data presented herewith further show that if Fe/ascorbate solutions are aged in the presence of O$_2$, Fe uptake by *in vitro* mucosal tissue behaves like that from Fe(NTA)$_2$ solutions (i.e., uptake is highly responsive to hypoxia and sensitive to metabolic inhibitors). This observation

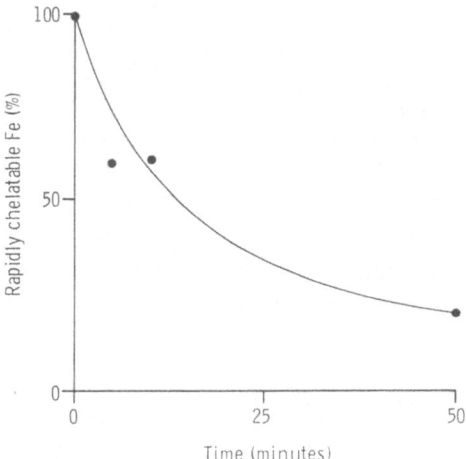

Figure 2. Availability of Fe in Fe/ascorbate solutions to chelator fer-rozine. Rapidly available ($t_{1/2}$ for complex formation $<$ 1-2 s) Fe in 100 μM Fe/ascorbate (1:20) in incubation mixture (see text). Mixture was prepared at t=0 and incubated at 37°C with O_2-bubbling. Samples were taken for availability assays at the indicated times.

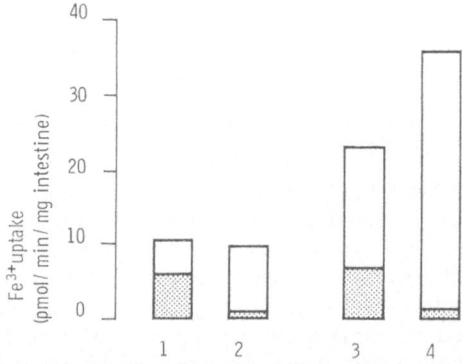

Figure 3. Mucosal uptake properties of two Fe uptake mechanisms. The open areas represent a Ca^{2+}-inhibitable uptake pathway, which is confined to the duodenum and responds to hypoxia. The hatched areas represent a Ca^{2+}-stimulable uptake pathway, present in all regions of intestine and not greatly responsive to hypoxia. 1) Normal mice, with Ca^{2+} in incubation mixture; 2) Normal, without Ca^{2+}; 3) Hypoxic mice, with Ca^{2+}; 4) Hypoxic, without Ca^{2+}. Adapted from Raja et al., 1987c.

demonstrates that our proposed, energy dependent, regulable Fe uptake mechanism (Raja et al., 1987c) previously observed with the unphysiological chelate $Fe(NTA)_2$ can also be observed using aged Fe/ascorbate, a physiological Fe source.

Aged Fe/ascorbate solutions, which contain predominantly polynuclear Fe^{3+} species (Dorey et al., 1987), are thus available for intestinal uptake by the same pathway as the complex $Fe(NTA)_2$. Fresh Fe/ascorbate solutions, containing predominantly Fe^{2+} and weak Fe^{3+} ascorbate complexes (Dorey et al., 1987) are available for intestinal uptake by a distinct pathway which also operates on destabilized $Fe(NTA)_2$ complex.

In conclusion these studies indicated that three mechanisms are important in *in vivo* Fe uptake by mouse duodenum. Firstly, paracellular uptake provides a non-regulated, low affinity process which should not be ignored in normal animals and may be important in certain pathological conditions. Two other cellular mechanisms of uptake involving brush border iron transport could be identified, namely, a partially regulated, passive transport and a high affinity highly regulated transport dependent on metabolic energy. The former process could be observed in isolated brush border membrane vesicles and may be explained by non-esterified fatty acid-dependent transport of Fe. The latter process is not observed in isolated membrane vesicles. Both mechanisms of uptake can be observed using both Fe/ascorbate and Fe/nitrilotriacetate solutions, under specific circumstances.

Acknowledgement

We thank Mrs. Sheila Kingsley for assistance in preparing the manuscript.

References

Acheson, L.S., & Schultz, S.G. (1972) *Biochim. Biophys. Acta* 255, 479-483.

Bjarnason, I., & Peters, T. J. (*1984*) *Gut* 25, 145-150.

Cox, T. M., & O'Donnell, M. W. (1982) *Br. J. Nutr.* 47, 251-258.

Crosby, W. H. (1966) *Seminars Haematol.* 3, 299-313.

Dorey, C., Dickson, D. P. E., St. Pierre, T. G., Pollard, R. F., Gibson, J. F., Simpson, R. J., & Peters, T. J. (1987) *Biochem. Soc. Trans.* 15, 688.

Garnett, E. S., Parsons, V., & Veall, N. (1967) *Lancet* i: 818-819.

Manis, J. G., & Schachter, D. (1962) *Am. J. Physiol.* 203, 73-80.

Marx, J. J. M., & Aisen, P. (1981) *Biochim. Biophys. Acta* 649, 297-304.

Moore, E. W., Linscher, W. G., & Keene, W. R. (1964) *J. Clin. Invest.* 43, 1282.

Muir, A. W., & Hopfer, U. (1985) *Am. J. Physiol.* 248, G376-G379.

O'Donnell, M. W., & Cox, T. M. (1982) *Biochem. J.* 202, 107-115.

Raja, K. B., Simpson, R. J., & Peters, T. J. (1987a) *Biochim. Biophys. Acta* 901, 52-60.

Raja, K. B., Bjarnason, I., Simpson, R. J., & Peters, T. J. (1987b) *Cell Biochem. Funct.* 5, 69-76.

Raja, K. B., Simpson, R. J., & Peters, T. J. (1987c) *Biochim. Biophys. Acta* 923, 46-51.

Raja, K. B., Simpson, R. J., Pippard, M. J., & Peters, T. J. (1988) *Br. J. Haematol.* 68, 373–378.

Royston, J. P. (1983) *J. Roy. Stat. Soc.* (Series C) 32, 121–133.

Sheehan, R. G. (1976) *Am. J. Physiol.* 231, 1438–1444.

Simpson, R. J., Moore, R., & Peters, T. J. (1988) *Biochim. Biophys. Acta* 941, 39–47.

Simpson, R. J., & Peters, T. J. (1984) *Biochim. Biophys. Acta* 772, 220–226.

Simpson, R. J., & Peters, T. J. (1985) *Biochim. Biophys. Acta* 814, 381–388.

Simpson, R. J., & Peters, T. J. (1986) *Biochim. Biophys. Acta* 856, 115–122.

Simpson, R. J., & Peters, T. J. (1987) *Biochim. Biophys. Acta* 898, 187–195.

Simpson, R. J., Raja, K. B., & Peters, T. J. (1986) *Biochim. Biophys. Acta* 860, 229–235.

Thomson, A. B. R., & Valberg, L.S. (1971) *Am. J. Physiol.* 223, 1327–1329.

Wetherill, G. B. (1967) in *Elementary Statistical Methods*, Methuen & Co. Ltd., London.

Wheby, M. S., Jones, L. G., & Crosby, W. A. (1964) *J. Clin. Invest.* 43, 1433–1442.

4

Trace Metal Interactions Involving the Intestinal Absorption Mechanisms of Iron and Zinc[1]

Peter R. Flanagan

The basis for absorptive trace element interactions is given by the statement of Hill & Matrone (1970) that "those elements whose physical and chemical properties are similar will act antagonistically to each other biologically". Although the direct antagonistic competition of chemically-alike metals is a straightforward concept, an important associated view is that dietary preconditioning with an excess or deficiency of an element may reveal interactions with the metabolism of chemically-similar metals.

I have reviewed elsewhere methods to demonstrate trace metal interactions (Flanagan, 1987). Since the present paper focuses on intestinal absorptive interactions, I will especially emphasize two methods to demonstrate them: 1) by simultaneous gastrointestinal presentation, e.g., in an oral dose or an intestinal perfusate, or; 2) by dietary preconditioning with subsequent absorptive studies. While the results of both kinds of studies often support each other, it is instructive that this is not always the case. For example in humans, an increased capacity to absorb Fe caused by diminished body Fe stores (preconditioning) did not result in increased Zn absorption (Valberg et al., 1984). This was in apparent contrast to the demonstration of a direct inhibition of Zn absorption by the simultaneous administration of an oral Zn dose containing a 10-fold molar excess of Fe (Valberg et al., 1984). The extent to which an interaction is demonstrable may be dependent on the degree to which a transport process is activated as well as its affinity for chemically-similar metals (Flanagan et al., 1980).

---

1 Financial support for the author's research was provided by the Medical Research Council of Canada.

Experimental Procedures

Mice were of the swiss-white strain. They were 6-7 weeks old at the time of study and groups of 8 mice were studied. Prior to study they were fed a semipurified Fe-deficient (FeD) or a similar Fe-normal (FeN) diet for 10-14 days as previously described (Flanagan et al., 1980). Some mice were fed semipurified Zn-deficient (ZnD) or Zn-normal (ZnN) diets for 5-7 days instead (Flanagan et al., 1983). Detailed procedures for the duodenal perfusion technique are given in these references. Briefly, mice were anaesthetised, a laparotomy performed and the proximal 4-5 cm of small intestine cannulated and ligated. Test solutions (5 ml) of 0.15 M NaCl containing 0.1 mM $ZnCl_2$, labelled with 10-20 kBq ^{65}Zn/ml, or 0.1 mM $FeCl_2$, labelled with 10-20 kBq/ml ^{59}Fe, were perfused over a 30 min period. A 2-fold molar excess of ascorbate was added to perfusates containing Fe to ensure its solubility. In some experiments $CuCl_2$ was added at concentrations of 0.05-1 mM (Tables I, III) or $CrCl_3$ at 1 mM (Table II). After killing the mouse, the carcass and the thoroughly-washed segment were counted. **Uptake** values were calculated from radioactivity in both the perfused segment and the carcass, whereas **transfer** measurements were from the carcass counts alone.

Results and Discussion

Interactions Involving the Absorption of Iron

Fe, Co, Mn, Zn. The studies of Pollack et al. (1965) examined the absorption of a series of nonferrous metals in rats preconditioned by Fe deficiency. They found that feeding an Fe-deficient diet increased the absorption of oral doses of not only Fe but also Co, Mn and Zn whereas absorption of Cu, Ca, Mg, Hg and Cs was unaffected. The reciprocal interactions of Fe, Co, Mn and Zn have been studied in detail by Flanagan et al. (1980). Whereas it was shown that each metal inhibited the intestinal uptake and transfer to the body of the others, Fe deficiency preconditioning profoundly affected the extent to which interactions were demonstrable. It is interesting to note that although these metals apparently can share a common absorptive transport mechanism, they differ with regards to excretion. Whereas Fe is retained by the body the others are excreted via pancreas and small intestine (Zn), bile (Mn) and urine (Co, Zn). The rapid urinary excretion of radiocobalt after an oral dose provides an indirect method to measure Fe absorption (Sorbie et al., 1975). Since a nutritional role for Co *per se* in monogastric species has yet to be demonstrated, its absorption is an oddity, due only to its affinity for the Fe absorption pathway. Mn, however, being a nutritionally-essential metal, requires a viable absorptive pathway and therefore may use that of Fe (Thomson et al., 1971; Davidsson et al., 1988).

The Fe-Zn interaction was briefly referred to above. Because inhibitory effects of Fe on Zn absorption have been demonstrated in studies with animals and humans, nutritional concern has focused on the possible dangerous effect of Fe supplementation on Zn metabolism (Anon., 1982). The interested reader is referred elsewhere for a discussion of this topic (Storey & Greger, 1987; Flanagan & Valberg, 1988; Solomons, 1988).

Fe, Cu. A synergistic interaction between Fe and Cu has been recognized from the classic studies of Hart et al. (1928). These workers showed that an anemia caused by the defective utilization of Fe was the result of Cu deficiency and that dietary Cu was required for normal Fe metabolism. This positive interaction is incompletely understood but probably involves the circulating Cu-binding protein ceruloplasmin. Ceruloplasmin has ferroxidase activity and Cu deficiency causes low plasma levels of this enzyme. If ceruloplasmin-ferroxidase is involved in the mobilization and incorporation of Fe into transferrin, this might explain the essentiality of Cu for normal Fe metabolism. However, other explanations for the interaction are possible (Cohen et al., 1985). Antagonistic interactions of Fe and Cu have also been demonstrated but usually at high dietary levels of the elements (Suttle & Mills, 1966; Humphries et al., 1983). The dietary approach has also been recently used to study the triple interaction between Fe, Cu and Zn (Gordon, 1987).

Absorptive interactions *per se* between Fe and Cu have not been studied extensively. The experiments of Pollack et al. (1965), referred to above, failed to show increased Cu absorption in Fe-deficient rats. El-Shobaki & Rummel (1979) confirmed this and showed that Fe did not inhibit Cu uptake and transfer in normal and Fe-deficient rats. This agrees with the work of Bremner & Young (1981) suggesting that high dietary Fe does not inhibit Cu absorption, although later work from this group did show an effect of Fe on Cu (Bremner & Price, 1985). El-Shobaki & Rummel (1979) also examined the other side of this interaction and found a profound inhibition of a 10-fold molar excess of Cu on Fe absorption. Our own studies in mice have confirmed the sensitivity of this interaction (Table I). Fe absorption (transfer) was inhibited by equimolar Cu regardless of dietary Fe pretreatment and by a Cu/Fe ratio of only 0.5 in Fe-deficient mice. The effect of Cu on Fe uptake differed with Fe pretreatment. No inhibitory effect was found in normal mice whereas Fe uptake was lowered in Fe-deficient mice at both levels tested. The results suggest that Cu may interact with the Fe absorption mechanism at usual dietary intakes of the metals and that the responsiveness of the animal is increased by Fe-deficiency. Cu is evidently a sensitive inhibitor of Fe absorption.

Fe, Cd. The electron configuration and position of Cd in the periodic table of elements most immediately suggest interactions with Zn. It is somewhat surprising, therefore, that Cd is a potent inhibitor of Fe absorption. The studies of Hamilton & Valberg (1974) showed that Cd competes for Fe at the uptake step of Fe absorption. Huebers et al. (1987) determined that Cd affected the intracellular processing of Fe. Hamilton & Valberg (1974) demonstrated the interaction with Fe pretreatment, by oral dosing of both metals and by duodenal perfusions. Cd absorption was also investigated; although normally low, it was increased in Fe-deficient animals. Flanagan et al. (1978) extended these findings to humans. Cd absorption in human subjects was shown to be variable but dependent on the level of Fe stores as measured by serum ferritin values. Fe-deficient individuals, with ferritin values < 20 ng/ml, absorbed significantly greater amounts of Cd than those with higher ferritin values. Thus it was not surprising that young female subjects, being on average more Fe-deficient, absorbed more Cd than their male counterparts. This difference may have significant public health implications for individuals exposed to Cd (Chmielnicka & Cherian, 1986).

Table I. Effect of Cu on the intestinal uptake and transfer of ^{59}Fe

Cu/Fe[a]	nmol ^{59}Fe (mean ± SE)	
	Uptake	Transfer
	FeN mice	
0.0	33.63 ± 3.68	8.89 ± 1.68
0.5	39.80 ± 4.30[b]	9.90 ± 1.50
1.0	35.16 ± 3.63	4.11 ± 0.83[b]
	FeD mice	
0.0	85.47 ± 5.32	38.70 ± 3.68
0.5	62.47 ± 4.88[b]	28.73 ± 2.59[b]
1.0	46.68 ± 4.61[b]	15.78 ± 1.90[b]

[a] 0.1 mM Fe was perfused for 30 min in the absence or presence of 0.05 or 0.1 mM Cu as indicated.

[b] Significant difference from value in absence of Cu, $P < 0.05$.

Fe, Pb. Many earlier studies in animals have demonstrated an absorptive interaction between Fe and Pb (Hamilton, 1978; Conrad & Barton, 1978; Flanagan et al., 1979). Compared to other interactions, the demonstration of the Fe-Pb interrelationship requires high molar ratios of one element over the other. Moreover, the existence of the interaction, and its demonstration, may depend on the extent to which the intestinal Fe absorption mechanism is activated (Flanagan et al., 1980; Morrison & Quarterman, 1987). Although dietary Fe deficiency clearly increased Pb absorption in the animal studies, a controversy exists as to whether this is the case in humans. Flanagan et al. (1982) showed that approximately 60% of a 0.1 mg aqueous oral dose of ^{203}Pb was absorbed in fasting subjects. Pb absorption was not related to the size of body Fe stores, nor was it affected by a 10-fold molar excess of oral Fe. On the other hand, Watson et al., (1986) showed a significant correlation between the absorption of dose ^{59}Fe and dose ^{203}Pb, when the isotopes were administered simultaneously as part of a 3-meal dietary regimen. Despite the correlation however, hyperabsorption of Fe was not invariably accompanied by increased Pb absorption. The mechanism of Pb absorption and the Fe connection in humans remains to be clarified satisfactorily.

Interactions Involving the Absorption of Zinc

Zn, Cr. Hahn & Evans (1975) examined the absorption of oral doses of radioisotopes of Fe, Zn, Cu, Cr, Co, Mn and Cd in rats preconditioned by feeding normal or Zn-deficient diets. Only increased absorption of Zn and Cr was demonstrated by this experiment. We recently confirmed this interaction from a different perspective (Table II). Using the murine duodenal perfusion technique, the absorption of 0.1 mM Zn was studied in the absence and presence of 1 mM

Table II. Effect of Cr on the intestinal uptake and transfer of ^{65}Zn

mM		nmol ^{65}Zn (mean ± SE)	
Zn	Cr	Uptake	Transfer
FeN mice			
0.1	—	20.12 ± 0.81	3.34 ± 0.33
0.1	1.0	30.54 ± 4.35[a]	1.28 ± 0.27[a]
FeD mice			
0.1	—	92.31 ± 7.48	32.54 ± 1.76
0.1	1.0	56.74 ± 4.98[a]	15.62 ± 0.87[a]

[a] Significant difference from value in absence of Cr, $P < 0.05$.

Cr. The experiment was performed in mice preconditioned by Fe-normal and Fe-deficient diets to determine whether or not a putative interaction was dependent on an increased capacity to absorb Fe. Cr reduced Zn transfer (absorption) in mice previously fed both the normal and Fe-deficient diets. Cr also reduced the uptake of Zn in the Fe-deficient mice but, paradoxically, increased the amount of Zn retained in the duodenal mucosa, and hence uptake, in the normal animals (Table II). The latter result is inexplicable at present. The transfer results might be explained most easily by hypothesizing two absorption pathways for Zn, one dependent on the Fe-absorptive mechanism and one independent of it (Flanagan et al., 1984). This is discussed below.

Zn, Cu. It is likely that these metals interact with at least two intestinal sites, firstly with transport carriers, and secondly with metallothionein. Each will be discussed in turn. Van Campen and coworkers some time ago demonstrated mutual antagonistic interactions between high ratios of Cu and Zn using ligated segments of rat intestine (Van Campen & Scaife, 1967; Van Campen, 1969). It is not yet certain that these interactions occur at intestinal membrane transport sites for the metals (Oestreicher & Cousins, 1985; Fischer & L'Abbe, 1985).

We recently examined this interaction using the duodenal perfusion technique (Table III). These experiments were carried out in mice preconditioned by brief dietary Zn- or Fe-deficiency. The results demonstrated two things: a) mice pretreated with either Zn-normal, Zn-deficient or Fe-normal diets absorbed only a basal amount of Zn, and a 10-fold molar excess of Cu was ineffective in inhibiting Zn absorption in any of these settings; b) Fe-deficiency stimulated Zn absorption approximately 3-fold, and only in this case did Cu inhibit Zn absorption. The results suggest that Cu is only an inhibitor of the Zn absorption due to the enhanced activity of the Fe absorption mechanism. Put another way, Zn may enter the body by its own transport process or, alternatively, by "piggy-backing" on the Fe-transport mechanism. Only the latter process appears to be inhibitable by Cu (Table III). The triple interaction of Zn, Cu and Fe is reminiscent of the Zn, Cd, Fe interaction discussed below. It may be noted that the absence of enhanced Zn absorption due to Zn-deficiency pretreatment (Table III) confirms

Table III.   Effect of Cu on intestinal ^{65}Zn transfer

Diet	nmol ^{65}Zn (mean ± SE)	
	Zn only[a]	Zn + Cu[a]
ZnN	4.78 ± 0.74	3.53 ± 0.50
ZnD	2.79 ± 0.38	2.63 ± 0.28
FeN	2.48 ± 0.30	3.48 ± 0.32
FeD	12.06 ± 1.78[b]	7.55 ± 0.89[b, c]

[a]   0.1 mM ^{65}Zn was perfused in the absence or presence of 1 mM Cu.

[b]   Significant difference from FeN, $P < 0.05$.

[c]   Significant difference from Zn only value, $P < 0.05$.

earlier results and may be a species-specific result (Flanagan et al. 1983; Cousins, 1985).

The now well-recognized inhibitory effect of high dietary Zn pretreatment on Cu absorption is not caused by simultaneous competition at transport sites. It is mediated by metallothionein within the intestinal absorptive cell. The work of Hall et al. (1979) and Fischer et al. (1981) demonstrated that dietary Zn induced increased levels of intestinal metallothionein because Zn is an excellent inducer of metallothionein. When Cu was subsequently given to the animals, it was taken up by the mucosa but bound to the metallothionein because Cu, having a higher affinity than Zn, displaced Zn from metallothionein binding sites. Metallothionein, in this situation, acts as a "mucosal block" for Cu absorption.

Dietary Zn has therapeutic value in lowering Cu hyperabsorption in certain clinical situations, e.g., Wilson's Disease (Brewer et al., 1983). Nonetheless, inappropriate use of Zn supplements can cause Cu deficiency (Hoffman et al., 1988). This is a concern because of the ready availability of Zn supplements in pharmacies and health food stores and the perception that Zn *per se* is relatively nontoxic (Fischer et al., 1984).

It is likely that "mucosal block" by metallothionein can also explain the potent inhibitory effect of dietary Cd on Cu absorption (Davies & Campbell, 1977; Bremner, 1979).

Zn, Cd.   Because both of these metals are inducers of metallothionein, the possible metal-trapping ability of the protein has dominated speculation on their intestinal interaction. This is particularly so in regard to studies employing dietary pretreatment with the metals (Foulkes & McMullen, 1986). The complexity of this aspect is attested to by the conflicting results of dietary Cd pretreatment on subsequent Zn absorption (Roberts et al., 1973; Oh & Whanger, 1981). Moreover, Zn-deficiency pretreatment did not increase Cd absorption (Foulkes & Voner, 1981; Hoadley & Cousins, 1985).

A direct competitive inhibition of Cd on Zn absorption has been difficult to demonstrate (Evans et al., 1974; Hamilton et al., 1978; Lyall et al., 1979). Using the duodenal perfusion technique *in vivo*, Hamilton et al. (1978) showed that a 2.5-10 fold excess of Cd failed to inhibit Zn uptake or transfer in mice fed a normal diet. However, when the mice were pretreated by feeding an Fe-deficient diet, Cd potently inhibited both uptake and transfer of Zn. This interesting finding points to a triple interaction of Fe, Zn and Cd in the intestine, and again suggests that Zn may be absorbed by more than one pathway. In particular, it suggests that the competitive interaction of two chemically-similar metals, Zn and Cd, is dependent on the absorption process of a third, not-so-similar, metal—Fe. Much more work is required to understand these complex interactions.

Conclusion

Although metal interactions are of obvious nutritional concern (Solomons, 1983; Mills, 1985), they are also of great interest in clarifying physiological and biochemical mechanisms of transport in animals. The remaining discussion will focus on this aspect.

Whereas the precise details of the mechanism of Fe absorption are not clear, there is much evidence that inorganic Fe is absorbed by a specific, carrier-mediated process in the upper intestine (Flanagan, 1988). The basic features of a two-step mechanism (Manis & Schachter, 1962) and the rate enhancement in Fe deficiency (Wheby et al., 1964) are well-recognized. Kinetic differences between the uptake and transfer steps in Fe-replete and in Fe-deficient animals are particularly noteworthy. Although both steps display saturation (i.e., carrier-mediated) kinetics, the transfer step from the mucosa to the body is more restricted to the duodenum and is more responsive to changes in body Fe stores and pretreatment with Fe (Wheby et al., 1964; Thomson & Valberg, 1971; Flanagan & Valberg, 1983). It is clear that a unique Fe-absorbing mechanism exists.

In contrast to Fe, most evidence suggests a diffusion-type mechanism for Zn absorption. Zn is absorbed throughout the small intestine (Antonson et al., 1979; Matseshe et al., 1980; Lee et al., 1987). Unlike Fe, its transport kinetics are not limited by increased amounts of metal, and "saturability" does not readily occur (Weigand & Kirchgessner, 1980; Flanagan et al., 1983; Steinhardt & Adibi, 1984; Hunt et al., 1987; Hoadley et al., 1987). Zn homeostasis is also very different to that of Fe, since excretion plays a significant role in its regulation. Indeed the degree to which Zn absorption adjusts according to dietary Zn level (Table III) and therefore contributes to homeostasis is still a matter for conjecture (Cousins, 1985).

Intestinal absorptive interactions between Fe, Zn and related metals confirm these differences. Whereas the interactions of Fe, Co, Mn, Cu, Cd and Zn support the concept of a distinctive Fe transport carrier(s), interactions with the absorption mechanism for Zn are not so dramatic and have been harder to demonstrate. More than that, the direct kinetic interactions between Zn and Cu (Table III) and Zn and Cd suggest that these occur on the Fe-absorbing mechanism rather than a specific Zn-absorbing site *per se*. This is shown by the fact that they are most-strikingly seen in Fe-deficient animals. The study of mineral interactions, therefore, is useful in clarifying absorptive mechanisms.

A further connection in this regard has come from an unlikely source—the study of Fe uptake mechanisms in bacteria. Several siderophores are synthesized by bacteria for trapping extracellular Fe prior to its uptake. The discovery of *fur* (*f*erric *u*ptake *r*egulation) mutants recently provided evidence for a Fe-regulated genetic element that controls siderophore gene expression (Bagg & Neilands, 1987a). The *fur* gene product has been purified and shown to repress expression of the aerobactin operon *in vitro* (Bagg & Neilands, 1987b). Furthermore, the *fur* protein was found to bind to and block the aerobactin promoter, but only in the presence of Fe(II). Of particular interest to the present discussion was the finding that the essential role of Fe(II) could be substituted by Mn, Co, Zn, Cu and Cd but not by Al. The similarity of this spectrum of active metals to the pattern interacting with the intestinal Fe absorption mechanism is striking. At present, however, the implications of the parallel are difficult to assess because of the apparent differences in the Fe uptake mechanisms of bacteria and animals (Flanagan, 1988).

References

Anonymous (1982) *Nutr. Rev.* 40, 76-77.

Antonson, D. L., Barak, A. J., & Vanderhoof, J. A. (1979) *J. Nutr.* 109, 142-147.

Bagg, A., & Neilands, J. B. (1987a) *Microbiol. Rev.* 51, 509-518.

Bagg, A., & Neilands, J. B. (1987b) *Biochemistry* 26, 5471-5477.

Bremner, I. (1979) *Proc. Nutr. Soc.* 38, 235-242.

Bremner, I., & Price J. (1985) in *Trace Elements in Man and Animals - TEMA 5,* (Mills, C. F., Bremner, I., Chesters, J. K., Eds.) pp 374-376, Commonwealth Agricultural Bureaux, Slough, U.K.

Bremner, I., & Young, B. W. (1981) *Proc. Nutr. Soc.* 40, 69A.

Brewer, G. J., Hill, G. M., Prasad, A. S., Cossack, Z. T., & Rabbani, P. (1983) *Ann. Int. Med.* 99, 314-320.

Chmielnicka, J., & Cherian, M. G. (1986) *Biol. Trace Element Res.* 10, 243-261.

Cohen, N. L., Keen, C. L., Lonnerdal, B., & Hurley, L. S. (1985) *J. Nutr.* 115, 633-649.

Conrad, M. E., & Barton J. C. (1978) *Gastroenterology* 74, 731-740.

Cousins, R. J. (1985) *Physiol. Rev.* 65, 238-309.

Davidsson, L., Cederblad, A., Hagebo, E., Lonnerdal, B., & Sandstrom, B. (1988) *J. Nutr.* in press.

Davies, N. T., & Campbell J. K. (1977) *Life Sci.* 20, 955-960.

El-Shobaki, F. A., & Rummel, W. (1979) *Res. Exp. Med.* (Berl.) 174, 187-195.

Evans, G. W., Grace, C. I., & Hahn, C. (1974) *Bioinorganic Chem.* 3, 115-120.

Fischer, P. W. F., Giroux, A., & L'Abbe, M. R. (1981) *Am. J. Clin. Nutr.* 34, 1670-1675.

Fischer, P. W. F., Giroux, A., & L'Abbe, M. R. (1984) *Am. J. Clin. Nutr.* 40, 743-746.

Fischer, P. W. F., & L'Abbe, M. R. (1985) *Nutr. Res.* 5, 759-767.

Flanagan, P. R. (1987) *AIN Symposium Proceedings. Nutrition '87*, 41-44.

Flanagan, P. R. (1989) in *Iron Transport and Storage* (Ponka, P., Schulman, H., Woodworth, R., & Richter, G., Eds.) CRC Press, Inc., Boca Raton, FL, in press.

Flanagan, P. R., Chamberlain, M. J., & Valberg, L. S. (1982) *Am. J. Clin. Nutr.* 36, 823-829.

Flanagan, P. R., Haist, J., MacKenzie, I., & Valberg, L. S. (1984) *Can. J. Physiol. Pharmacol.* 62, 1124-1128.

Flanagan, P. R., Haist, J., & Valberg. L. S. (1980) *J. Nutr.* 110, 1754-1763.

Flanagan, P. R., Haist, J., & Valberg. L. S. (1983) *J. Nutr.* 113, 962-972.

Flanagan, P. R., Hamilton, D. L., Haist, J., & Valberg, L. S. (1979) *Gastroenterology* 77, 1074-1081.

Flanagan, P. R., McLellan, J. S., Haist, J., Cherian, M. G., Chamberlain, M. J., & Valberg, L. S. (1978) *Gastroenterology* 74, 841-846.

Flanagan, P. R., & Valberg, L. S. (1988) in *Essential and Toxic Trace Elements in Human Health and Disease* (Prasad A. S., Ed.) pp 501-507, Alan R. Liss, Inc., New York.

Foulkes, E. C., & McMullen, D. M. (1986) *Toxicol.* 38, 285-291.

Foulkes, E. C., & Voner, C. (1981) *Toxicol.* 22, 115-22.

Gordon, D. T. (1987) *AIN Symposium Proceedings. Nutrition '87* 27-31.

Hahn, C. J., & Evans, G. W. (1975) *Am. J. Physiol.* 228, 1020-1023.

Hall, A. C., Young, B. W., & Bremner, I. (1979) *J. Inorg. Biochem.* 11, 57-66.

Hamilton, D. L. (1978) *Toxicol.* 46, 1-11.

Hamilton, D. L., Bellamy, J. E. C., Valberg, J. D., & Valberg, L. S. (1978) *Can. J. Physiol. Pharmacol.* 56, 384-389.

Hamilton, D. L., & Valberg, L. S. (1974) *Am. J. Physiol.* 227, 1033-1037.

Hart, E. B., Steenbock, H., Waddell, J., & Elvehjem, C. A. (1928) *J. Biol. Chem.* 77, 797-812.

Hill, C. H., & Matrone, G. (1970) *Fed. Proc.* 20, 1474-81.

Hoadley, J. E., & Cousins, R. J. (1985) *Proc. Soc. Exp. Biol. Med.* 180, 296-302.

Hoadley, J. E., Leinart, A. S., & Cousins, R. J. (1987) *Am. J. Physiol.* 252, G825-831.

Hoffman, H. N., Phyliky, R. L., & Fleming, C. R. (1988) *Gastroenterology* 94, 508-512.

Huebers, H. A., Huebers, E., Csiba, E., Rummel, W., & Finch, C. A. (1987) *Am. J. Clin. Nutr.* 45, 1007-1012.

Humphries, W. R., Phillippo, M., Young, B. W., & Bremner, I. (1983) *Br. J. Nutr.* 49, 77-86.

Hunt, J. R., Johnson, P. E., & Swan, P. B. (1987) *J. Nutr.* 117, 1427-1433.

Lee, H. H., Owyang, C., Brewer, G. J., & Prasad, A. S. (1987) *Gastroenterology* 92, 1497.

Lyall, V., Mahmood, A., & Nath, R., (1979) *Ind. J. Biochem. Biophys.* 16, 80-83.

Manis, J. G., & Schachter, D. (1962) *Am. J. Physiol.* 203, 73-80.

Matseshe, J. W., Phillips, S. F., Malagelada, J. R., & McCall, J. T. (1980) *Am. J. Clin. Nutr.* 33, 1946-1953.

Mills, C. F. (1985) *Ann. Rev. Nutr.* 5, 173-193.

Morrison, J. N., & Quarterman, J. (1987) *Biol. Tr. El. Res.* 14, 115-126.

Oestreicher, P., & Cousins, R. J. (1985) *J. Nutr.* 115, 159-166.

Oh, S. H., & Whanger, P. D. (1981) *Environ. Res.* 26, 130-135.

Pollack, S., George, J. N., Reba, R. C., Kaufman, R. M., & Crosby W. H. (1965) *J. Clin. Invest.* 44, 1470-1473.

Roberts, K. R., Miller, W. J., Stake, P. E., Gentry, R. P. & Neathery, M. W. (1973) *Proc. Soc. Exp. Biol. Med.* 144, 906-908.

Solomons, N. W. (1983) *Nutr. Today* 38, 603–606.

Solomons, N. W. (1988) in *Essential and Toxic Trace Elements in Human Health and Disease* (Prasad A. S., Ed.) pp 509–511, Alan R. Liss, Inc., New York.

Sorbie, J., Valberg, L. S., Corbett, W. E. N., & Ludwig, J. (1975) *Can. Med. Assoc. J.* 112, 1173–1178.

Steinhardt, H. J., & Adibi, S. A. (1984) *Am. J. Physiol.* 247, G176–182.

Storey, M. L., & Greger, J. L. (1987) *J. Nutr.* 117, 1434–1442.

Suttle, N. F., & Mills, C. F. (1966) *Br. J. Nutr.* 20, 135–148.

Thomson, A. B. R., Olatunbosun, D., & Valberg, L. S. (1971) *J. Lab. Clin. Med.* 78, 642–655.

Thomson, A. B. R., & Valberg, L. S. (1971) *Am. J. Physiol.* 220, 1080–1085.

Valberg, L. S, Flanagan, P. R., & Chamberlain, M. J. (1984) *Am. J. Clin. Nutr.* 40, 536–541.

Valberg, L. S., & Flanagan, P. R. (1983) in *Biological Aspects of Metals and Metal-Related Diseases* (Sarkar, B., Ed.) pp 41–66, Raven Press, New York.

Van Campen, D. R. (1969) *J. Nutr.* 97, 104–8.

Van Campen, D. R., & Scaife, P. U. (1967) *J. Nutr.* 91, 473–475.

Watson, W. S., Morrison, J., Bethel, M. I. F., Baldwin, N. M., Lyon, D. T. B., Dobson, H., Moore, M. R., & Hume, R. (1986) *Am. J. Clin. Nutr.* 44, 248–255.

Weigand, E., & Kirchgessner, M. (1980) *J. Nutr.* 110, 469–480.

Wheby, M. S., Jones, L. G., & Crosby, W. H. (1964) *J. Clin. Invest.* 43, 1433–1442.

5

On the Molecular Mechanism of Intestinal Calcium Transport

Robert H. Wasserman and Curtis S. Fullmer

The calcium concentration in blood, presumably similar to the calcium concentration in ancient seas during evolution, is a relatively stable biological "constant", averaging about 2.5 mM (10 mg/dl) in the normal individual. The maintenance of blood calcium concentrations is primarily the function of the calcium regulating hormones, namely, parathyroid hormone (PTH), calcitonin and the vitamin D hormone, 1,25-dihydroxyvitamin D_3 ($1,25(OH)_2D_3$) (Bronner & Coburn, 1982; Lawson, 1978). The main organ systems involved in systemic calcium homeostasis are the intestine, kidney and skeleton. Parathyroid hormone, secreted during periods of hypocalcemia, exerts three main effects: (a) increases bone resorption, (b) decreases phosphate reabsorption by renal tubules and (c) stimulates the synthesis of $1,25(OH)_2D_3$ by the renal $25(OH)D_3$-1-hydroxylase system. The vitamin D hormone: (a) synergizing with parathyroid hormone, increases the bone resorptive process, (b) increases the intestinal absorption of calcium, and (c) increases the reabsorption of calcium by the distal renal tubules (Figure 1). The net effect of the dual action of parathyroid hormone and $1,25(OH)_2D_3$ is to assure that normal levels of blood Ca^{2+} are maintained. Phosphate absorption by the intestine is also stimulated by vitamin D and $1,25(OH)_2D_3$ (Wasserman & Taylor, 1973; Peterlik & Wasserman, 1978). Calcitonin, on the other hand, is secreted during periods of hypercalcemia and, by inhibiting osteoclastic bone resorption, brings blood Ca^{2+} levels down to within the normal range (Mac Intyre, 1986).

As Fujita (1986) stated, "Life does not exist without calcium", a provocative and true statement, and a view that accentuates the significant and numerous roles of calcium in biological systems. Calcium, with phosphate and other ions, comprises the mineral phase of bone. In soft tissues, calcium participates in a wide variety of processes, including stimulus-secretion coupling, stimulus-contraction coupling, and nerve impulse transmission. Within many or all cells, Ca^{2+} serves a "second messenger" function, connecting receptor occupancy by specific hormones with the ultimate physiological response, the latter possibly in association with other "second messengers", such as diacylglycerol, the prostaglandins, cyclic AMP and cyclic GMP.

The "second messenger" function requires that intracellular Ca^{2+} concentrations are maintained at a reasonably "constant" level in the non-stimulated basal state.

The factors controlling intracellular Ca^{2+} levels at about 10^{-7} M are shown in Figure 2 and the various Ca^{2+}-regulating features of this typical cell are described in the figure legend. Upon stimulation, the intracellular free Ca^{2+} concentration is elevated by a factor of 2-10. This calcium is derived from intracellular stores or from the influx of Ca^{2+} from the extracellular fluid, or both. The higher Ca^{2+} concentration, through calcium-receptor proteins (e.g., calmodulin, troponin C), stimulates the activity of Ca^{2+}-dependent enzymes and Ca^{2+}-dependent processes (Campbell, 1983).

The only source of Ca^{2+} to meet these many essential functions is ultimately from the diet and special mechanisms have evolved to assure an adequate and proper transfer of dietary calcium across the intestinal membrane. Although the physiological description of processes of calcium absorption are available, the details of their operation at the biochemical and molecular level requires further definition. There is an active process of calcium transport as demonstrated a number of years ago, using *in vitro* everted gut sac preparations (Schachter & Rosen, 1959) and *in situ* biophysical techniques (Wasserman et al., 1961). When present in the intestinal lumen at concentrations above 5-10 mM, calcium is absorbed by a non-saturable process, i.e., the absorption of Ca^{2+} becomes directly related to intraluminal Ca^{2+} concentration (Wasserman & Taylor, 1969; Pansu et al., 1983a; Toverud & Dostal, 1986). Further, the possibility that Ca^{2+} traverses the epithelial membrane by vesicular flow (an endocytotic-exocytotic process) has also been proposed (Nemere et al., 1986). Thus, as depicted in Figure 3, three processes are potentially available to move Ca^{2+} from the intestinal lumen, through or across the intestinal cell layer, and into the circulatory system draining the intestinal region.

Brief Description of the Intestinal Ca Transport Processes

The calcium ion, required for many cellular processes, can elicit toxic effects in cells when present at abnormally high concentrations. For example, the excessive accumulation of Ca^{2+} by mitochondria compromises ATP production, activates Ca^{2+}dependent proteases and phospholipases, inhibits the activity of Na^+, K^+-Mg ATPase (the sodium pump), and decreases cell-cell communication by effects on gap junctions (Campbell, 1983). A significant premise pertinent to the transport of Ca^{2+} across epithelial tissues is that the cytosolic concentration of free Ca^{2+} does not reach toxic levels. The three mechanisms of calcium absorption mentioned below are in line with this premise.

Diffusion-active transport process. This process is depicted as (A) in Figure 3. Intraluminal Ca^{2+} is considered to enter the enterocyte by diffusion-type processes, both facilitated and non-facilitated, down a considerable electropotential gradient comprised of a concentration difference of about 10,000-fold and a negative intracellular potential of -30 to -50 millivolts. After entering the cytosolic compartment of the enterocyte, calcium translocates to the basolateral membrane. During transfer through the cytosol, Ca^{2+} ions might be transiently sequestered by the endoplasmic reticulum, Golgi apparatus and other membranous structures, in addition to binding to proteins and other macromolecules. The basolateral membrane contains an ATP-dependent calcium pump and a sodium/calcium exchange

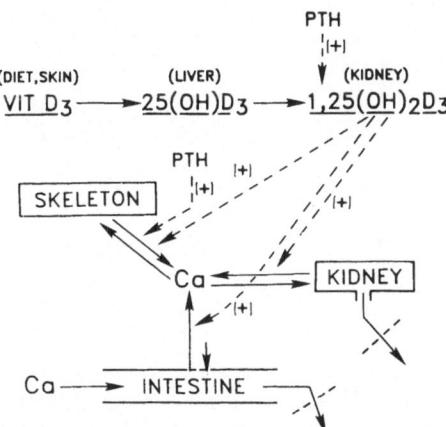

Figure 1. Vitamin D and systemic calcium homeostasis. See text for description.

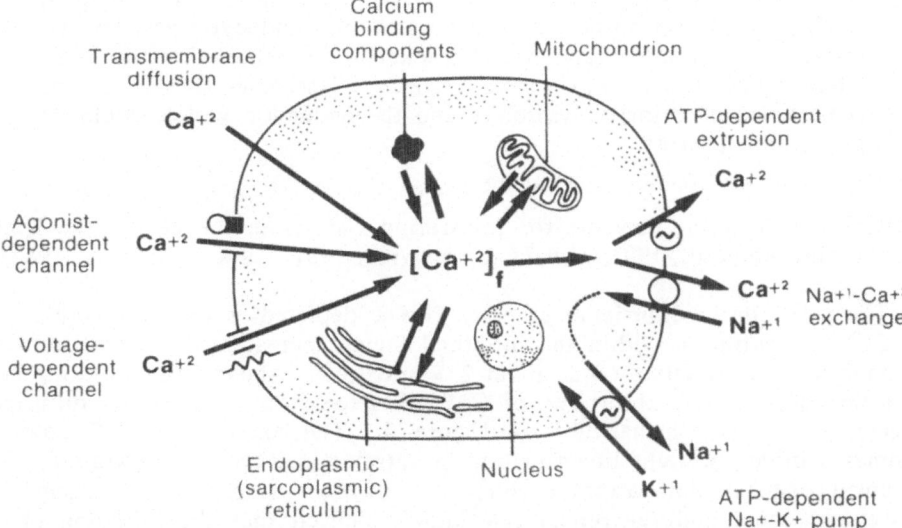

Figure 2. Cellular controls of cytosolic free calcium concentration. The cytosolic free calcium concentration is determined by the rate of influx by diffusion across the plasma membrane, through agonist-dependent and voltage-dependent channels; the rate of efflux by ATP-dependent extrusion (the calcium pump) and Na^+/Ca^{2+} exchange; and the intracellular sequestration by endoplasmic reticulae, mito-chondria, Golgi membranes and binding components.

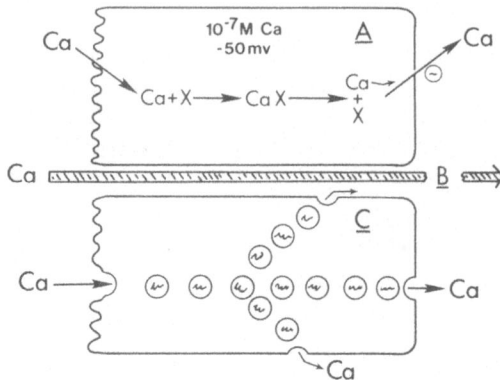

Figure 3. Proposed calcium absorptive processes. (A) The transcellular route in which Ca^{2+} associates with a diffusional translocator (calbindin-D), thereby increasing the rate of transfer of Ca^{2+} from the brush border membrane to the basolateral membrane. Entry into the cell is by diffusion and exit from the cell by primary and secondary active transport mechanisms. (B) At higher concentrations of luminal Ca^{2+}, the evidence indicates that the paracellular route is taken. (C) A proposed vesicular flow mechanism is depicted in which luminal Ca^{2+}, at the brush border, is incorporated into endocytic vesicles and transferred in a membrane-bound "packet" to be extruded at the basolateral membrane by exocytosis. Secondary lysosomes formed by the coalescence of primary lysosomes and the endocytic vesicle could be part of this process.

mechanism that are responsible for transfering Ca^{2+} from the cell to the lamina propria (Ghijsen et al., 1982; Nellans & Popovich, 1981; Hildemann et al., 1982).

The paracellular diffusional process. This is depicted as (B) in Figure 3. As the Ca^{2+} concentration within the intestinal lumen increases, the active transport mechanism becomes saturated at about 2-5 mM Ca^{2+}. Above this saturating concentration of Ca^{2+}, the absorption of Ca^{2+} takes the form of a strictly diffusional process, as shown schematically in Figure 4. The amount of Ca^{2+} absorbed becomes a direct, straight line function of intraluminal Ca^{2+} concentration. It is presumed that the non-saturable component of Ca^{2+} absorption is through the paracellular route and theoretical calculations showed that the initiation of the non-saturable process coincides with the luminal Ca^{2+} concentration ($Ca^{2+} > 5$ mM) at which the energetics favor diffusion directly from lumen to blood (Wasserman & Taylor, 1969).

Endocytotic-exocytotic-vesicular flow process. This is depicted as (C) in Figure 3. Earlier histological and electron microprobe studies (Warner & Coleman, 1975; Davis & Jones, 1981; Jande & Brewer, 1974) provided evidence suggesting that Ca^{2+} was translocated in association with vacuoles or in "packets". Rubinoff & Nellans (1985) isolated an endoplasmic reticular-enriched fraction from rat

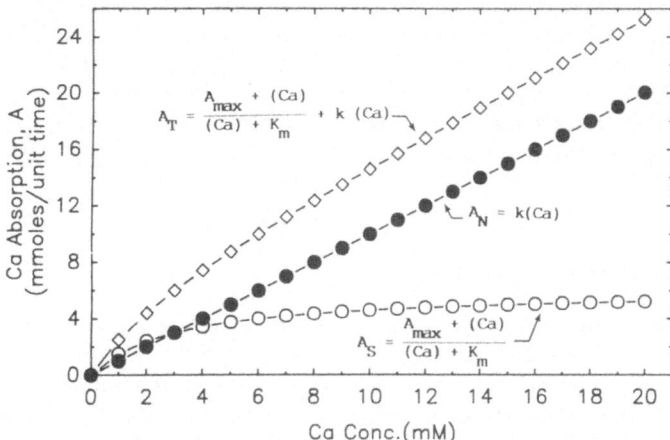

Figure 4. The relation between the rate of calcium absorption and intraluminal calcium concentration. As the calcium concentration within the intestinal lumen increases, a two phase relationship is observed. At lower concentrations, the primary process is a saturable, active process mechanism (A_s) and attains a maximal rate (o). Further increases in luminal calcium yields a straight-line relation (A_n), characteristic of a strictly diffusional process (•). The saturable phase is considered to be via the intracellular route and the non-saturable phase, by the paracellular route. □ = total rate of calcium absorption (A_t).

intestine that accumulated Ca^{2+} by an ATP-dependent mechanism possibly involved in Ca^{2+} absorption. The more recent studies by Nemere et al. (1986) have provided biochemical evidence for the presence of absorbed Ca^{2+} in vesicular components. Such a vesicular-flow process could move Ca^{2+} from the brush border membrane (endocytosis) to the basolateral membrane (exocytosis) without Ca^{2+} entering the cell proper.

Vitamin D & Calcium Absorption

The major factor influencing Ca^{2+} absorption is vitamin D and, more specifically, the hormonal form of this steroid, $1,25(OH)_2D_3$. Vitamin D deficiency in the young, growing individual results in rickets, a disease character-ized by undermineralized bone and a decreased absorption of calcium. Vitamin D deficiency in the adult, termed osteomalacia, is characterized by a lack of re-mineralization of the skeleton during the course of bone turnover. The absorption of Ca^{2+} is also depressed.

The source of vitamin D is from the diet or from the conversion of 7-dehydrocholesterol in the skin to vitamin D by ultraviolet light. Vitamin D is transported in blood primarily in association with the vitamin D binding protein (DBP). In liver, vitamin D is converted to the 25-hydroxylated derivative and, in kidney, $25(OH)D_3$ is converted to $1,25(OH)_2D_3$. During periods of calcium need, $1,25(OH)_2D_3$ is preferably synthesized and, during periods of calcium adequacy, $24,25(OH)_2D_3$ is preferably made, the latter having a considerably lesser activity than $1,25(OH)_2D_3$ on calcium absorption. Parathyroid hormone, secreted as a consequence of hypocalcemia, stimulates the synthesis of $1,25(OH)_2D_3$ and thereby constitutes a significant feature of feed-back control on systemic calcium homeostasis (Figure 1).

The Genomic Action of Vitamin D

Present within the intestinal cell (and in other tissues and organs) is a receptor for $1,25(OH)_2D_3$ (Haussler, 1986). This polypeptide receptor, upon binding $1,25(OH)_2D_3$, interacts with the genetic components of the nucleus of the enterocyte to induce the synthesis of an mRNA coded for the vitamin D-dependent calcium-binding protein, named calbindin-D. Other responses of intestinal cells to $1,25(OH)_2D_3$ have been documented and these include an increase in the activities of alkaline phosphatase-low affinity Ca ATPase, phospholipase A2 (O'Doherty, 1979), adenylate cyclase (Corradino, 1977; Wasserman et al., 1977; Long et al., 1986), guanylate cyclase (Vesely & Juan, 1984), and S-adenosylmethionine decarboxylase (Steeves & Lawson, 1985). The increase in the activity of the various enzymes listed above might represent either their increased synthesis, a more direct effect of $1,25(OH)_2D_3$ on enzyme activity, or an indirect effect due to elevated levels of intracellular calcium.

The stimulatory effect of $1,25(OH)_2D_3$ has a lag period of 3-4 hr in vitamin D-deficient animals at which time there is an increase in Ca^{2+} absorption and the simultaneous appearance of calbindin D (Figure 5).

Non-Genomic Actions of $1,25(OH)_2D_8$

The administration of $1,25(OH)_2D_3$ appears to stimulate an early event that apparently precedes the synthesis of the $1,25(OH)_2D_3$-induced gene product. For example, we have shown that $1,25(OH)_2D_3$ given to chicks maintained on a suboptimal dietary level of vitamin D_3 (one-third the recommended level) results in a significant increase in Ca^{2+} absorption in 1-2 hr (Figure 6). A longer lag period (3-4 hr) is required to elicit an absorptive response in vitamin D-deficient animals (Figure 5). Recently, Nemere & Norman (1986, 1987), using an isolated dual intestinal-vascular perfusion preparation, reported that $1,25(OH)_2D_3$ or PTH increases Ca^{2+} absorption in a matter of minutes but only in preparations derived from vitamin D-replete animals. The molecular nature of these early responses is not known although it is possible that the direct stimulation of cAMP and/or cGMP synthesis or activation of phospholipase A2 might be involved. Further, Brasitus et al. (1986) demonstrated that the fluidity of the brush border membrane is increased by 1 hr after D is given to vitamin D-deficient animals. However, Ca^{2+} absorption did not increase until 5 hr post-$1,25(OH)_2D_3$, sufficient time for the induction of the synthesis of calbindin D.

Thus, current evidence suggests that $1,25(OH)_2D_3$ exerts multiple effects on the enterocyte to optimize calcium absorption, and these include an apparent non-

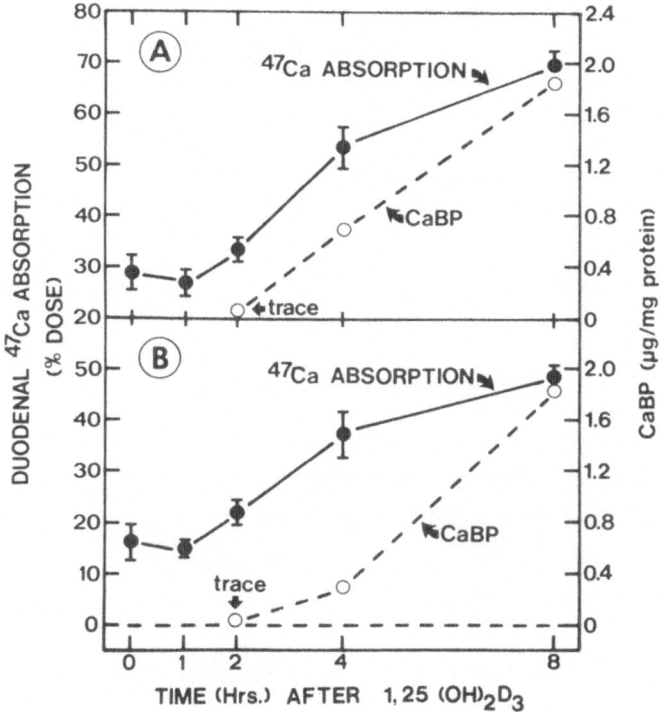

Figure 5. Temporal relation of calbindin-D to the stimulation of calcium absorption by $1,25(OH)_2D_3$ in vitamin D-deficient chicks. The effect of $1,25(OH)_2D_3$ on duodenal absorption of ^{47}Ca and on CaBP synthesis in rachitic chicks is shown. (A) Absorption period, 30 min; $1,25(OH)_2D_3$; 1 μg per chick. (B) Absorption period, 15 min; $1,25(OH)_2D_3$, 0.3 μg per chick. The data represent the mean ± SEM for ^{47}Ca absorption for five or six chicks per group. $1,25(OH)_2D_3$ significantly increased ^{47}Ca absorption at 4 and 8 hr above the zero time control; $(P < 0.01)$. From Wasserman et al. (1982) and reproduced with permission.

genomic effect on the entry of luminal Ca^{2+} into the intestinal tissue, and a genomic effect on the transfer of Ca^{2+} through the cell proper and into the circulatory system.

The Basolateral ATP-Dependent Ca Pump

The extrusion of Ca^{2+} across the basolateral membrane of the enterocyte, as mentioned, is the function of an energy-dependent Ca pump and a Na/Ca exchange process. The vitamin D-dependency of the activity of the Ca pump has been shown by several groups (Ghijsen & Van Os, 1982; Meyer & Wasserman, 1983; Meyer et al., 1984; Walters & Weiser, 1987) but whether this effect of

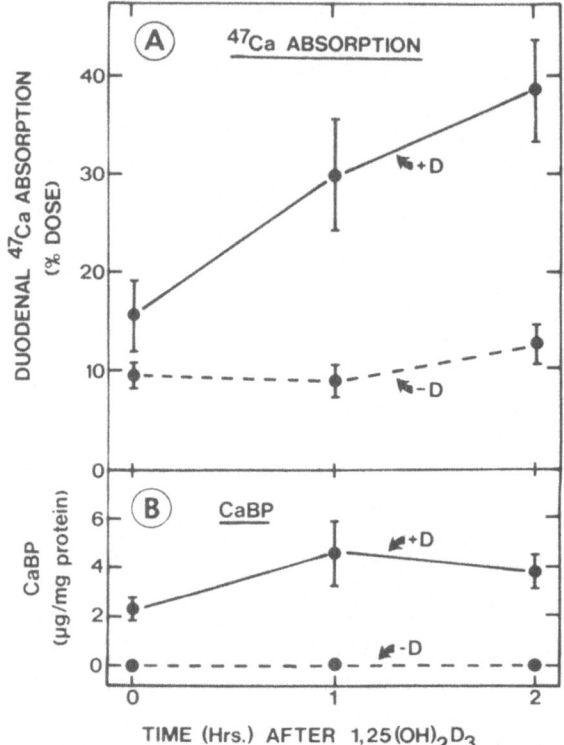

Figure 6. Effect of partial vitamin D_3 repletion in rachitic chicks on the stimulation of ^{47}Ca absorption by $1,25(OH)_2D_3$. Half (+D) of the group of rachitic chicks was given 2 IU of D_3 for 6 days prior to the $1,25(OH)_2D_3$ injection (intracardially, 0.3 μg per chick) at time zero. The other half served as vitamin D-deficient controls (-D). Each point represents the mean ± SEM of five or six chicks per group. Note the lack of significant response of the -D chicks to $1,25(OH)_2D_3$ over the time period examined whereas the +D chicks responded within 2 hr. CaBP was present in the +D chicks but not detectable in the -D chicks. From Wasserman et al. (1982) and reproduced with permission.

$1,25(OH)_2D_3$ is direct or indirect needs be sorted out (Van Corven et al., 1986). There is evidence that calbindin D and calmodulin directly stimulate pump activity (Nellans & Popovich, 1981; Chandler & Wasserman, 1987; Walters, 1987).

The Relation of Calbindin D to Calcium Absorption

A high correlation exists between the concentration of calbindin D in the intestine and the efficiency or rate of Ca^{2+} absorption, and this relationship seems to pertain more to the active transport of calcium than to the non-saturable

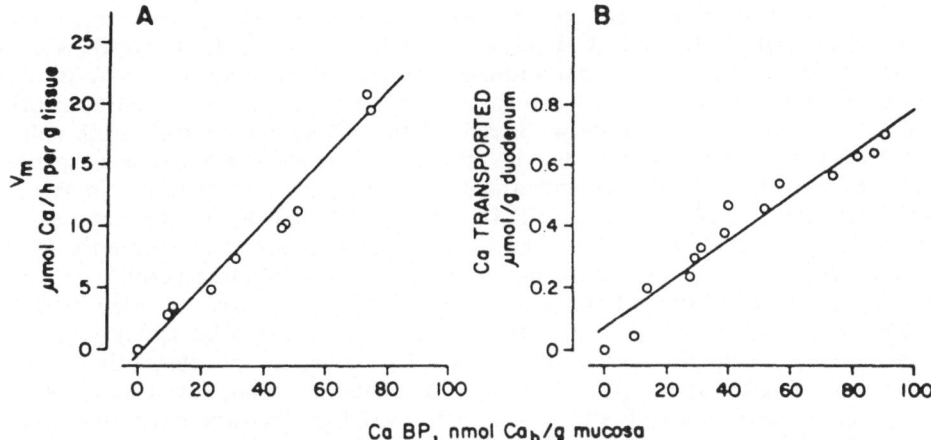

Figure 7. Relation between intestinal calcium transport and calbindin D (CaBP). A: Vm (maximum rate of transport) was calculated from *in situ* duodenal, jejunal and ileal loop experiments shown as a function of CaBP content. B: calcium transport, as evaluated from everted duodenal sac experiments shown as a function of CaBP content. In Figure 5B, the rats were of varying age (70-150 g body wt) and fed high calcium diets with or without vit. D. Groups of -D and +D rats at 4 or 9 hr before experiment, respectively, were given varying doses of $1,25(OH)_2D_3$. From Bronner et al. (1986) and reproduced with permission.

diffusional component (Bronner et al., 1986). Correlations between calcium absorption and intestinal calbindin-D concentration are shown in the Figures 7-9. These correlations were observed: (a) when the rate of calcium absorption by the saturable component of the process was plotted against the calbindin D content of the intestine, using the *in situ* ligated loop technique with duodenal, jejunal and ileal segments of rats (Pansu et al., 1983a,b; Bronner et al., 1986), (Figure 7A); (b) when the transport of calcium across the everted gut sacs of rats fed vitamin D-deficient and vitamin D-sufficient diets were given varying doses of $1,25(OH)_2D_3$ at 9 or 4 hr, respectively, before experiment (Roche et al., 1986; Bronner et al., 1986) (Figure 7B); (c) when calcium absorption was determined in vitamin D-deficient chicks given cortisone and repleted with either $1,25(OH)_2D_3$ or vitamin D_3, using the *in situ* ligated duodenal loop procedure (Figure 8) (Feher & Wasserman, 1979a,b); (d) when calcium absorption was determined in chicks fed a low calcium diet containing varying concentrations of lead chloride, again using the *in situ* ligated loop technique (Figure 9) (Fullmer, 1988). This correlation also holds for other experimental situations, including the direct relationship between the concentration of calbindin D in the uterus of the laying hen and egg shell thickness (Bar et al., 1984) and the calbindin D content of duodenal mucosa and calcium absorption in chicks fed diets containing different levels of calcium and phosphate (Morrissey & Wasserman, 1971).

In the cortisone experiment, the chicks given hydrocortisone were made vitamin D-replete with either 1,25(OH)$_2$D$_3$ or vitamin D$_3$ (Figure 8) (Feher & Wasserman, 1979a,b). The amount of calbindin-D present in the intestine was less when 1,25(OH)$_2$D$_3$ was administered as compared to vitamin D$_3$ although the absorption of Ca^{2+} was of similar magnitude with each vitamin D source. Within each subset, i.e., 1,25(OH)$_2$D$_3$ versus vitamin D$_3$ dosages, high correlations between absorption of calcium and calbindin D concentrations were evident. The question remains as to why Ca^{2+} absorption after 1,25(OH)$_2$D$_3$ administration is about the same as that after vitamin D$_3$ repletion, despite significantly different levels of calbindin D. In this same study, a high correlation between alkaline phosphatase activity and calcium absorption was observed (Figure 10), no matter the source of vitamin D (D$_3$ or 1,25(OH)$_2$D$_3$). This latter observation points to the potential function of this enzyme, known to be influenced by vitamin D$_3$ status, in the absorptive process and as considered by others (cf. Wasserman & Chandler, 1985, for references). In this regard, an early effect of vitamin D$_3$ is to alter the electrophoretic mobility of alkaline phosphatase due to a modification of the carbohydrate moiety associated with this enzyme (Moriuchi et al., 1977).

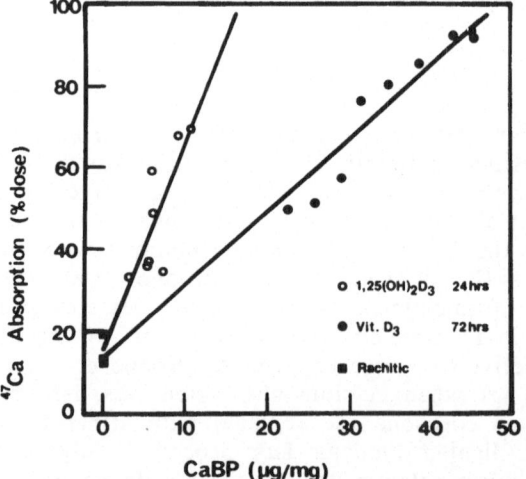

Figure 8. Relation between intestinal calcium absorption and calbindin-D (CaBP) in chicks as influenced by cortisone. The chicks were fed a rachitogenic diet for 22-24 days and given vehicle, vitamin D$_3$ 72 hr. or 1,25(OH)$_2$D$_3$ 24 hr. before experiment. The different degrees of calcium absorption were produced by the administration of cortisol acetate i.m. at various dosages. From Feher & Wasserman (1979a) & reproduced with permission.

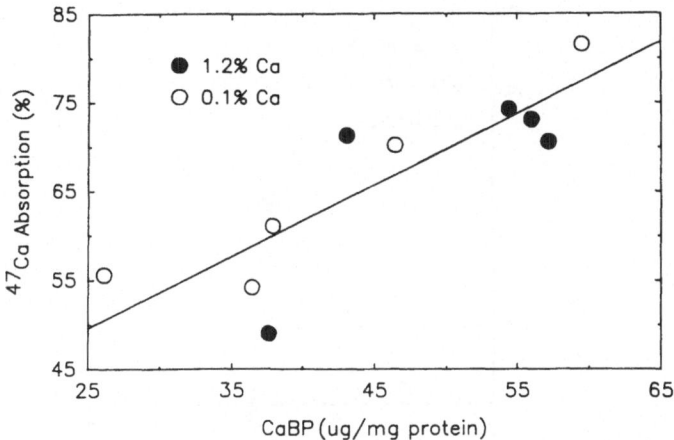

Figure 9. Relation between intestinal calcium absorption and calbindin-D concentrations in chicks fed diets containing varying levels of PbCl$_2$. The chicks were fed a semi-synthetic diet containing 0.1% Ca; the lead concentrations as the chloride varied from 0-0.8% of the diet. Based on data of Fullmer (1988).

Properties of Calbindin D

The vitamin D-induced calcium-binding protein from chick intestine and that from mammalian intestine have been isolated and their properties studied by a number of groups (cf. Wasserman & Fullmer, 1982, for review). The avian type has a molecular weight of about 30,000 daltons and binds four calcium ions per molecule with an affinity of about 2 x 10^6 M^{-1}. The molecular weight of the mammalian type (bovine, in this case) has a molecular weight of about 10,000 daltons and binds two calcium ions with about the same affinity as the avian type. Both proteins have been sequenced (Fullmer & Wasserman, 1981, 1987; Hofman et al., 1979; Desplan et al., 1983; Wilson et al., 1985; Hunziker, 1986). The calcium-binding regions contain the EF hand configuration homologous to that in parvalbumin and other members of the troponin C superfamily. The bovine protein is the only calbindin D for which the crystal structure has thus far been determined (Szebenyi et al., 1981; Szebenyi & Moffat, 1986).

These are acidic proteins (pI ~4.3) and no covalent modification of the calbindins has been detected.

The calbindins are, for the most part, soluble in aqueous solutions and about 90% of the intracellular protein in intestinal mucosa is readily released upon homogenization. The remainder (5-10%) is bound to structures within the cells and is releasable by detergent (Feher & Wasserman, 1978). A brush border protein of about 60,000 daltons was shown to bind calbindin D selectively (Shimura & Wasserman, 1984) and, more recently, the association of the protein with microtubules (Nemere et al., 1988) and lysosomal particles (Nemere et al., 1986) has been reported.

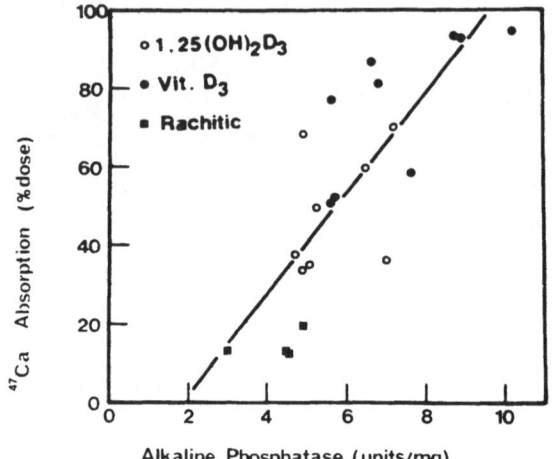

Figure 10. Relation between total homogenate alkaline phosphatase activity and calcium absorption as influenced by cortisone. Chicks were given vitamin D_3 or $1,25(OH)_2D_3$. Varying degrees of calcium absorption were produced by administering cortisol acetate at varying dose levels. Values given are the mean of at least six animals per group. From Feher & Wasserman (1979a) and reproduced with permission.

The Function of Calbindin D in Calcium Absorption

The definitive role of cytosolic calbindin-D in the calcium absorptive process has been difficult to assess. Factors important to consider in any hypothesis are, as follows: (a) the concentration of the calbindins in the chick and rat intestinal mucosa is rather high and about 0.3-0.4 mM; (b) the disassociation constant of these proteins is about 5×10^{-7} M; (c) the disassociation constant of the basolateral ATP-dependent calcium pump is about 2×10^{-7} M and (d) most of the protein is apparently soluble in the cytosolic compartment or loosely bound to components of the cell.

Theoretical analysis of a possible function of calbindin in calcium absorption was put forth by Kretsinger et al. (1982). The essence of the theory is, as follows: Ca^{2+}, after entering the cell, binds to calbindin and the diffusion of absorbed Ca^{2+} from the microvillar region to the basolateral membrane occurs in the forms of "free" Ca^{2+} and calbindin-bound Ca^{2+}. At the basolateral membrane, "free" Ca^{2+} is rapidly extruded from the cell and the "free" Ca^{2+} concentration is replenished by Ca^{2+} disassociating from calbindin. The latter can occur because of the respective disassociation constants of calbindin and the Ca pump, 5×10^{-7} M and 2×10^{-7} M, respectively. As the Ca^{2+} concentration in the micro-region adjacent to the basolateral Ca pump is decreased, bound Ca^{2+} is released from calbindin. Thereby the Ca pump, considered to be "starved" for calcium during non-absorptive periods, is provided sufficient Ca^{2+} from calbindin to account for the accelerated absorption of Ca^{2+} in the vitamin D-replete animal. The profile of Ca^{2+} concentration of a

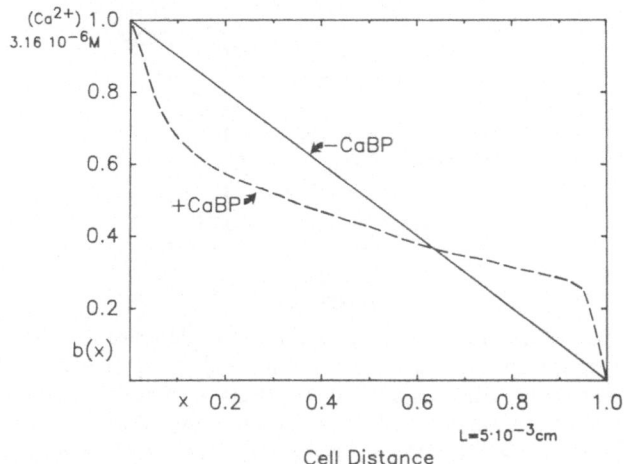

Figure 11. The steady state concentration of free Ca²⁺ over the length of a hypthetical intestinal cell in the presence or absence of calbindin D (CaBP). Luminal Ca²⁺ enters at the brush border (left), diffuses through the cell and is extruded by the basolateral Ca pump (right). In the absence of CaBP, the gradient is linear (—). In the presence of CaBP (- - - -), the Ca²⁺ entering the cell is bound by CaBP and diffuses in the bound form to the region of the basolateral membrane containing the ATP-dependent calcium pump. In the presence of CaBP, available for active extrusion are Ca²⁺ ions that diffused in the unbound form and that disassociated from CaBP. Modified from Kretsinger et al. (1982) and reproduced with permission.

hypothetical intestinal cell with or without calbindin, as modified from Kretsinger et al. (1982), is shown in Figure 11.

Bronner et al. (1986) estimated that the rate of free diffusion of Ca²⁺ through the cytosol of the epithelial cell was much too slow to account of the maximal rate of active transport. When the presence of intracellular calbindin is taken into account, this "paradox" can be resolved with the calbindin serving as a diffusional facilitator in accordance with Kretsinger's analysis.

A test of the theoretical approach of Kretsinger was made by Feher (1983), using an *in vitro* diffusion system comprised of three chambers, separated by semi-permeable membranes (Figure 12). The transfer of ⁴⁵Ca from the precursor compartment (intestinal lumen), through the center compartment (enterocyte) containing calbindin or buffer or bovine serum albumin, to the product compartment (circulatory system) was determined. An essential feature of this system was the continuous flow of buffer through the product compartment to maintain a continuous concentration gradient of Ca²⁺ between the center compartment and the product compartment. As shown in Figure 13, the replacement of buffer in the center compartment by buffer containing calbindin results in an immediate decrease in Ca²⁺ diffusivity, an effect due to binding to calbindin. After steady state was achieved, the rate of entry of ⁴⁵Ca into the product compartment from the calbindin containing compartment was greater than when either buffer alone or

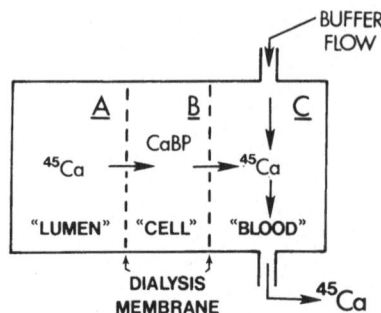

Figure 12. The *in vitro* apparatus to determine the effect of calbindin-D on calcium diffusion. Radiocalcium, placed in the "luminal" compartment, diffuses across one dialysis membrane into the "cell" compartment containing CaBP or buffer, and then across the other membrane into the "blood" compartment. To maintain a concentration gradient, the ^{45}Ca entering the "blood" compartment is removed by buffer flow. Modified from Feher (1983) and reproduced with permission.

when buffer containing bovine serum albumin was in the center compartment. Thus, the experiments of Feher support the theoretical analysis of Kretsinger et al. (1982) and provide a basis for a mechanism by which calbindin increases calcium absorption in the vitamin D-replete animal. However, further proof is required to demonstrate that, in fact, this is the manner by which calbindin affects an increase in calcium absorption within the intestine *in situ*. The latter constitutes a difficult problem. As pointed out by Feher & Fullmer (1988), the facilitated transfer of Ca^{2+} by the presence of calbindin should be bidirectional and, interestingly, earlier studies on calcium absorption have already borne out this prediction (Wasserman & Kallfelz, 1962). Further, Pansu et al. (1988) reported that theophylline inhibits the binding of Ca^{2+} by rat calbindin and inhibits Ca^{2+} transport by an *in vitro* everted gut sac preparation. Although these observations tend to verify a role of calbindin in calcium absorption, other effects of theophylline (e.g., inhibition of phosphodiesterases) might account for its inhibitory effect on the physiological response.

Factors Other Than Calbindin Potentially Involved in Vitamin D-Dependent Calcium Absorption

The discussion thus far has accentuated the possible role or roles of calbindin in the calcium absorptive process. Other significant contributions to our understanding of the function of vitamin D in stimulating calcium transport have been made. Although the concentration of another calcium-binding protein, calmodulin, is not affected by vitamin D (Thomasset et al., 1981; Christakos et al., 1984), a vitamin D-dependent redistribution of enterocyte calmodulin from the cytosol to the brush border region was reported (Bikle & Munson, 1985). Calmodulin apparently associates with a brush border protein with a molecular weight of about 105,000 daltons, and this complex might be involved in altering the permeability

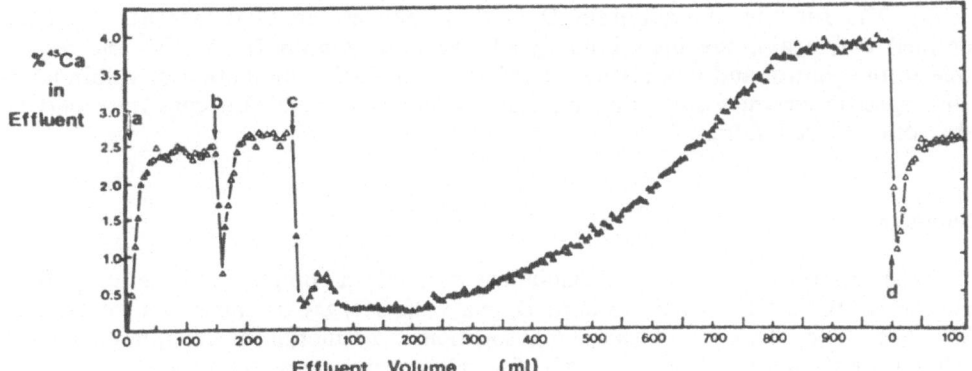

Figure 13. Effect of calbindin-D (CaBP) on the ^{45}Ca diffusional flux. The *in vitro* apparatus schematically depicted in Figure 12 was used. The left compartment was perfused with ^{45}Ca-containing buffer, while the right compartment was perfused with an identical solution lacking ^{45}Ca. The middle compartment was filled with buffer (a); the middle compartment was emptied and again filled with buffer (b); the middle compartment was emptied and then filled with buffer containing 1.6 mg/ml CaBP (c); and middle compartment was emptied, washed twice, and then filled with buffer (d). From Feher (1983) and reproduced with permission.

of the brush border membrane to Ca^{2+}. Likewise, the early alteration of the fluidity of the brush border membrane, as noted by Brasitus et al. (1986), might also result in an increased entry of Ca^{2+} into the cell. Further, 1,25(OH)$_2$D$_3$ stimulated increase of cAMP (Corradino, 1977; Wasserman et al, 1977; Long et al., 1986) and cGMP (Veseley & Juan, 1984) in enterocytes through kinase catalyzed phosphorylation of Ca "channels", might also affect the increased entry of luminal Ca into the enterocytes.

The Role of Calbindin in Non-Intestinal Tissues

Calbindin D is present in other epithelial-type membranes, including kidney (Kendrick et al., 1984; Pansini et al., 1984; Taylor & Wasserman, 1972; Thomasset et al., 1983), placenta (Warembourg et al., 1986; Bruns et al., 1986; Bruns et al., 1985; Garel et al., 1981) and the egg shell gland of the laying hen (Corradino et al., 1968; Lippiello & Wasserman, 1975). Whatever Ca^{2+} transport mechanism occurs in the intestine probably pertains to these other epithelial membranes.

Calbindin D has also been localized in non-epithelial tissues, including the central nervous system (Garcia et al., 1984; Pasteels et al., 1986; Baimbridge et al., 1982; Feldman et al., 1983; Roth et al., 1981; Taylor, 1977; Jande et al., 1981; Thomasset et al., 1984), in peripheral nerve (Lee et al., 1987), tibia growth cartilage cells (Balmain et al., 1986), cells of the cochlea and vestibula (Oberholtzer et al., 1986; Legrand et al., 1988; Rabie et al., 1983), the visual system (Pasteels et al., 1987; Verstappen et al.. 1986), and other organs and tissues (Christakos et al.,

1979). The function of calbindin D in these non-epithelial tissues has not been defined but, again, the high binding affinity of calbindin D for Ca^{2+} suggests a role in the control and modulation of intracellular Ca^{2+}. Interaction of calbindin D with specific enzymes and other cellular components could also constitute part of the action of calbindin.

Summary

The intestinal absorption of calcium is certainly a complex process, dependent on several factors of which vitamin D, via $1,25(OH)_2D_3$, is the major controlling hormone. The efficiency of calcium absorption is a function of calcium status and calcium need. As the body's demand for calcium increases, the process commonly termed, adaptation, is activated in which the synthesis of $1,25(OH)_2D_3$ from precursor is increased, resulting in the stimulation of the rate of calcium absorption. The increased demand for calcium might result from the ingestion of a diet deficient in calcium, from growth, pregnancy, lactation and egg shell formation in the laying hen. Accompanying the change in calcium absorptive efficiency are molecular modifications of the transporting enterocytes, some mentioned herein and elsewhere (Wasserman & Chandler, 1985; Wasserman, 1980; Wasserman et al., 1984). Highly correlated with the rate of calcium absorption under a wide variety of conditions is the concentration of the vitamin D-induced calcium-binding protein, calbindin-D28K (avian type) and calbindin-D9K (mammalian intestinal type). The role of calbindin-D in this transport process is not precisely known but is considered to act at the present time as a cytosolic facilitator of Ca^{2+} diffusion from the brush border membrane to the basolateral membrane.

In addition to the induction of calbindin-D synthesis, $1,25(OH)_2D_3$ exerts other effects on the intestinal epithelium that can have consequences on the calcium absorptive process. Some of these effects are summarized in Figure 14. Vitamin D-dependent reactions might be either direct effects of $1,25(OH)_2D_3$ or indirect effects due to elevated intracellular Ca^{2+} concentrations. These include changes in the fluidity of the brush border membrane, an increase in microvillar alkaline phosphatase-low affinity Ca-activated ATPase activity, an association of calmodulin with the 105 kD brush border cytoskeletal protein and, following calbindin D synthesis, the binding of calbindin D to a 60 kD brush border protein and to microtubules. The latter has been suggested to be related to the proposed transfer of Ca^{2+} by an endocytotic-exocytotic mechanism. In addition, a vitamin D-dependent intestinal membrane calcium-binding protein has been identified (Kowarski & Schachter, 1980). Playing into this multi-component system is a stimulation of cyclic nucleotide synthesis by $1,25(OH)_2D_3$ which, through activation of cyclic nucleotide-dependent protein kinases, might modify membrane Ca^{2+} "channels" by phosphorylation reactions.

Intracellular organelles, i.e., the endoplasmic reticulum, mitochondria, the Golgi apparatus, are potent sequesters of Ca^{2+} and could contribute to the protection of the cell from excessively high Ca^{2+} concentrations by transiently storing absorbed Ca^{2+}. The vitamin D stimulation of the uptake of Ca^{2+} by a membrane fraction identified primarily of Golgi origin was reported (Freedman et al., 1977; MacLaughlin et al., 1980).

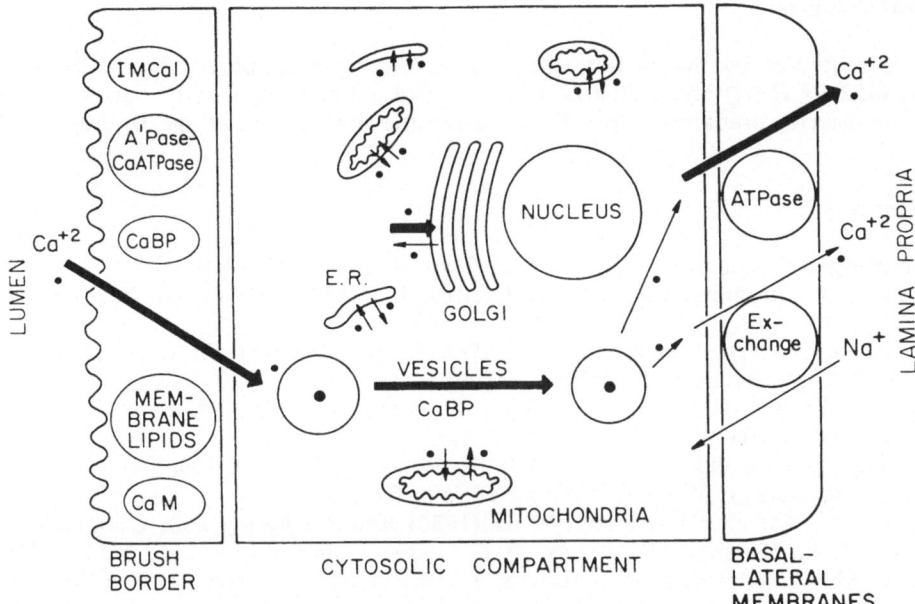

Figure 14. A summary of molecular aspects of intestinal calcium absorption. See text for discussion. The abbreviations are defined as follows: IMCal, intestinal membrane calcium-binding protein; A'Pase-CaATPase, alkaline phosphatase-low affinity CaATPase; CaBP, the vitamin D-induced calcium-binding protein, i.e., calbindin D; CaM, calmodulin; E.R., endoplasmic reticulum.

At the basolateral membrane, Ca^{2+} is extruded against an electropotential gradient by an ATP-dependent calcium pump and sodium/calcium exchange mechanism.

In addition to the transcellular path, luminal Ca^{2+} at higher concentrations seemingly moves through the paracellular path. The evidence for this mode of absorption is indirect.

Over the past few years, a considerable amount of pertinent and valuable information has become available on describing the Ca^{2+} absorptive process. Much is yet to be learned to define this process in detail. In addition to the intellectual satisfaction derived from the study of this biological process, there are practical, medically oriented applications. One is the debilitating disease of osteoporosis in which there is an age related depression in calcium absorption. Knowledge of the physiological, biochemical and molecular basis of the calcium absorptive process could provide a rational therapeutic approach to offset the defect in this and other diseases in which there is an inadequate absorption of Ca^{2+} from the diet.

Acknowledgements

The studies by the authors included herein were supported by N.I.H. Grants DK04652 (R.H.W.) and ES04072 (C.S.F.). We acknowledge with thanks N. Jayne for manuscript preparation and F. Davis for the preparation of the figures.

References

Baimbridge, K. G., Miller, J. J. (1982) *Brain Res.* 245, 223-229.

Balmain, N., Brehier, A., Cuisinier-Gleizes, P. (1986) *Cell Tissue Res.* 245, 331-335.

Bar, A., Rosenberg, J. & Hurwitz, S. (1984) *Comp. Biochem. Physiol.* 78B, 75-79.

Bikle, D. D., & Munson, S. (1985) *J. Clin. Invest.* 76, 2312-2316.

Brasitus, T. A., Dudeja, P. K., Eby, B., Lau, K. (1986) *J. Biol. Chem.* 261, 16404-16409.

Bronner, F., & Coburn, J. W. (1982) *Disorders of Mineral Metabolism. Calcium Physiology,* Vol. 11, Academic Press, New York.

Bronner, F., Pansu, D., & Stern, W. D. (1986) *Am. J. Physiol.* 250, G561-G569.

Bruns, M. E., Kleeman, E., Bruns, D. E. (1986) *J. Biol. Chem.* 261, 7485-7490.

Bruns, M. E., Kleeman, E., Mills, S. E., Bruns, D. E., Herr, J. C. (1985) *Anat. Rec.* 213, 514-517.

Campbell, A. K. (1983) *Intracellular Calcium. Its Universal Role as a Regulator,* John Wiley, New York.

Chandler, J. S., & Wasserman, R. H. (1987) in *Calcium-Binding Proteins in Health and Disease* (Norman, A. W., Vanaman, T. C., & Means, A. R., Eds.) pp 110-112, Academic Press, New York.

Christakos, S., Bruns, M. E., Mehra, A. S., Rhoten, W. B., Van Eldik, L. J. (1984) *Arch. Biochem. Biophys.* 231, 38-47.

Christakos, S., Friedlander, E. J., Frandsen, B. R., Norman, A. W. (1979) *Endocrinology* 104, 1495-1503.

Corradino, R. A. (1977) in *Vitamin D: Biochemical, Chemical and Clinical Aspects Related to Calcium Metabolism* (Norman, A. W. et al., Eds.) pp 231-240, de Gruyter, Berlin.

Corradino, R. A., Wasserman, R. H., Pubols, M. H., & Chang, S. I. (1968) *Arch. Biochem. Biophys.* 125, 378-380.

Davis, W. L., & Jones, R. G. (1981) *Tissue Cell* 13, 381-391.

Desplan, C., Heidmann, D., Auffray, C., Lillie, J. & Thomasset, M. (1983) in *Calcium-Binding Proteins* (de Bernard et al., Eds.) pp 301-302, Elsevier, New York.

Feher, J. J. (1983) *Am. J. Physiol.* 244, C303-C307.

Feher, J. J., and Fullmer, C. S. (1988) in *Cellular Calcium and Phosphate Transport* (Bronner, F., & Peterlik, M., Eds.) pp 121-126, Alan R. Liss, New York.

Feher, J. J., & Wasserman, R. H. (1978) *Biochim. Biophys. Acta* 540, 134-143.

Feher, J. J., & Wasserman, R. H. (1979a) *Endocrinology* 104, 547-551.

Feher, J. J., & Wasserman, R. H. (1979b) *Am. J. Physiol.* 236, 556-561.

Feldman, S. C., & Christakos, S. (1983) *Endocrinology* 112, 290-302.

Freedman, R. A., Weiser, M. M., Isselbacher, K. J. (1977) *Proc. Natl. Acad. Sci. USA* 74, 3612-3616.

Fujita, T. (1986) *Miner. Electrolyte Metab.* 12, 149-156.

Fullmer, C. S. (1988) *FASEB J.* 2, A1632.

Fullmer, C. S., & Wasserman, R. H. (1981) *J. Biol. Chem.* 256, 5669-5674.

Fullmer, C. S., & Wasserman, R. H. (1987) *Proc. Natl. Acad. Sci. USA* 84, 4772-4776.

Garcia Segura, L. M., Baetens, D., Roth, J., Norman, A. W., & Orci, L. (1984) *Brain Res.* 296, 75-86.

Garel, J. M., Delorme, A. C., Marche, P., NGuyen, T. M., & Garabedian, M. (1981) *Endocrinology* 109, 284-289.

Ghijsen, W. E. J. M., DeJong, M. D., & Van Os, C. H. (1982) *Biochim. Biophys. Acta* 689, 327-336.

Ghijsen, W. E. J. M., & Van Os, C. H. (1982) *Biochim. Biophys. Acta* 689, 170-172.

Haussler, M. R. (1986) *Ann. Rev. Nutrition* 6, 527-562.

Hofman, T., Kawakami, M., Hitchman, A. J. W., Harrison, J. E. & Dorrington, K. H. (1979) *Can. J. Biochem.* 57, 737-748.

Hunziker, W. (1986) *Proc. Natl. Acad. Sci. USA* 83, 7578-7582.

Hildemann, B., Schmidt, A., & Murer, H. (1982) *J. Membr. Biol.* 65, 55-62.

Jande, S. S., & Brewer, L. M. (1974) *Z. Anat. Entwicklungsgesch.* 144, 249-265.

Jande, S. S., Maler, L., & Lawson, D. E. (1981) *Nature* 294, 765-767.

Kendrick, N. C., Bishop, C. W., & DeLuca, H. F. (1984) *J. Biol. Chem.* 259, 12691-12695.

Kowarski, S., & Schachter, D. (1980) *J. Biol. Chem.* 255, 10834-10840.

Kretsinger, R. H., Mann, J. E., & Simmonds, J. G. (1982) in *Vitamin D: Chemical, Biochemical and Clinical Endocrinology of Calcium Metabolism* (Norman, A. W. et al., Eds.) pp 233-248, de Gruyter, New York.

Lawson, D. E. M. (1978) *Vitamin D,* Academic Press, New York.

Lee, Y. S., Taylor, A. N., Reimers, T. J., Edelstein, S., Fullmer, C. S., & Wasserman, R. H. (1987) *Proc. Natl. Acad. Sci. USA* 84, 7344-7348.

Legrand, C., Brehier, A., Clavel, M. C., Thomasset, M., & Rabie, C. (1988) *Brain Res.* 466, 121-129.

Lippiello, L., & Wasserman, R. H. (1975) *J. Histochem. Cytochem.* 23, 111-116.

Long, R. G., Bikle, D. D., & Munson, S. J. (1986) *Endocrinology* 119, 2568-2573.

Mac Intyre, 1. (1986) *British Med. Bulletin* 42, 343-352.

MacLaughlin, J. A., Weiser, M. M., & Freedman, R. H. (1980) *Gastroenterology* 78, 325-332.

Meyer, S. A., Chandler, J. S., & Wasserman, R. H. (1984) in *Endocrine Control of Bone and Celcium Metabolism* (Cohn, D. V., Potts, J. T. Jr., & Fujita, T.,Eds.) pp 324-326, Elsevier, Amsterdam.

Meyer, S. A., & Wasserman, R. H. (1983) *Fed. Proc.* 42, 1367.

Moriuchi, S., Yoshizawa, S., & Hosoya, N. (1977) *J. Nutr. Sci. Vitaminol.* 23, 497-504.

Morrissey, R. L. & Wasserman, R. H. (1971) *Am. J. Physiol.* 220, 1509-1515.

Nellans, H. N., & Popovitch, J. E. (1981) *J. Biol. Chem.* 256, 9932-9936.

Nemere, I., Leathers, V., & Norman, A. W. (1986) *J. Biol. Chem.* 261, 16106-16114.

Nemere, I., Leathers, V. L., Jones, G. I., Luben, R. A., & Norman, A. W. (1988) *J. Bone and Mineral Res.* 3(suppl. 1), S153.

Nemere, I., & Norman, A. W. (1986) *Endocrinology* 119, 1406-1408.

Nemere, I., & Norman, A. W. (1987) *J. Bone and Mineral Res.* 2, 99-107.

Nemere, I., Yoshimoto, Y., & Norman, A. W. (1984) *Endocrinology* 119, 2568-2573.

Oberholtzer, J. C., Schneider, M. E., Summers, M. C., Saunders, J. C., and Matschinsky, F. M. (1986) *Hear. Res.* 23, 161-168.

O'Doherty, P. J. A. (1979) *Lipids* 14, 75-77.

Pansini, A. R., & Christakos, S. (1984) *J. Biol. Chem.* 259, 9735-9741.

Pansu, D., Bellaton, C., & Bronner, F. (1983a) *Am. J. Physiol.* 244, G20-G26.

Pansu, D., Bellaton, C., Roche, C., & Bronner, F. (1983b) *Am. J. Physiol.* 244, G695-G700.

Pansu, D., Ballaton, C. & Roche, C. (1988) in *Cellular Calcium and Phosphate Transport in Health and Disease* (Bronner, F. & Peterlik, M., Eds.) pp 115-120, Alan R. Liss, New York.

Pasteels, B., Parmentier, M., Lawson, D. E. M., Verstappen, A., & Pochet, R. (1987) *Invest. Ophthalmol. Vis. Sci.* 28, 658-664.

Pasteels, J. L., Pochet, R., Surardt, L., Hubeau, C., Chirnoaga, M., Parmentier, M., & Lawson, D. E. (1986) *Brain Res.* 384, 294-303.

Peterlik, M., & Wasserman, R. H. (1978) *Am. J. Physiol.* 234, E379-E388.

Rabie, A., Thomasset, M., & Legrand, C. (1983) *Cell Tissue Res.* 232, 691-696.

Roche, C., Bellaton, C., Pansu, D., Miller, A. 3d., & Bronner, F. (1986) *Am. J. Physiol.* 251, G314-G320.

Roth, J., Baetens, D., Norman, A. W., & Garcia Segura, L. M. (1981) *Brain Res.* 222, 452-457.

Rubinoff, M. J., & Nellans, H. N. (1985) *J. Biol. Chem.* 260, 7824-7828.

Schachter, D., & Rosen, S. M. (1959) *Am. J. Physiol.* 196, 357-362.

Shimura, F., & Wasserman, R. H. (1984) *Endocrinology* 115, 1964-1972.

Steeves, R. M., & Lawson, D. E. (1985) *Biochim. Biophys. Acta* 841, 292-298.

Szebenyi, D. M. E., & Moffat, K. (1986) *J. Biol. Chem.* 261, 8761-8777.

Szebenyi, D. M. E., Obendorf, S. K., & Moffat, K. (1981) *Nature* (London) 294, 327-332.

Taylor, A. N. (1977) *J. Nutr.* 107, 480-486.

Taylor, A. N., & Wasserman, R. H. (1972) *Am. J. Physiol.* 223, 110-114.

Thomasset, M., Desplan, C., & Parkes, O. (1983) *Eur. J. Biochem.* 129, 519-524.

Thomasset, M., Molla, A., Parkes, O., & Demaille, J. G. (1981) *FEBS. Lett.* 127, 13-16.

Thomasset, M., Rabie, A., Parkes, O., Desplan, C., Henin, D., & Cuisinier Gleizes, P. (1984) *Dev. Pharmacol. Ther.* 7, 6-10.

Toverud, S. U., & Dostal, L. A. (1986) *J. Pediatr. Gastroenterol. Nutr.* 5, 688-695.

Van Corven, E. J. J. M., DeJong, M. D., & Van Os, C. H. (1986) *Cell Calcium* 7, 89-99.

Verstappen, A., Parmentier, M., Chirnoaga, M., & Lawson, D. E. (1986) *Opthalmic. Res.* 18, 209-214.

Vesely, D. L., & Juan, D. (1984) *Am. J. Physiol.* 246, E115-E120.

Walters, J. R. F. (1987) in *Calcium-Binding Proteins in Health and Disease* (Norman, A. W., Vanaman, T. C., & Means, A. R., Eds.) pp 122-124, Academic Press, New York.

Walters, J. R. F., & Weiser, M. M. (1987) *Am. J. Physiol.* 252, G170-G177.

Warembourg, M., Perret, C., & Thomasset, M. (1986) *Endocrinology* 119, 176-184.

Warner, R. R., & Coleman, J. R. (1975) *J. Cell Biol.* 64, 54-74.

Wasserman, R. H. (1980) in *Pediatric Diseases Related to Calcium* (DeLuca, H. F., & Anast, C. S., Eds.) pp 107-132, Elsevier, New York.

Wasserman, R. H., Brindak, M. E., Meyer, S. A., & Fullmer, C. S. (1982) *Proc. Natl. Acad. Sci. USA* 79, 7939-7943.

Wasserman, R. H., & Chandler, J. S. (1985) in *Bone and Mineral Research/3* (Peck, W. A., Ed.) pp 181-211, Elsevier, Amsterdam.

Wasserman, R. H., Corradino, R. A., Feher, J. J., & Armbrecht, H. J. (1977) in *Vitamin D: Biochemical, Chemical and Clinical Aspects Related to Calcium Metabolism* (Norman, A. W., Schaefer, K., Coburn, J. W., De Luca, H. F., Fraser, D., Grigoleit, H. G., & Herrath, D. v., Eds.) pp 331-340, de Gruyter, Berlin.

Wasserman, R. H., & Fullmer, C. S. (1982) in *Calcium and Cell Function* (Cheung, W. Y., Ed.) Vol. 11, pp 175-216, Academic Press, N.Y.

Wasserman, R. H., Fullmer, C. S. & Shimura, F. (1984) in *Vitamin D: Basic and Clinical Aspects* (Kumar, R., Ed.) pp 233-257, Martinus Nijhoff, Boston.

Wasserman, R. H., & Kallfelz, F. A. (1962) *Am. J. Physiol.* 203, 221-224.

Wasserman, R. H., Kallfelz, F. A. & Comar, C. L. (1961) *Science* 133, 883-884.

Wasserman, R. H. & Taylor, A. N. (1969) in *Mineral Metabolism, An Advanced Treatise* (Comar, C. L., & Bronner, F., Eds.) pp 321-403, Academic Press, New York.

Wasserman, R. H., & Taylor, A. N. (1973) *J. Nutrition* 103, 586-599.

Wilson, P. W., Harding, M. & Lawson, D. E. M. (1985) *Nucleic Acids Res.* 13, 8867-8881.

6

Equilibrium Constants for the Complexation of Metal Ions by Serum Transferrin

Wesley R. Harris

In mammals iron is transported through blood as ferric ion bound tightly to serum transferrin, which is one member of a small family of iron binding proteins that includes ovotransferrin and lactoferrin (Brock, 1985; Chasteen, 1983; Aisen & Listowsky, 1980). The distinguishing characteristic of the transferrins is the requirement of a synergistic anion to achieve strong metal binding. In the body bicarbonate serves this function. Binding of the anion precedes metal binding (Kojima & Bates, 1981). In the absence of bicarbonate, metal binding is not strong enough to prevent hydrolysis of ferric ion, so that bicarbonate serves as an "all-or-nothing" switch for iron binding.

Serum transferrin (Tf) is a single-chain glycoprotein with a MW of 80,000 (MacGillavrey et al., 1982). The overall dimensions of diferric transferrin are approximately 95 x 60 x 50 Å (Gorinsky et al., 1979). It is a bilobal protein, with a single high-affinity iron binding site located in each lobe. The structure of lactoferrin has been determined at 3.2 Å resolution (Anderson et al., 1987). In this protein the two lobes are connected by a three turn segment of helix with few additional points of interaction. Although the structure of transferrin is not as well established, it appears that the lobes are also relatively independent in this protein as well (Gorinsky et al., 1979; Bailey et al., 1988). Each lobe can be isolated by limited proteolysis and retains its iron binding affinity (Evans & Williams, 1978; Lineback-Zins & Brew, 1980; Zak et al., 1983).

The degree of homology in the amino acid sequences of the two lobes strongly suggests that the modern protein evolved from a single-site ancestor (MacGillavrey et al., 1982), and indeed a protein with a MW of 41,000 and only a single iron binding site has recently been isolated from the ascidian *Pyura stolonifera* and tentatively identified as a member of the transferrin family (Martin et al., 1984). Iron binding produces a significant conformational change (Kilar & Simm, 1985; Krysteva et al., 1976; Rosseneu-Motreff et al., 1971), which may be important in controlling access to the iron (Cowart et al., 1982, 1986).

The identity of the iron-binding ligands in transferrin has been a controversial issue for many years. Difference uv spectra of metallo-transferrins clearly indicate the coordination of tyrosines (Luk, 1971; Gelb & Harris, 1980; Tan & Woodworth,

67

1969; Pecoraro et al., 1981). Comparisons of the difference uv spectra of metal-transferrin complexes with the spectra of corresponding metal complexes of the phenolate ligand ethylenebis(o-hydroxyphenylglycine) show that the protein spectra are consistent with the coordination of two tyrosines per metal ion (Pecoraro et al., 1981).

Early EPR studies on Cu^{2+}-Tf established the coordination of at least one histidine at the Tf binding site (Zweier et al., 1979; Zweier & Aisen, 1977). More recently both the ENDOR spectrum (Roberts et al., 1983) and the low frequency EPR spectrum (Froncisz & Aisen, 1982) of cupric transferrin have shown coordination of only a single nitrogen. It is also accepted that the synergistic bicarbonate anion occupies one coordination site (Zweier et al., 1979; Harris & Gelb, 1980; Scheider et al., 1984). Proton exchange studies show coordination of one solvent molecule either as water or hydroxide (Koenig & Schillinger, 1969).

Recent crystallographic studies on both transferrin (Bailey et al., 1988) and lactoferrin (Anderson et al., 1987) appear to have settled the issue of the metal binding ligands from the protein. The crystal structures confirm coordination of two tyrosines and one histidine. They also reveal the coordination of the carboxylate group of an aspartate residue which had not been identified by spectroscopic studies. Coordination of the water/hydroxide and the synergistic anion could not be confirmed at the present state of structure refinement.

The synergistic anion is thought to form a bridge between the metal ion and the protein by coordinating one oxygen directly to the metal ion while simultaneously hydrogen bonding to cationic groups on the protein (Bates, et al., 1987). One proposed variation on this structure involves the bridging of the carbonate anion and the coordinated water molecule by an uncoordinated imidazole (Woodworth, 1986).

The two specific metal-binding sites of transferrin are commonly identified as N-terminal and C-terminal, corresponding to the lobe of the protein in which the site resides. If one allows for the possibility of cooperativity between the two transferrin binding sites, then four microconstants describe the iron-binding equilibrium system (Aisen et al., 1978), as shown in the scheme.

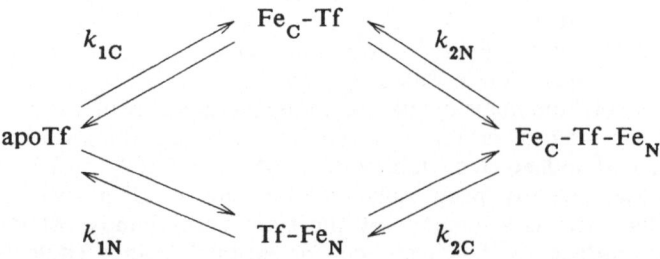

The subscript for each microconstant denotes whether it corresponds to the first or second iron to bind to the protein and whether the binding is at the N-terminal or C-terminal site. Macroscopic iron binding constants are given by the equations

$$K_1 = k_{1C} + k_{1N} \tag{1}$$

$$\frac{1}{K_2} = \frac{1}{k_{2C}} + \frac{1}{k_{2N}} \tag{2}$$

There have been conflicting reports on the magnitude and heterogeneity of the two transferrin iron binding constants (Davis et al., 1962; Aasa et al., 1963). However, Aisen et al. (1978) have now determined accurate macroscopic iron binding constants of log $K_1^* = 20.7$ and log $K_2^* = 19.4$ at pH 7.4 and ambient bicarbonate. They have also shown that the separations between k_{1C} and k_{2C} and between k_{1N} and k_{2N} are about 0.3 log units. Chasteen & Williams (1981) have measured relative iron binding constants and reported a negative cooperativity of about 0.2 log units for the N-terminal site. Since the precision of the reported equilibrium constants is probably around 0.2 to 0.3 log units, it appears that cooperativity, if it exists, is of the same order of magnitude as the uncertainties in the equilibrium constants.

Under normal conditions serum transferrin is only about 30% saturated with iron (Chasteen, 1983), leaving a high binding capacity for other metal ions. Thus there has been considerable interest in the role of transferrin in the serum transport of metals other than iron. In some cases the involvement of transferrin in the metabolism of a metal ion can be demonstrated rather easily. For example, plutonium(IV) binds quite strongly to transferrin and can be readily traced due to its radioactivity (Stevens et al., 1968; Durbin, 1975; Boocock & Popplewell, 1965). This is not the case with the complexes of most divalent metal ions. Stability constants are frequently so low that procedures used to separate and identify proteins can lead to the dissociation of the complex. Thus one must study the stability of these weak complexes *in vitro*, and attempt to make reasonable extrapolations to the species that would be expected *in vivo*.

An added impetus for the study of a variety of metal ions with transferrin is the information to be gained about the protein itself. This principle is well established for spectroscopic probes. Lanthanide-transferrin complexes have been used to estimate the distance between metal binding sites (O'Hara et al., 1981) and the depth of each site below the surface of the protein (Yeh & Meares, 1980). This paper reports on thermodynamic studies of metal ion complexation to serum transferrin. One objective is to illustrate the use of equilibrium data on a variety of metal ions to derive fundamental information about transferrin and its iron complexes.

Experimental Section

Materials. Human apotransferrin was purchased from Calbiochem and purified as previously described to remove any chelating agents (Harris, 1986b). The molar absorptivity of each batch of apotransferrin was measured by spectrophotometric titration at 465 nm with a pH 4 solution of bis(nitrilotriacetato)ferrate(III). Stock metal ion solutions were prepared from reagent grade salts and standardized by atomic absorption spectroscopy. Stock metal ion solutions typically contained 0.1 M to 0.001 M HCl, depending on the hydrolytic tendencies of the metal ion. The competitive chelating agents nitrilotriacetic acid (NTA), ethylenediamine-N,N'-diacetic acid, triethylenetetramine tetrahydrochloride (trien), iminodiacetic acid, and N-(2-hydroxyethyl)iminodiacetic acid were purchased and used as received. A variety of ligands have been used to provide an adequate match between the competing ligand and Tf. All metal ion titrations were conducted in 0.1 M N-(2-hydroxyethyl)-piperazine-N'-ethanesulfonic acid (Hepes) buffer. Anion titrations were conducted in both 0.1 M and 0.01 M Hepes.

C-terminal monoferric transferrin was prepared by the addition of one equiv of bis(nitrilotriacetato)ferrate(III) to apoTf in 0.1 M Hepes/0.1 M perchlorate. This solution was eluted through a 1.5 x 23 cm sephadex G-15 column using 0.1 M Hepes to remove the NTA and the perchlorate. N-terminal monoferric transferrin was prepared by two methods. In some cases freshly prepared ferrous ammonium sulfate was added to apoTf in 0.1 M Hepes/0.1 M perchlorate/15 mM sodium bicarbonate at pH 7.4. In other cases, iron was selectively removed from the C-terminal site of diferric transferrin using the procedure of Baldwin & de Sousa (1981). In both cases, the initial product was eluted through a 1.5 x 23 cm Sephadex G-15 column using 0.1 M Hepes, pH 7.4. The ratios of the absorbances at 280 and 465 nm indicated approximately 45% saturation of the transferrin binding sites.

The distribution of iron between the two transferrin binding sites was evaluated by urea-polyacrylamide gel electrophoresis as described by Makey & Seal (1976). The gels were 7% acrylamide containing 6.5 M urea in pH 8.4 tris buffer. Samples were run at 120 V for approximately 20 h.

Methods. Equal volumes of a 1.5 x 10^{-4} M apoTf solution were added to dry sample and reference cuvettes, and a baseline of protein vs. protein was recorded from 320 nm to 240 nm. To measure anion binding constants, the sample cuvettes were titrated with 5 to 50 mM solutions of the sodium salts of either bicarbonate, hydrogen phosphate, sulfate, or arsenate. To measure metal binding constants, a known concentration of sodium bicarbonate was added to the apoTf solution, which was then titrated with solutions containing the metal ion and a suitable competing ligand. The cell holder was maintained at 25 °C by an external circulating water bath.

The nonlinear least squares method for calculating transferrin binding constants has been previously described in detail (Harris & Pecoraro, 1983). Briefly, initial guesses of the metal-Tf binding constants are used to solve the system mass balance equations. The resulting concentrations of the 1:1 and 2:1 metal-Tf complexes are used to calculate the expected absorptivity for each titration point. The squares of the residuals between observed and calculated absorptivities are used to adjust the values of the transferrin binding constants. This program has been used to calculate binding constants for both the binary HCO_3-Tf species as well as the ternary metal-HCO_3-Tf complexes. The anion-binding constants are defined as

$$K_1 = \frac{[A-Tf]}{[A^-][Tf]} \tag{3}$$

$$K_2 = \frac{[A-Tf-A]}{[A^-][A-Tf]} \tag{4}$$

Table I. Equilibrium constants for the binding of anions to human serum transferrin

Anion	ApoTf			Monoferric Tf		
	Log K_1	Log K_2	$\Delta\varepsilon_M$	Log K_C	Log K_N	$\Delta\varepsilon_M$
Phosphate	4.25(17)	3.50(16)	7,500(900)	3.79(8)	3.99(13)	7,600
Sulfate	3.74(18)	2.86(12)	8,000(600)	3.37(3)	3.43(15)	7,600
Carbonate	2.96(5)	2.33(36)	4,400(500)	2.74(5)	2.67(16)	4,300
Arsenate	4.07(16)	3.36(6)	6,900(500)			

Conditional metal binding constants are defined as

$$\log K_1{}^* = \frac{[M\text{-}Tf]}{[M][Tf]} \tag{5}$$

$$\log K_2{}^* = \frac{[M\text{-}Tf\text{-}M]}{[M][M\text{-}Tf]} \tag{6}$$

where [M-Tf] and [M-Tf-M] represent the 1:1 and 2:1 metal-bicarbonate-protein complexes, and [Tf] represents the sum of all free transferrin, which includes apo-transferrin and the binary bicarbonate-transferrin species shown in eqns (3) and (4). Since terms for hydrogen ion are omitted from eqns (5) and (6), these equations define effective binding constants which are valid only at pH 7.4. Because the distribution of the binary HCO_3-Tf species which comprise [Tf] is a function of the free bicarbonate concentrations, the value of K^* varies with the bicarbonate concentration.

Results and Discussion

Anion binding. It has been shown recently that the binding of bicarbonate, sulfate, and phosphate to apoTf can be followed by difference uv spectroscopy (Harris, 1985). Typical spectra for phosphate are shown in Figure 1. The spectra show a strong minimum at 245 nm, along with a weaker, broader minimum around 290 nm. These spectra are essentially inverted forms of the metal-induced difference uv spectra, which show positive peaks around 245 nm and 290 nm. No spectra are observed when the anions are added to diferric transferrin, which suggests that the spectra reflect an interaction between the anion and the tyrosines which also serve as ligands to the iron.

The absorbance at 245 nm is converted to an apparent absorptivity ($\Delta\varepsilon$) by dividing by the analytical transferrin concentration. This normalizes the data from different experiments. Titration curves of $\Delta\varepsilon$ vs. molarity of anion for phosphate, sulfate, arsenate, and bicarbonate are shown in Figure 2. Successive macroscopic anion binding constants are shown in Table I. The binding constants and molar absorptivities of sulfate, arsenate and phosphate are very similar. Both the binding constant and molar absorptivity for the bicarbonate-Tf complex are significantly

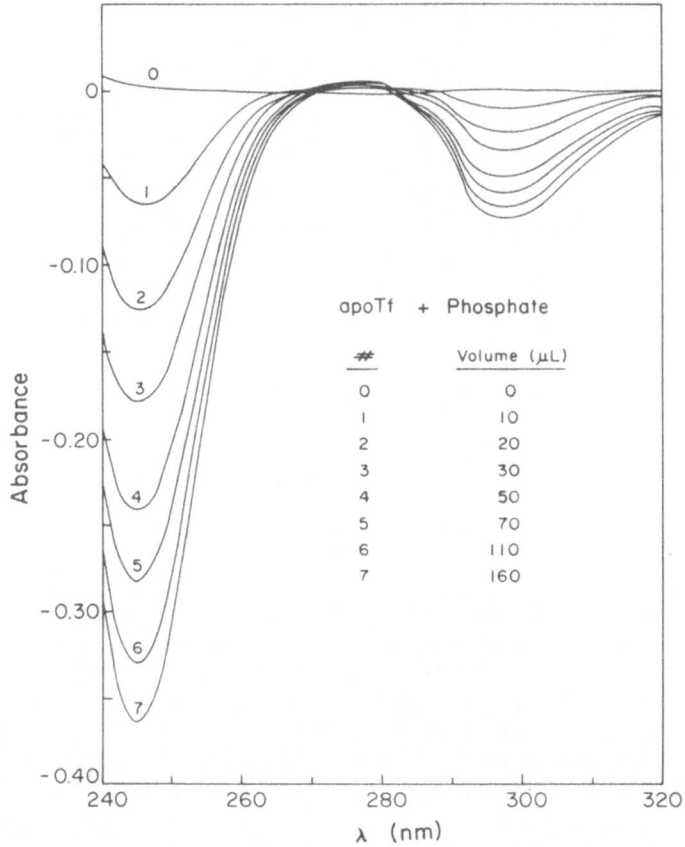

Figure 1. Difference uv spectra generated by the addition of aliquots of a 5.0 mM, pH 7.4 phosphate solution to 2.0 mL of 1.28 x 10^{-5} M apoTf in 0.010 M, pH 7.4 Hepes buffer at 25 °C.

smaller. It is not clear whether this is due to the different geometry of bicarbonate or to its lower charge.

Titration curves for apoTf and both N-terminal and C-terminal monoferric transferrin with phosphate are shown in Figure 3. These data have been used to calculate binding constants for the vacant binding sites of the monoferric transferrins. These constants are listed in Table I. The values for the two monoferric transferrins are virtually identical, indicating that the two sites are equivalent with regard to the binding of anions. Similar results have been obtained for the binding of sulfate.

Figure 4 shows titration curves for bicarbonate with apoTf and both forms of monoferric transferrin. The titrations of the monoferric species confirm the lower molar absorptivity of the bicarbonate complexes. Once again, the binding at the two sites appears to be equivalent.

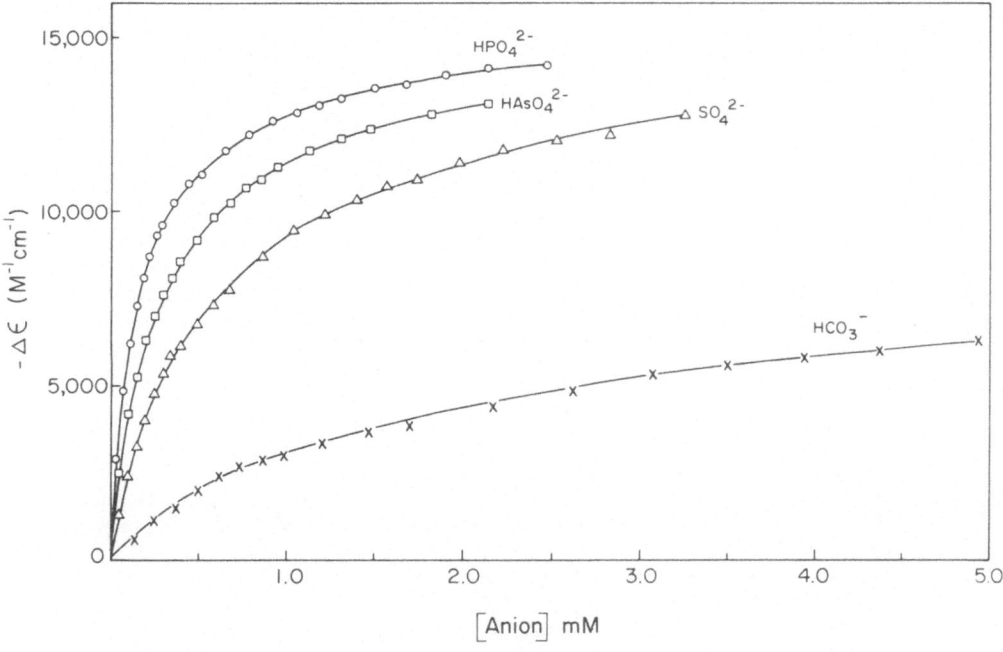

Figure 2. Titration curves for addition of anions to ~1.3 x 10^{-5} M apoTf in 0.010 M pH 7.4 Hepes buffer. Phosphate titrant: 15 mM, pH 7.4; Arsenate titrant: 20 mM, pH 7.4; Sulfate titrant: 20 mM, pH 7.4; Bicarbonate titrant, 50 mM, pH 8.0.

Bicarbonate-dependence of metal binding. Diferric transferrin can also bind anions at "nonsynergistic" binding sites (Folajtar & Chasteen, 1982). Thus one needs to demonstrate that the difference uv spectra correspond to the binding of the synergistic anion. This can be done by establishing the thermodynamic relationship between anion binding and metal binding. One can describe the overall process of metal binding in terms of two reactions

$$HCO_3^- + apoTf \underset{\longleftarrow}{\overset{K_C}{\longrightarrow}} HCO_3\text{-Tf} \tag{7}$$

$$M^{n+} + HCO_3\text{-Tf} \underset{\longleftarrow}{\overset{K_M}{\longrightarrow}} M\text{-}HCO_3\text{-Tf} \tag{8}$$

A set of equations can be written for each binding site. The K_C values appear to be the same for each site. In general the K_M values will be different for the two sites. A total of two or three protons are released during the reactions shown in eqns (7) and (8). Since they are not shown in the equilibria, both K_C and K_M are conditional constants for pH 7.4.

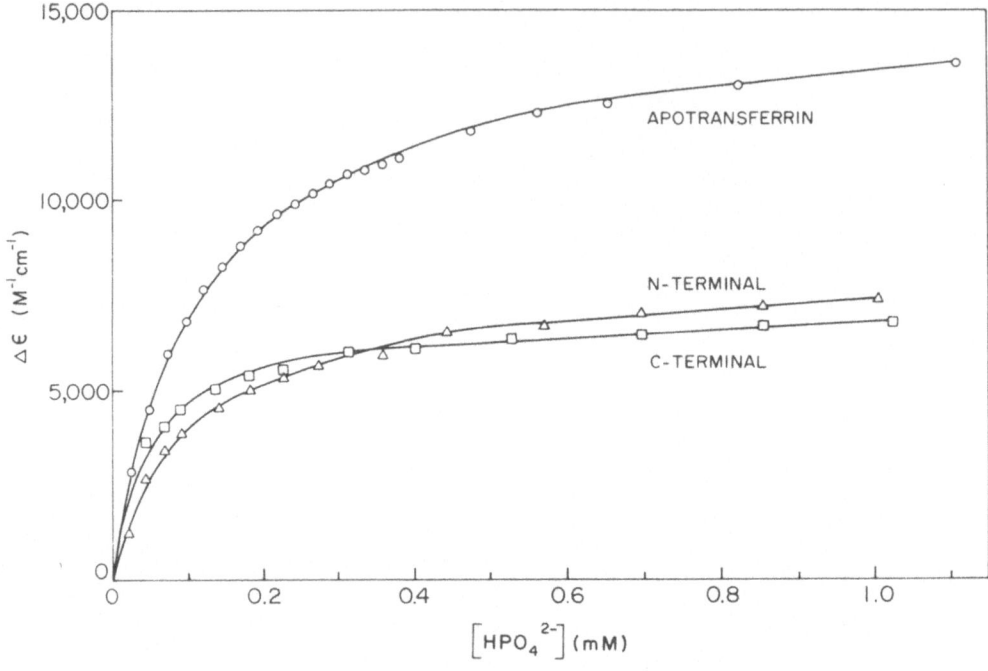

Figure 3. Titration curves from the addition of phosphate to apoTf and to both N-terminal and C-terminal monoferric transferrins. Experimental conditions are given with Figure 2.

Eqns (7) and (8) can be used to predict the bicarbonate dependence of the effective metal binding constant for a particular metal ion. The effective binding constant is defined by eqn (5). The percent saturation of each binding site with bicarbonate can be calculated as

$$\alpha = \frac{K_C[HCO_3]}{1 + K_C[HCO_3]} \tag{9}$$

One can then substitute $[HCO_3\text{-}Tf]/\alpha$ for $[Tf]$ in eqn (5) to give

$$K_1{}^* = \frac{[M\text{-}HCO_3\text{-}Tf]\alpha}{[M][HCO_3\text{-}Tf]} \tag{10}$$

Taking the log of both sides of eqn (10) yields

$$\log K_1{}^* = \log K_M + \log \alpha \tag{11}$$

Thus if the bicarbonate binding constants measured spectrophotometrically correspond to the binding of the synergistic anions, then one should be able to use the bicarbonate K_C values to obtain linear plots of $\log K^*$ for a metal ion vs. $\log \alpha$.

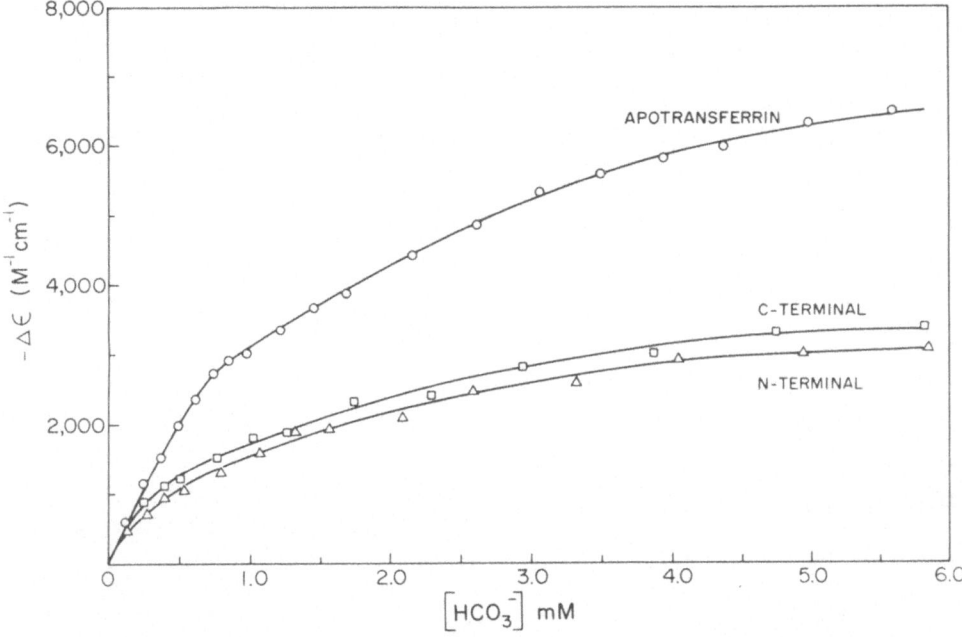

Figure 4. Titration curves for the addition of bicarbonate to apoTf and to both N-terminal and C-terminal monoferric transferrins. Experimental conditions are given with Figure 2.

The relationship between the bicarbonate binding constants and metal binding has been evaluated using the Zn^{2+} ion. The difference uv spectra produced by the addition of aliquots of Zn^{2+} to apoTf are shown in Figure 5. The titration curves for apo-, C-terminal monoferric, and N-terminal monoferric transferrin are shown in Figure 6. The titration curves for apoTf are typically linear from r = 0 to r = ~0.5 (r = ratio of $[Zn]/[Tf]_{tot}$), with the actual linear range depending on the bicarbonate concentration. This linearity results from the complete binding of all the added Zn. Therefore the slope of this linear segment is equal to the molar absorptivity of the Zn-Tf complex. The observed molar absorptivities for a series of bicarbonate concentrations are listed in Table II.

ApoTf has also been titrated with Zn solutions containing various concentrations of trien as a competing ligand. Value for two successive macroscopic Zn binding constants, K_1^* and K_2^*, have been calculated from a least squares fit of the absorbance data. The resulting values of log K_1^* and log K_2^* for a series of bicarbonate concentrations are listed in Table II.

The microscopic reactions for the Zn system are identical to the scheme shown above for iron. The separation between successive macroscopic Zn-binding constants is so great at all bicarbonate concentrations that if one assumes noncooperativity, then calculations using eqns (1) and (2) show that there is no significant difference between the macroscopic and microscopic zinc constants. Titrations of both forms of monoferric transferrin indicate that the larger Zn-binding constant can be assigned to the C-terminal site, while the smaller binding constant

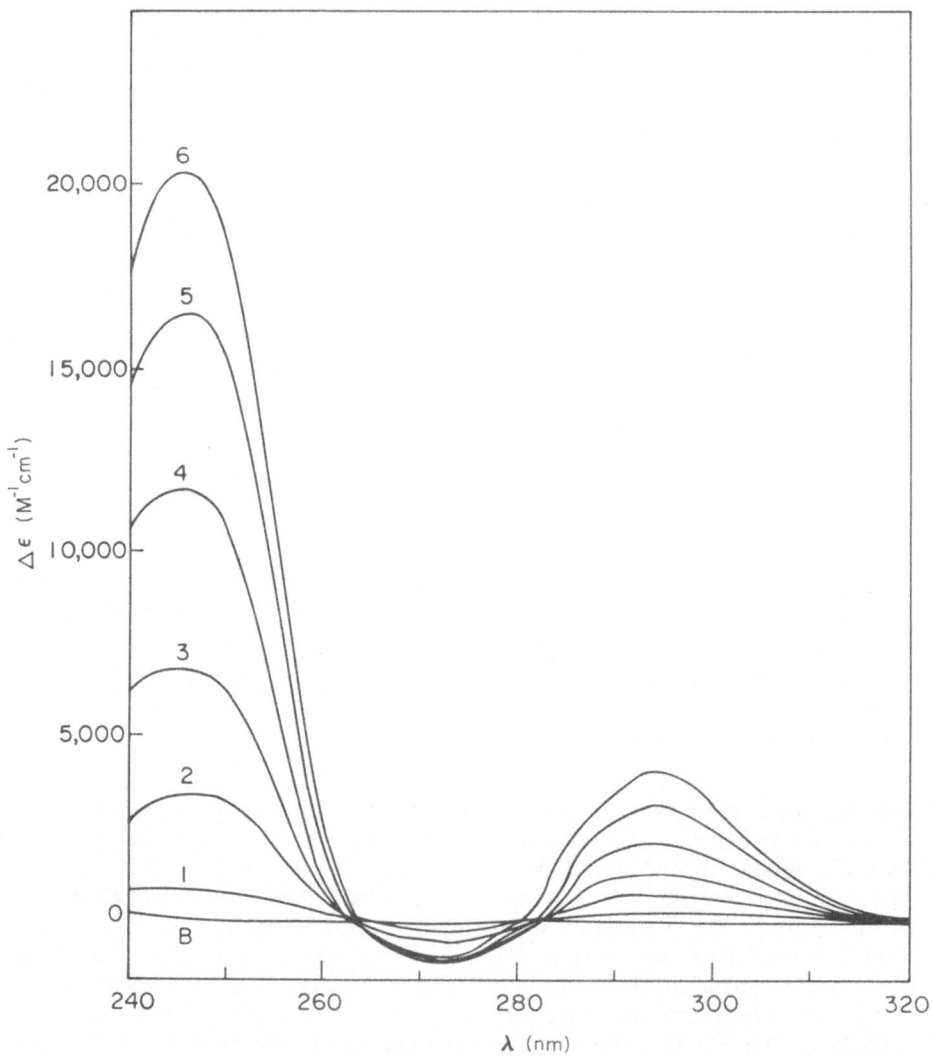

Figure 5. Difference uv spectra generated by the addition of 2.934 x 10^{-4} M zinc(II) to 2.0 mL of 1.518 x 10^{-5} apoTf in 100 mM Hepes/15 mM bicarbonate pH 7.4 buffer. Spectrum #1, 5 μL zinc; #2, 25 μL; #3, 50 μL; #4, 90 μL; #5, 140 μL; #6, 240 μL.

corresponds to the N-terminal site (Harris, 1983). Thus one can evaluate the effects of bicarbonate in terms of a single site.

A plot of log K_1^* vs. log α for bicarbonate concentrations from ambient to 15 mM is shown in Figure 7. The slope of 1.24 ± 0.16 is close to the value of 1.0 predicted by eqn (11). The intercept gives a log K_M value of 7.42 ± 0.18. Excessive losses of CO_2 from the solutions preclude measurements of log K^* at higher bicarbonate concentrations. Nevertheless, there is a good fit of the Zn-binding data to

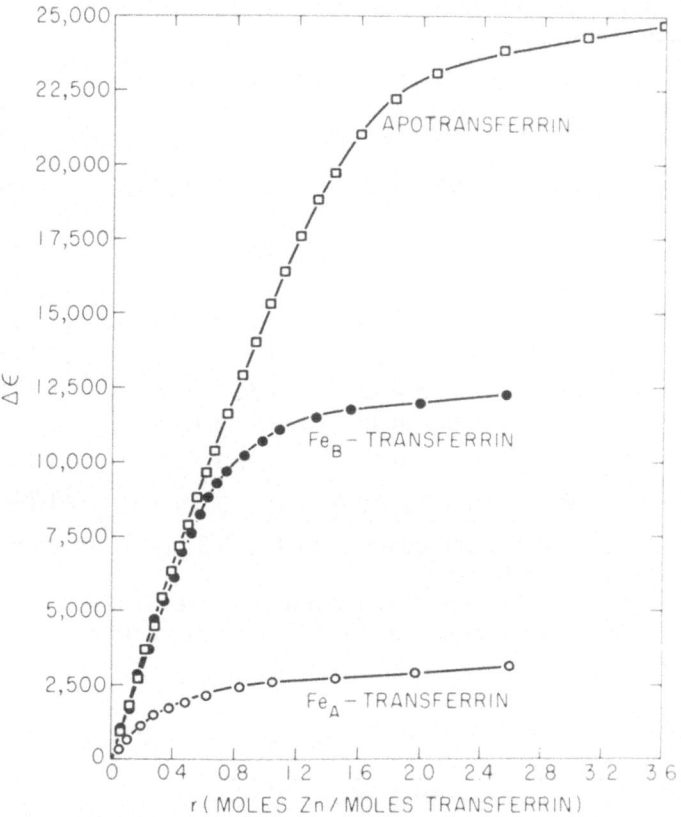

Figure 6. Titration curves from addition of $ZnCl_2$ to apoTf and to both forms of monoferric transferrin in 0.1 M Hepes/15 mM bicarbonate at pH 7.4.

eqn (11). The data are consistent with the binding mechanism shown in eqns (7) and (8).

The bicarbonate dependence of the Zn-Tf molar absorptivity provides additional evidence that the difference uv spectra shown in Figure 1 correspond to binding of the synergistic anion. Changes in the molar absorptivity can be explained on the basis of competitive binding between Zn and bicarbonate. The binding of an aliquot of Zn produces a positive absorbance in the difference uv spectrum which is equal to $\Delta\varepsilon_{Zn}[Zn\text{-}HCO_3\text{-}Tf]$, where $\Delta\varepsilon_{Zn}$ is the true molar absorptivity of the ternary Zn-Tf complex. However, this Zn complex replaces an equimolar concentration of transferrin which had existed as an equilibrium mixture of apoTf and HCO_3-Tf. The negative absorbance of the HCO_3-Tf complex, equal to $\Delta\varepsilon_C[HCO_3\text{-}Tf]$, is lost concomitantly with the generation of the positive absorbance of the Zn-Tf complex. Thus the apparent absorptivity of the Zn complex ($\Delta\varepsilon_M$) will depend on the fraction of free transferrin that exists as the binary bicarbonate complex. This dependence is described by the equation

Table II. Zinc-transferrin binding constants measured at different bicarbonate concentrations

[HCO$_3^-$] (mM)[a]	n[b]	Log K_1^* ± 2 SEM	Log K_2^* ± 2 SEM	$\Delta\varepsilon$ (M^{-1}cm^{-1})
0.2	8	5.84 ± 0.25	4.44 ± 0.23	9,300[c] 10,400[d]
0.7	10	6.69 ± 0.34	4.66 ± 0.11	10,900 ± 300
1.2	10	6.77 ± 0.13	4.54 ± 0.08	11,600 ± 960
2.2	7	6.65 ± 0.20	4.92 ± 0.46	11,800 ± 600
3.2	8	6.98 ± 0.31	4.43 ± 0.10	13,200 ± 900
5.2	20	7.12 ± 0.15	4.85 ± 0.18	13,300 ± 500
10.2	8	7.29 ± 0.30	5.17 ± 0.75	14,300 ± 1000
15.2	8	7.47 ± 0.17	5.91 ± 0.17	14,200 ± 400
25.2	4	—	—	14,900 ± 700

[a] Values represent total bicarbonate, including 0.2 mM from ambient CO_2.
[b] Number of replicate titrations.
[c] Calculated from initial slope of the titration curves at 0.2 mM.
[d] Calculated from equation (12) and used in the calculations of K_1^* and K_2^*.

$$\Delta\varepsilon_M = \Delta\varepsilon_{Zn} - \alpha(\Delta\varepsilon_C) \tag{12}$$

A plot of $\Delta\varepsilon_M$ vs. α is shown in Figure 8. The data are linear for solutions that contain at least 0.5 mM bicarbonate. At ambient bicarbonate concentrations, the effective binding constant is so low that the assumption of complete binding of the initial aliquots of Zn is no longer valid. Thus the $\Delta\varepsilon_M$ value at ambient bicarbonate lies below the extrapolated least squares line. The extrapolated value of 10,400 M^{-1}cm^{-1} was used to calculate the Zn-Tf binding constants.

The fit of the variation in apparent molar absorptivity to eqn (12) strongly supports the hypothesis that the initial binding of the synergistic anion to apoTf involves hydrogen bonding interactions with the same tyrosine residues that are eventually involved in metal binding. These interactions are lost when the metal enters the binding site and deprotonates the tyrosines. One can calculate a value of $\Delta\varepsilon_C = -5,400 \pm 400$ from the slope of the plot in Figure 8. This is in good agreement with the molar absorptivity of $-4,200 \pm 300$ determined from difference uv titrations of apoTf with free bicarbonate.

Metal-binding constants. Most of the available thermodynamic data on metal complexation by transferrin are summarized in Table III. As one expects, ferric ion forms the most stable complex, followed by the other trivalent ions Ga^{3+} and Al^{3+}. There is a big decrease in the log K values for the divalent metal ions and the large trivalent lanthanides, with typical log K values of 6 to 8. The binding

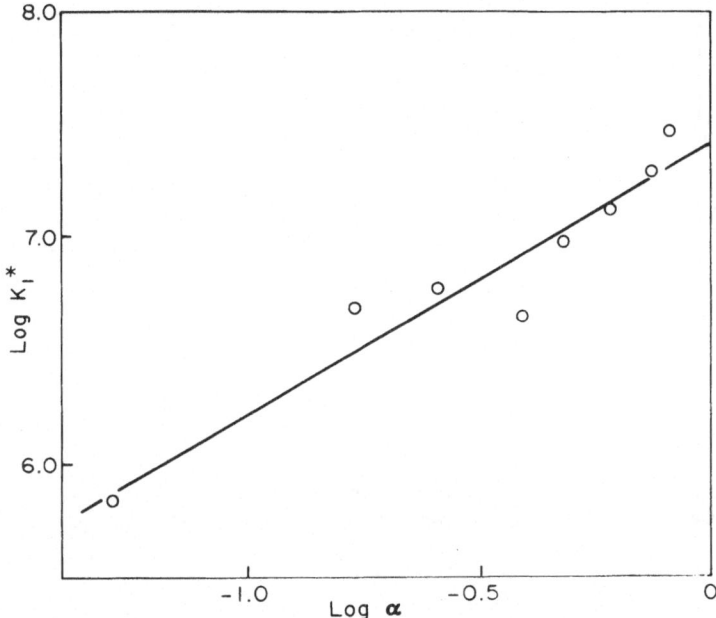

Figure 7. Plot of the effective zinc(II)-Tf binding constant as a function α, defined by equation (9) as the degree of saturation of the free transferrin binding site with bicarbonate.

constants for Ni^{2+} are unusually low, which may be due to crystal field effects (Harris, 1986c).

Experimentally it is easier to measure log K_1^* than it is to measure log K_2^*. The weaker binding at the second site leads to greater interferences from side reactions such as hydrolysis and formation of carbonate complexes. It is not uncommon to make equilibrium measurements on solutions that are supersaturated with respect to the metal-carbonate. Actual precipitation appears to be retarded by the low metal ion concentrations, since good isosbestic points are maintained throughout the titrations. However, these complications do result in a larger standard deviation for log K_2^* for most metal ions.

The separation between successive macroscopic binding constants (Δlog K) provides an indication of the heterogeneity between the two binding sites. For a protein with two identical binding sites, statistical effects would lead to a Δlog K of 0.6 log units. Thus separations in excess of 0.6 may indicate site heterogeneity in metal binding. This is illustrated by the detailed study of Aisen et al., (1978) on iron binding. The microscopic binding constants for the two sites differ by 0.8 log units, while the macroscopic binding constants are separated by 1.3 log units.

For the metal ions studied thus far, the separation between macroscopic constants varies from 0.6 to 1.7 log units. A serious problem in analyzing the Δlog K values is that they have a very high uncertainty, since they are calculated as the difference between two numbers that each have standard deviations of 0.2 to 0.3

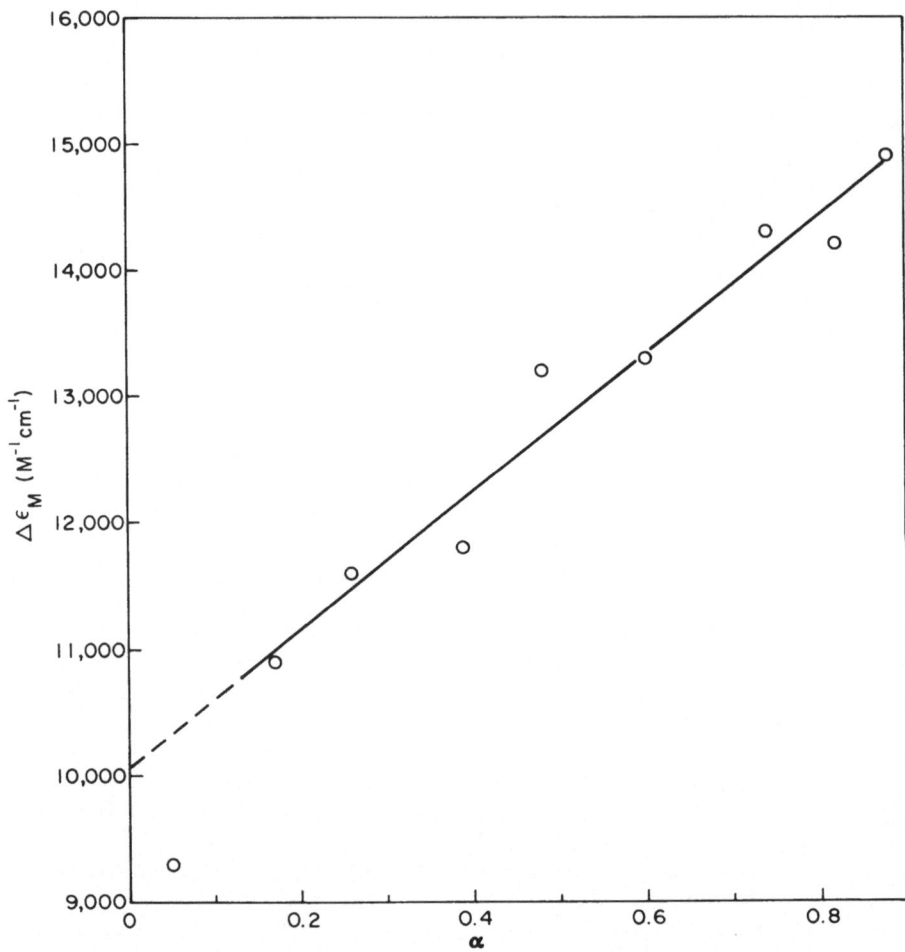

Figure 8. Plot of the apparent molar absorptivity of the ternary Zn–HCO$_3$-Tf complex as a function of α, defined by eqn (9) as the degree of saturation of the free transferrin binding site with bicarbonate.

log units. Nevertheless, the $\Delta\log K$ values are consistently greater than 0.6, and it appears that there is a slight difference between the metal binding affinities of the two sites. The average $\Delta\log K$ value is about 1.1 log units, which would correspond to a three-fold difference in binding affinities for the two sites.

It is usually not possible to measure equilibrium constants for the binding of metal ions at the vacant binding site of monoferric transferrins because addition of a competitive chelating agent may scramble the iron between the sites. However, titrations of both forms of monoferric transferrin with another metal ion in the absence of any chelating agent will usually identify the weaker and stronger

Table III. Summary of transferrin binding constants

Metal Ion	[HCO_3^-] (mM)	Log K_1^* ± 2 SEM	Log K_2^* ± 2 SEM	ΔLog K	References
Al^{3+}	15	15.4			a
Al^{3+}	27	12.9	12.3	0.6	b
Cd^{2+}	5	5.95 ± 0.10	4.86 ± 0.13	1.09	c
Fe^{3+}	0.2	20.67	19.38	1.29	d
Ga^{3+}	5	19.53 ± 0.25	18.58 ± 0.25	0.95	e
Gd^{3+}	0.2	6.83			f
Nd^{3+}	0.2	6.09 ± 0.15	5.04 ± 0.46	1.05	g
Ni^{2+}	5	4.10 ± 0.15	3.23 ± 0.31	0.87	h
Sm^{3+}	0.2	7.13 ± 0.24	5.39 ± 0.32	1.74	g
VO_2^+	0.2	7.45 ± 0.10	6.60 ± 0.30	0.85	i
Zn^{2+}	15	7.80 ± 0.20	6.4 ± 0.4	1.4	j

[a] Cochran et al., 1984.
[b] Martin, 1986.
[c] Harris & Madsen, 1988.
[d] Aisen et al., 1978.
[e] Harris & Pecoraro, 1983.
[f] Zak & Aisen, 1988.
[g] Harris, 1986b.
[h] Harris, 1986c.
[i] Harris, 1985.
[j] Harris, 1983.

binding sites due to obvious differences in the intensities of the difference uv peaks. Studies on Fe^{3+}, Zn^{2+}, Cd^{2+}, Nd^{3+}, and Sm^{3+} all indicate that the C-terminal binding site forms the most stable complex. (Aisen et al., 1978; Harris, 1983; Harris, 1986b; Harris & Madsen, 1988)

The site selectivity for Ni^{2+} may be unique. Because of the small binding constants for Ni^{2+}, one can measure the equilibrium between free Ni^{2+} and Ni-Tf even in the absence of any competing ligand. Thus it is possible to measure binding constants for the vacant binding sites of both forms of monoferric transferrin of log K_N = 4.39 ± 0.21 and log K_C = 4.11 ± 0.14 (Harris, 1986c). The separation of 0.9 log units between the successive macroscopic Ni-Tf binding constants listed in Table III is consistent with a site selectivity of 0.3 log units. Thus the empty N-terminal site of Fe_C-Tf may form the more stable Ni^{2+} complex. However, the standard deviations of the log K values precludes any definitive conclusions regarding Ni^{2+} site selectivity.

Linear free energy relationships. Linear free energy relationships (LFER) have been widely used in inorganic chemistry. Such relationships are typically presented as a plot in which the log K for a "reference" metal ion is used as the x-coordinate for a data point, while the log K of a "sample" metal ion with the same ligand is used as the y-coordinate. LFER have been used to evaluate the relative "hardness" of two metal ions (Hancock et al., 1974; Marsicano & Hancock, 1978; Irving & Rossotti, 1956; Misono & Saito, 1970). It is well established that one obtains linear plots only when using a set of ligands of comparable hardness.

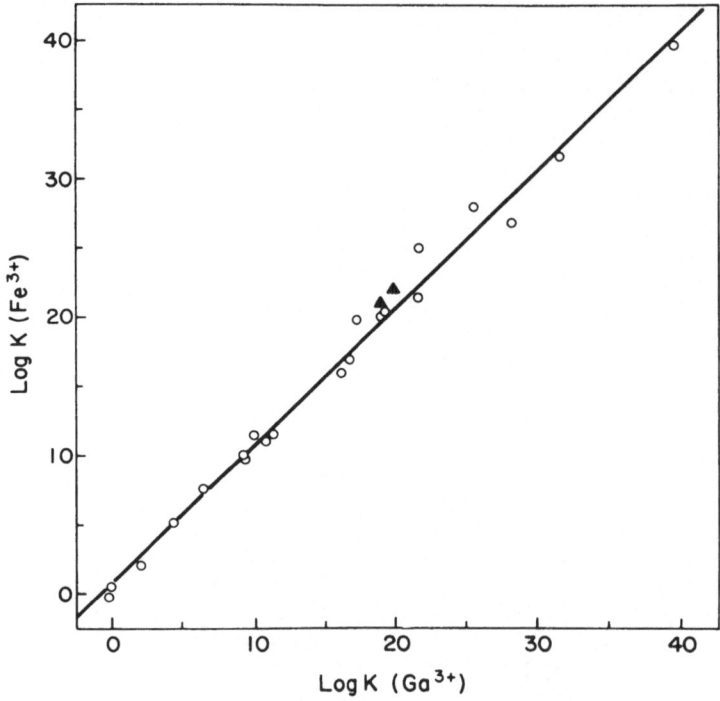

Figure 9. Linear free energy relationship for the complexation of Fe^{3+} and Ga^{3+}. Each data point represents the stability constant of a given ligand with Ga^{3+} as the x-coordinate and the Fe^{3+} stability constant with the same ligand as the y-coordinate. The points for human serum transferrin are shown as closed triangles.

The use of LFER has now been extended to include binding constants for the transferrins (Harris, 1986a). Figure 9 shows the LFER between Ga^{3+} and Fe^{3+}. These ions are ideally suited for an LFER, since they are both trivalent and have virtually identical ionic radii. Unfortunately there are relatively few ligands for which both the Fe^{3+} and the Ga^{3+} binding constants are known. The LFER has been constructed using equilibrium constants for 21 low-molecular-weight (LMW) ligands and is described by the equation

$$\log K_{Fe} = (1.00 \pm 0.02) \log K_{Ga} + (0.7 \pm 1.2) \tag{13}$$

The transferrin binding constants have been measured for both Fe^{3+} (Aisen et al., 1978) and Ga^{3+} (Harris & Pecoraro, 1983). Since the constants were measured at different bicarbonate concentrations, the reported effective binding constants (K^*'s) have been converted to bicarbonate-independent metal binding constants (K_M's), which correspond to eqn (8). The successive macroscopic binding constants for transferrin are represented as closed triangles in Figure 9. The transferrin binding constants are in excellent agreement with the LFER. This demonstrates that when metal ions are properly matched for size, charge, and crystal field stabilization energy, transferrin conforms to LFER which are constructed from data for LMW ligands.

Size restrictions to metal binding. Because of the role of Tf in the serum transport of the large tri- and tetravalent actinides, there is considerable interest in size restrictions to metal binding. LFER offer an excellent way to probe for such steric effects. Since the LFER are constructed from flexible LMW ligands, they are not expected to be very sensitive to variations in the ionic radii of the two metal ions. When a metal binds to Tf, however, it presumably must fit into a site whose dimensions are largely predetermined by the tertiary structure of the protein. Thus metal ions which are too large will fit poorly and will not bind as tightly to the protein.

Figure 10 shows a LFER for Cd^{2+} vs. Zn^{2+}. The LMW data on these two metals have been restricted to ligands that bind through some combination of nitrogen and oxygen donors. A total of 243 complexes have been included in the LFER, including some bis and tris complexes of tri- and bidentate ligands. The LFER is described by the equation

$$\log K_{Cd} = (0.874 \pm 0.010) \log K_{Zn} - (0.07 \pm 0.68) \tag{14}$$

Because of the larger number of data points, the uncertainty in estimated cadmium binding constants is about half of that for the Ga-Fe LFER.

The ionic radii for Zn^{2+} and Cd^{2+} are 0.74 Å and 0.95 Å respectively. If there are significant steric restrictions to the binding of the larger Cd^{2+} ion, one would expect the data points corresponding to the Cd^{2+}-Tf binding constants to fall below the LFER. The experimental Cd^{2+}-Tf binding constants are shown as the closed triangles in Figure 10. There is an excellent fit of the Tf binding constants to the LFER. This indicates that there are no significant steric effects up to an ionic radius of 0.95 Å. The radii of Th^{4+} and Pu^{4+} are 0.94 Å and 0.86 Å respectively. Thus is appears that steric strain is not an important factor in the binding of these tetravalent actinides.

Previous studies had indicated that steric effects were important for the binding of Th^{4+}, Nd^{3+} (r = 0.98 Å) and Pr^{3+} (r = 0.99 Å). Difference uv titrations for Nd^{3+} and Pr^{3+} leveled off at absorptivities much less than those observed for the smaller lanthanides, and it was concluded that these larger cations were binding to only one site (Luk, 1971). Similarly, a lower absorptivity for the Th^{4+}-Tf complex led to the suggestion that only one tyrosine was bound at one of the two sites (Harris et al., 1981). However, it now has been shown that binding of the lanthanides to Tf is in competition with formation of sparingly soluble lanthanide carbonate complexes (Harris, 1986b; Zak & Aisen, 1988). Lanthanide titrations consistently leveled off prior to saturation of both binding sites. The original study by Luk (1971) on the lanthanides included 5 mM bicarbonate in the buffer, which exacerbated this problem. Similarly, formation of $Ga(OH)_4^-$ caused the Ga titrations to level off prior to saturation of the protein (Harris & Pecoraro, 1981). It now seems likely that hydrolysis was also responsible for the low absorptivity in the Th-Tf system.

Molar absorptivities for a series of lanthanide-Tf complexes have been determined from the initial slopes of the titration curves, so that it is not necessary to make any assumptions about the ultimate degree of saturation of the protein. The

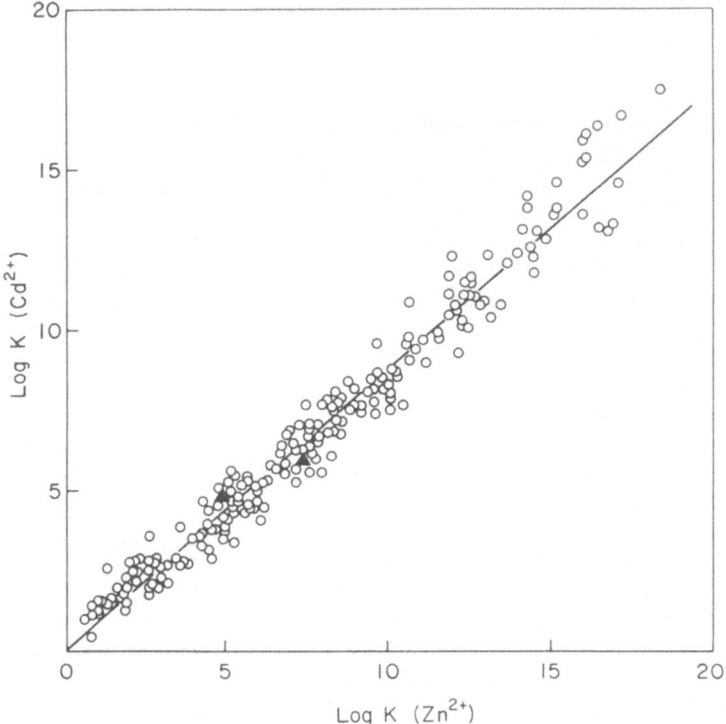

Figure 10. Linear free energy relationship for the complexation of Zn^{2+} and Cd^{2+}. Each data point consists of the stability constant of a given ligand with Zn^{2+} as the x-coordinate and the stability constant of the same ligand with Cd^{2+} as the y-coordinate. The data points corresponding to the log K_1^* and log K_2^* for human serum transferrin are shown as the closed triangles.

results are shown in Table IV. There is no obvious change in molar absorptivity until one reaches Pr^{3+}. Thus steric effects appear to be important only for the very largest trivalent lanthanides.

More subtle changes in binding affinity as a function of size are indicated by lanthanide LFER. A LFER for Nd^{3+} and Sm^{3+} based on 88 LMW complexes is shown in Figure 11. The equation corresponding to this plot is

$$\log K_{Sm} = (1.033 \pm 0.003) \log K_{Nd} + (0.013 \pm 0.18) \tag{15}$$

Because of the great chemical similarity among the lanthanides, the quality of this LFER is outstanding, with an uncertainty of only about 0.2 log units in the estimated log K values. The experimental Sm^{3+} and Nd^{3+} binding constants are given in Table III. Using the LFER and the Nd-Tf binding constants, one estimates Sm binding constants of log $K_1^* = 6.32 \pm 0.28$ and log $K_2^* = 5.23 \pm 0.52$. There is no significant difference between the observed and estimated log K_2^* values. However, the difference between the log K_1^* values is 0.8 log units, which

Table IV. Molar absorptivities of lanthanide transferrin complexes

Metal Ion	Ionic Radius (Å)	$\Delta\varepsilon_M$	n[a]
Lu^{3+}	0.861	19,900 ± 1200	1.98
Er^{3+}	0.890	20,800 ± 1000	1.90
Ho^{3+}	0.901	20,300 ± 1300	1.87
Tb^{3+}	0.923	20,600 ± 1600	1.82
Gd^{3+}	0.938	19,800 ± 1700	1.77
Sm^{3+}	0.958	21,000	1.57
Nd^{3+}	0.983	18,700	1.50
Pr^{3+}	0.990	12,300	1.71

[a] Average number of metal ions bound to transferrin at saturation.

is considered to be significant due to the high quality of the Nd-Sm LFER. It appears that the Tf complex of the larger Nd^{3+} ion is slightly destabilized relative to that of the smaller Sm^{3+} ion, but only for binding at the C-terminal site. Thus the thermodynamically more stable C-terminal site may be more susceptible to steric strain than the less stable N-terminal site.

Estimates of log K values for ferrous ion. One value of LFER is their ability to make predictions of the chemistry of species that are difficult to study experimentally. Ferrous-Tf falls in this category because of the oxidative instability of this complex (Kojima & Bates, 1981) and its poorly behaved electrochemistry (Harris et al., 1985). Ni^{2+} has been selected as a reference ion for Fe^{2+}, since it is a good match in terms of size and charge and exists in a single oxidation state (Harris, 1986c).

A LFER for Ni^{2+} and Fe^{2+} is shown in Figure 12. The scatter is somewhat greater than for the Zn-Cd LFER, and this is reflected in the larger standard deviations of the slope and intercept for this plot. The equation describing the plot in Figure 12 is

$$\log K_{Fe} = (0.761 \pm 0.018) \log K_{Ni} + (0.07 \pm 0.83) \tag{16}$$

This equation leads to estimates of $\log K_1^* = 3.2 \pm 0.8$ and $\log K_2^* = 2.5 \pm 0.9$ for ferrous transferrin. These constants are lower than the average value of 3.7 previously determined from kinetic studies (Kojima & Bates, 1981).

In principle, the ferrous-Tf binding constant can be determined from the ferric-Tf reduction potential and the ferric-Tf binding constants. This is difficult in practice because of the slow heterogeneous reduction kinetics of ferric-Tf at electrode surfaces and dissociation of the ferrous complex. However, it is possible to evaluate the consistency between electrochemical data and ferrous binding constants.

By using very long equilibration times, it was possible to determine that 50% of the iron from diferric transferrin was reduced at a potential of -400 mV vs. the normal hydrogen electrode (NHE) (Harris et al., 1985). This observed potential does not correspond to the formal reduction potential of ferric-Tf because the

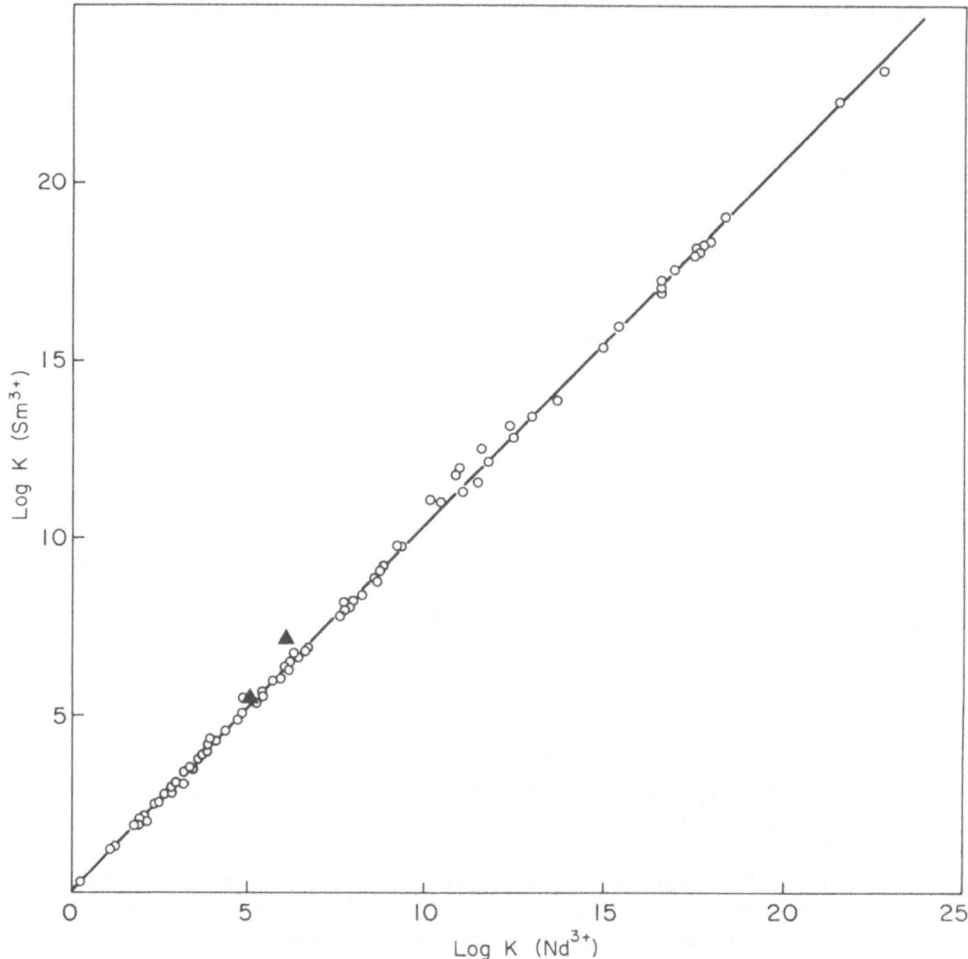

Figure 11. Linear free energy relationship for the complexation of Nd^{3+} and Sm^{3+}. Each data point consists of the stability constant of a given ligand with Nd^{3+} as the x-coordinate and the stability constant of the same ligand with Sm^{3+} as the y-coordinate. The data points corresponding to the log K_1^* and log K_2^* for human serum transferrin are shown as closed triangles.

reduced iron exists as an equilibrium mixture of ferrous-Tf and free ferrous ion. Since no ferrous-Tf binding constants were available, this study was not able to partition the reduced iron between ferrous-Tf and free ferrous ion. Using the average of the ferrous transferrin binding constants determined from the Ni-Fe LFER (Harris, 1986c), one can now calculate that 91% of the reduced iron would have existed as free ferrous ion. This would shift the observed potential for 50% reduction 62 mV positive of the formal reduction potential for ferric-Tf. This

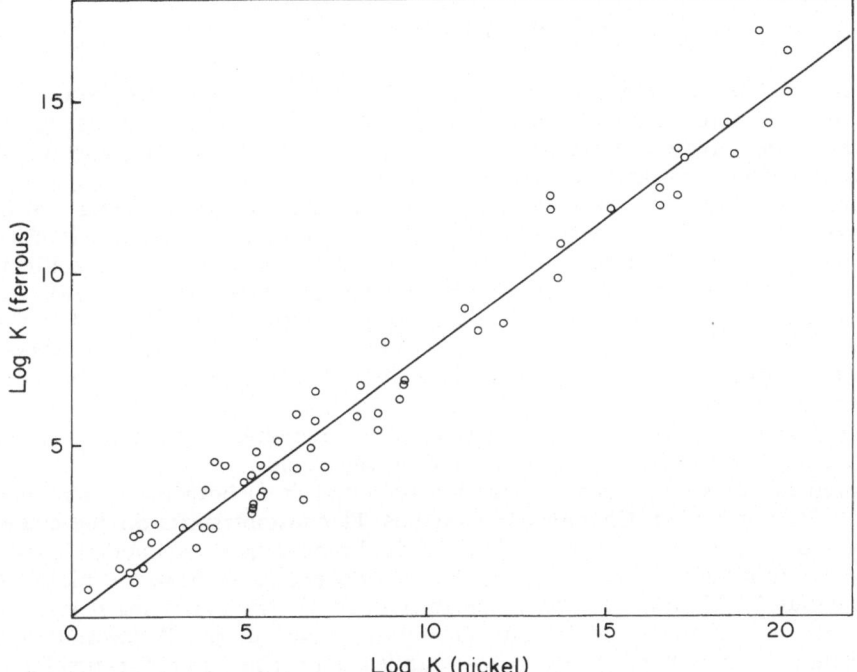

Figure 12. Linear free energy relationship for the complexation of Ni^{2+} and Fe^{2+}. Each data point consists of the stability constant of a given ligand with Ni^{2+} as the x-coordinate and the stability constant of the same ligand with Fe^{2+} as the y-coordinate.

gives an average reduction potential of about -460 mV for the two sites of diferric transferrin at 0.1 M ionic strength and 20 mM bicarbonate.

Kretchmar et al. (1988) have recently reported a spectroelectrochemical study of ferric-Tf in 2.0 M KCl and 0.14 mM (ambient) bicarbonate. Since ferrous transferrin should be completely dissociated under these conditions, the results are interpretted in terms of the chemical equilibrium

$$Fe^{3+}\text{-Tf} + e^- \rightleftharpoons Fe^{2+}(aq) + \text{apoTf} \qquad (17)$$

The observed potential for this reaction is -640 mV vs. NHE. After accounting for a junction potential and the ΔG for dissociation of ferrous-Tf, Kretchmar et al. (1988) obtain a formal reduction potential for ferric-Tf of -520 ± 80 mV. Given the difference in experimental conditions, the agreement between the two electrochemical studies is quite good.

One can also calculate a formal reduction potential directly from the Nernst equation and the binding constants for ferric and ferrous ion.

$$E_x = 0.770 - 0.059 \log \frac{K_x{}^{III}}{K_x{}^{II}} \tag{18}$$

where the x subscript denotes the N-terminal or C-terminal binding site, E is the formal reduction potential of ferric transferrin, 0.770 V is the formal reduction potential of the aquated ferric ion, and $K_x{}^{III}$ and $K_x{}^{II}$ are the site-specific binding constants for ferric and ferrous ion, respectively.

Using the site-selectivity factor of 2 calculated from the data on nickel monoferric transferrins (Harris, 1986c), one can estimate site-specific ferrous-transferrin binding constants of log K_C = 2.7 and log K_N = 3.0. Site specific ferric transferrin binding constants have been reported by Aisen et al. (1978), so that one can use eqn (18) to calculate potentials of -340 mV vs. NHE for the C-terminal site and -280 mV for the N-terminal site. The average of these two values is -310 mV, which is significantly higher than the values determined from electrochemical data.

The discrepancy between reported ferric-Tf reduction potentials can not be resolved merely by changing the estimated ferrous binding constant. This constant is required to calculate a formal reduction potential from both the electrochemical data and from eqn (18). Changing the ferrous-Tf constant shifts all the calculated reduction potentials in the same direction. Differences in experimental conditions may be an important factor. In particular, we do not know how the bicarbonate-Tf or ferrous-Tf binding constants change with ionic strength. Thus it may not be appropriate to use the same ferrous-Tf binding constant in all cases. It appears that further work will be required to establish a precise value for the ferric-Tf reduction potential.

Species distribution calculations. The role of transferrin in the serum transport of zinc has been a matter of some disagreement. Almost 100% of serum zinc is bound to proteins (Prasad & Oberleas, 1970). About 30 to 40% of serum zinc is tightly bound to α_2-macroglobulin and does not exchange with free serum zinc (Parisi & Vallee, 1970). There have been reports that transferrin binds some zinc in serum (Boyett & Sullivan, 1970; Evans & Winter, 1975) and that transferrin is more effective than albumin at accepting zinc from the intestinal basolateral plasma membrane (Evans, 1976). However, several recent studies have shown that albumin is the major carrier of labile serum zinc, and that less than 10% of serum zinc is bound to transferrin (Chesters & Will, 1981; Smith et al., 1978; Failla et al., 1982).

Both Chesters & Will (1981) and Charlwood (1979) have presented data that suggests that the Zn-Tf binding constant is too small to allow transferrin to bind significant amounts of zinc in serum. However, our data on Zn-Tf indicate stronger complexation of this metal, with a log $K_1{}^*$ of about 7.4 at serum bicarbonate levels (Harris, 1983). This is comparable to the reported Zn-albumin binding constant of log K = 7.0 (Giroux & Henkin, 1972).

To evaluate the competition between these two proteins, species distribution calculations were performed using a computer program (ECCLES) and a model for human serum developed by May et al. (1977). Our initial calculation included only LMW ligands. It differed from the model of May et al. (1977) in that the ternary complex of zinc, citrate, and cysteinate was not included in our calculations. This model resulted in the following distribution of LMW zinc: 41% Zn(cysteine)$_2$; 29%

Zn(cysteine)(histidine); 9% Zn(cysteine); and 6% Zn(histidine). The addition to this model of serum albumin with a single binding site and a log K of 7.0 resulted in 99% of the zinc binding to albumin. This was consistent with the accepted view that only ~2% of serum zinc exists as LWM complexes (Prasad & Oberleas, 1970; Failla et al., 1982)

If one adds the $Zn-HCO_3-Tf$ complex to the model, the results change dramatically. Assuming 30% saturation of Tf with iron, the calculations now indicate that 63% of the zinc is bound to transferrin, with only 37% bound to albumin. This clearly conflicts with the biological studies which have convincingly shown that at least 90% of the labile zinc is bound to albumin (Chesters & Will, 1981; Failla et al., 1982; Smith et al., 1978). Thus the speciation model appears to fail.

If one now includes the binary HCO_3-Tf complex as a species, the distribution shifts to 84% Zn-albumin and 15% Zn-Tf. If one includes anion complexes with sulfate and phosphate, one obtains the species distribution shown in Table V, which shows that Tf binds only 11% of the loosely bound zinc. Given the errors in this type of calculation, we doubt whether 11% can be considered significantly different from 0%.

One can easily rationalize the effects of the binary HCO_3-Tf complex on the zinc distribution. Computer programs such as ECCLES require that each species be described in terms of simple components. Thus the Zn-Tf complex is entered as the quarternary complex of zinc, apoTf, CO_3^{2-}, and H^+. The concentration of this complex would thus increase linearly with increasing bicarbonate concentration. However, the actual equilibria are shown in eqns (7) and (8). The bicarbonate dependence of the zinc binding constants shows that the effective binding ability depends not on the actual free bicarbonate concentration, but on the degree of saturation of apoTf to form the binary HCO_3-Tf species. By including the binary species in the calculation, the effective thermodynamic driving force for the binding of zinc is no longer the overall stability constant for the zinc complex, but rather the net difference between the stability constant for zinc-Tf and the stability constant for HCO_3-Tf.

There is also a slight reduction in the calculated concentration of Zn-Tf due to phosphate and sulfate, even though these do not form a reactive intermediate such as the HCO_3-Tf complex. One can view these anions as being in direct competition with the zinc. By occupying almost 30% of the free transferrin binding sites, they reduce the effective concentration of sites available for binding of zinc, and thus decrease the calculated concentration of Zn-Tf in serum.

One should not conclude that bicarbonate destabilizes the Zn-Tf complex. Quite the contrary is true. The zinc distribution calculations have been repeated for models in which the total carbonate concentration has been decreased from 25 mM to 10 mM, 1 mM, and 0.2 mM. The concentrations of sulfate and phosphate have been reduced in proportion to the carbonate concentration. The results are shown in Table VI. Going from 25 mM to 10 mM total carbonate has virtually no effect on the calculated zinc distribution. This is because the anion concentrations are still high enough to bind 80% of the total available transferrin binding sites. The fraction of transferrin that exists as the reactive HCO_3-Tf species is still determined primarily by competition among the anions, and thus only changes from 60% to 54%.

Table V. Distribution of zinc and transferrin species in a serum model

Zinc Distribution		Transferrin Distribution	
	(%)		(%)
Zn–Albumin	88	HCO_3-Tf	60
Zn–Tf	11	PO_4-Tf	22
$Zn(cys)_2$	0.5	apoTf	8.6
Zn(cys)(his)	0.3	SO_4-Tf	7.4
Zn(cys)	0.1	Zn-HCO_3-Tf	2.2
Zn(his)	0.1		

Table VI. Distribution of zinc and transferrin as a function of anion concentration

	% of Total Zinc		% of Total Tf				
$[CO_3]_{tot}$ [a]	Zn-Albumin	Zn-Tf	Zn-Tf	HCO_3-Tf	PO_4-Tf	SO_4-Tf	apoTf
24.5 mM	88	11	2.2	60	22	7.4	8.6
10 mM[b]	89	10	2.0	54	19	6.5	19
1 mM[b]	95	4.1	0.8	20	6.0	2.2	71
0.2 mM[b]	98	1.1	0.2	5.3	1.5	0.6	92

[a] Total concentration of free carbonate. Calculation also includes 3.81×10^{-4} M total phosphate and 2.11×10^{-4} M total sulfate.
[b] Total phosphate and sulfate reduced by same factor as total carbonate.

Going from 10 mM to 1 mM total carbonate causes a substantial dissociation of the rather weak HCO_3-Tf complex, which now only accounts for 20% of total transferrin. This decrease in the reactive species for formation of the zinc complex leads directly to a decreased zinc binding affinity. Thus the distribution of zinc changes to 95% bound to albumin and only 4% bound to transferrin.

Further dilution to 0.2 mM carbonate, which approximates an air-saturated pH 7.4 buffer, results in almost complete dissociation of all transferrin-anion complexes. The reactive bicarbonate complex now represents only 5% of total transferrin. Under these conditions, transferrin is essentially incapable of competing with albumin and binds only 1% of the zinc.

These calculations are interesting because they mimic procedures that are routinely used to prepare serum samples for analysis, i.e., washing samples in ultrafiltration cells, dialysis, and gel chromatography. In all cases the proteins are maintained at relatively high concentrations, while the LMW components such as bicarbonate, sulfate, and phosphate are replaced by a buffer. We would suggest that workers measuring the distribution of metal ions among serum proteins might wish to consider the ionic composition of their buffers. If transferrin is a suspected transport agent, it appears to be quite important that at least the bicarbonate level be maintained at several mM.

We would also point out the preliminary nature of these calculations. One factor which has not been assessed is the impact of relatively high concentrations of NaCl on the anion binding. Chloride itself does not generate the difference uv spectrum characteristic of the oxo-anions like bicarbonate and phosphate. However, its effect on the magnitude of the bicarbonate-Tf binding constants has not been evaluated.

References

Aisen, P., & Listowsky, I. (1980) *Ann. Rev. Biochem.* 49, 357-393.

Aisen, P., Leibman, A., & Zweier, J. (1978) *J. Biol. Chem.* 253, 1930-1937.

Anderson, B. F., Baker, H. M., Dodson, E. J., Norris, G. E., Rumball, S. V., Waters, J. M., & Baker, E. N. (1987) *Proc. Natl. Acad. Sci.* (USA) 84, 1769-1773.

Bailey, S., Evans, R. W., Garratt, R. C., Gorinsky, B., Hasnain, S., Horsburgh, C., Jhoti, H., Lindley, P. F., Mydin, A., Sarra, R., & Watson, J. L. (1988) *Biochemistry* 27, 5804-5812.

Baldwin, D. A., & de Sousa, D. M. R. (1981) *Biochem. Biophys. Res. Commun.* 99, 1101-1107.

Bates, G. W., Graybill G., & Chidambraram, M. V. (1987) in *Control of Animal Cell Proliferation* (Boynton, A. L., & Leffert, H. L., Eds.) vol II, pp 153-202, Academic Press, New York.

Boocock, G., & Popplewell, D. S. (1965) *Nature* (London) 208, 282-283.

Boyett, J. D., & Sullivan, J. F. (1970) *Metabolism* 19, 148-157.

Charlwood, P. A. (1979) *Biochim. Biophys. Acta* 581, 260-265.

Chasteen, N. D. (1983) *Adv. Inorg. Biochem.* 5, 201-233.

Chasteen, N. D., & Williams, J. (1981) *Biochem. J.* 193, 717-727.

Chesters, J. K., & Will, M. (1981) *Br. J. Nutr.* 46, 111-118.

Cochran, M., Coates, J., & Neoh, S. (1984) *FEBS* 176, 129-132.

Cowart, R. E., Kojima, N., & Bates, G. W. (1982) *J. Biol. Chem.* 257, 7560-7565.

Cowart, R. E., Swope, S., Loh, T. T., Chasteen, N. D., & Bates, G. (1986) *J. Biol. Chem.* 261, 4607-4614.

Durbin, P. W. (1975) *Health Physics* 29, 495-510.

Evans, G. W. (1976) *Proc. Soc. Exp. Biol. Med.* 151, 775-778.

Evans G. W., & Winter T. W. (1975) *Biochem. Biophys. Res. Commun.* 66, 1218-1224.

Evans, R. W., & Williams, J. (1978) *Biochem. J.* 173, 543-552.

Failla, M. L., van de Veerdonk, M., Morgan, W. T., & Smith, J. C. (1982) *J. Lab. Clin. Med.* 100, 943-952.

Folajtar, D. A., & Chasteen, N. D. (1982) *J. Amer. Chem. Soc.* 104, 10314-10316.

Froncisz, W., & Aisen, P. (1982) *Biochem. Biophys. Acta* 700, 55-58.

Gelb, M. H., & Harris, D. C. (1980) *Arch. Biochem. Biophys.* 200, 93-98.

Giroux, E. L., & Henkin, R. I. (1972) *Biochim. Biophys. Acta* 273, 64-72.

Gorinsky, B., Horsburgh, C., Lindley, P. F., Moss, D. S., Parker, M.,, & Watson, J. L. (1979) *Nature* 281, 157-158.

Hancock, R. D., Finkelstein, N. P., & Evers, A. (1974) *J. Inorg. Nucl. Chem.* 36, 2539-2543.

Harris, D. C., & Gelb, M. H. (1980) *Biochim. Biophys. Acta* 623, 1-9.

Harris, D. C., Rinehart, A. L., Herald, D., Schwartz, R. W., Burke, F. P., & Salvador, A. P. (1985) *Biochim. Biophys. Acta* 838, 295-301.

Harris, W. R. (1983) *Biochemistry* 22, 3920-3926.

Harris, W. R. (1985) *Biochemistry* 24, 7412-7418.

Harris, W. R. (1986a) *Biochemistry* 25, 803-808.

Harris, W. R. (1986b) *Inorg. Chem.* 25, 2041-2045.

Harris, W. R. (1986c) *J. Inorg. Biochem.* 27, 41-52.

Harris, W. R., & Pecoraro, V. L. (1983) *Biochemistry* 22, 292-299.

Harris, W. R., & Madsen, L. J. (1988) *Biochemistry* 27, 284-288.

Harris, W. R., Carrano, C. J. Pecoraro, V. L., & Raymond, K. N. (1981) *J. Amer. Chem. Soc.* 103, 2231-2237.

Irving, H., & Rossotti, H. (1956) *Acta Chem. Scand.* 10, 72-93.

Kilar, F., & Simon, I. (1985) *Biophys. J.* 48, 799-802.

Koenig, S. H., & Schillinger, W. E. (1969) *J. Biol. Chem.* 244, 6520-6526.

Kojima, N., & Bates, G. W. (1981) *J. Biol. Chem.* 256, 12034-12039.

Kretchmar, S. A., Reyes, Z. E., & Raymond, K. N. (1988) *Biochim. Biophys. Acta* in press.

Krysteva, M. A., Mazurier, J., & Spik, G. (1976) *Biochim. Biophys. Acta* 453, 484-493.

Lineback-Zins, J., & Brew, K. (1980) *J. Biol. Chem.* 255, 708-713.

Luk, C. K. (1971) *Biochemistry* 10, 2830-2843.

MacGillivray, R. T. A., Mendez, E., Sinha, S. K., Sutton, M. R., Linebeck-Zins, J., & Brew, K. (1982) *Proc. Natl. Acad. Sci.* (USA) 79, 2504-2508.

Makey, D. G., & Seal, U. S. (1976) *Biochim. Biophys. Acta* 870, 250-256.

Marsicano, F., & Hancock, R. D. (1978) *J. Chem. Soc. Dalton* 228-233.

Martin, A. W., Huebers, E., Huebers, H., Webb, J., & Finch, C. A. (1984) *Blood* 64, 1047-1052.

Martin, R. B. (1986) *Clin. Chem.* 32, 1797-1806.

May, P. M., Linder, P. W., & Williams, D. R. (1977) *J. Chem. Soc. Dalton* 588-595.

Misono, M., & Saito, Y. (1970) *Bull. Chem. Soc. Jpn.* 43, 3680-3684.

O'Hara, P., Yeh, S. M., Meares, C. F., & Bersohn, R. (1981) *Biochemistry* 20, 4704-4708.

Parisi, A. F., & Vallee, B. L. (1970) *Biochemistry* 9, 2421-2426.

Pecoraro, V. L., Harris, W. R., Carrano, C. J., & Raymond, K. N. (1981) *Biochemistry* 20, 7033-7039.

Prasad, A. S., & Oberleas, D. (1970) *J. Lab. Clin. Med.* 76, 416-425.

Roberts, J. E., Brown, T. G., Hoffman, B. M., & Aisen, P. (1983) *Biochim. Biophys. Acta* 747, 49-54.

Rosseneu-Motreff, M. Y., Soetewey, F., Lamote, R., & Peeters, H. (1971) *Biopolymers* 10, 1039-1048.

Scheider, D. J., Roe, A. L., Mayer, R. J., & Que, L. (1984) *J. Biol. Chem.* 259, 9699-9703.

Smith, K. T., Failla, M. L., & Cousins, R. J. (1978) *Biochem. J.* 184, 623-633.

Stevens, W., Breunger, F. W., & Stover, B. J. (1968) *Radiat. Res.* 33, 490-500.

Tan, A. T., & Woodworth, R. C. (1969) *Biochemistry* 8, 3313-3316.

Woodworth, R. C. (1986) *J. Inorg. Biochem.* 256, 12034-12039.

Yeh, S. M., & Meares, C. F. (1980) *Biochemistry* 19, 5057-5062.

Zak, O., Leibman, A., & Aisen, P. (1983) *Biochim. Biophys. Acta* 742, 490-495.

Zak, O., & Aisen, P. (1988) *Biochemistry* 27, 1075-1080.

Zweier, J., & Aisen, P. (1977) *J. Biol. Chem.* 252, 6090-6096.

Zweier, J., Peisach, J., & Mims, W. B. (1982) *J. Biol. Chem.* 257, 10314-10316.

Zweier, J., Aisen, P., Peisach, J., & Mims, W. B. (1979) *J. Biol. Chem.* 254, 3512-3515.

Section II

Dietary Influences on Mineral Uptake

7

Protein Digestion and the Absorption of Mineral Elements

Raul A. Wapnir

Our understanding of the chemical processes leading to the digestion and absorption of proteins has undergone significant changes in the last century. Although the existence of gastric and pancreatic "ferments" predates any published notions of the form in which protein was assimilated, the identification of peptones as soluble breakdown products of proteins, produced as a result of the action of proteases, made those poorly defined products candidate substrates for absorption.

Soon after the turn of the century, the work of Cohnheim, Van Slyke and other pioneering physiologists established the concept that amino acids appearing in the circulation were the end products of protein ingestion and, therefore, amino acids themselves were the form in which proteins were absorbed (Van Slike & Meyer, 1912; Matthews, 1977). This concept appears to have been reached more out of consensus than out of experimentation. However, the site of ultimate hydrolysis of small peptides remained obscure, and whether it occurred as a result of the action of soluble peptidases present in the lumen, or of brush border enzymes remained unclear. If the final hydrolytic step occurred in the enterocyte, the possibility remained for fragments larger than single amino acids, i.e., di-, tri- or polypeptides, to be absorbed as such by the intestinal mucosa. The latter concept was actually built on by the work of Newey & Smith (1962), Nixon & Mawer (1970), Adibi (1971), Burston et al., (1977), Silk (1973), and other investigators (Matthews, 1977).

An understanding of the absorption of mineral elements has generally lagged behind that of major dietary components. The exceptions, to a certain extent, are calcium and iron, which by virtue of their quantitative importance in body composition and in dietary requirements have attracted the interest of researchers for almost as long as proteins and other macronutrients. With calcium, the intimate relationship between its intestinal absorption and the hormonal form of vitamin D is an unique feature which stands this element aside from all other minerals. The singular properties of calcium as an intracellular messenger and its involvement in hormonal regulation, as well as its role as a major constitutive component of the body have been extensively reviewed and will not be dealt with here (DeLuca &

Schones, 1976; Schuette & Linkswiler, 1984). Iron, as a key constituent of the heme molecule, has similar critical importance (Hallberg, 1984; Lynch, 1984). Both elements are among those whose daily requirements are most often not met in normal diets. The efficacy of their intestinal absorption plays a fundamental role in the determination of the nutritional requirements of man. Dietary, physiological and pathological alterations can have severe effects on their bioavailability, as well as on the availability of all other essential elements.

How, where and why do protein and mineral nutrition intersect? The answers are complex and vary from one element to the other. In general terms, some reasons are presented in the following non-exhaustive list:

[1] Protein nutritional status may affect the integrity of the intestinal mucosa and, hence, the synthesis of hydrolytic enzymes, absorption mediators and fluid exchanges between the lumen and the enterocyte.

[2] Proteins may have constitutive trace elements which can become a key portion of the dietary daily intake. Dietary protein content may be reflected in a proportional accumulation of mineral elements in tissues, which is a good index of nutritional sufficiency. In contrast, specific element deficiencies can ensue from inadequate protein sources.

[3] Digestion fragments of proteins may either bind and make unavailable certain essential metals, or, conversely, these hydrolytic breakdown products can complex with some transition elements and render them more bioavailable.

[4] Intestinal membrane turnover products of proteinaceous nature could have the same effects as those attributed to dietary proteins or their degradation products.

[5] A greater renal excretion of amino acids may be linked to the level of protein intake and, therefore, to losses of essential minerals resulting in possible deficiency states.

This review will be limited to a few mineral elements of quantitative major importance for man and animals, and will attempt to support the thesis of the importance of the protein-mineral linkage. In the following sections we will provide examples which may justify the postulates listed above as they apply to some mineral elements particularly essential in human nutrition.

Calcium and Magnesium

These two elements are required in far larger dietary amounts than other divalent minerals of nutritional significance. Due to their chemical characteristics they are less prone to be influenced by protein intake. However, in spite of chemical similarities, magnesium, the element with the lower atomic weight and ionic radius, is a cofactor for many enzymes of intermediary metabolism (Garfinkel & Garfinkel, 1985), and can be mobilized through cell membranes with a greater ease than calcium, which in most cases goes through specialized channels which are subject to metabolic and pharmacologic controls (Birge & Avioli, 1986).

While magnesium is widely distributed in foods of plant and animal origin, good calcium sources are more restricted. Dairy products are rich in calcium and are primary protein sources as well. Nevertheless, an additional factor in calcium absorption is related to the phosphorus content of diets and its ratio to calcium. Much of the available phosphorus is of organic origin and associated with nitrogen sources. Phosphorus plays an important role in the maintenance of calcium balance. The second key factor in calcium absorption is the active form of vitamin D, 1,25-dihydroxy-cholecalciferol, which is synthesized in the kidney and acts as a hormone on the small intestine (DeLuca & Schones, 1976), regulating the activity of a calcium-binding protein present in the mucosal brush border (Alpers et al., 1972), following the attachment of the hormone to a cytosolic receptor in the enterocyte.

There is no evidence that the level of dietary protein intake may have an effect on the mucosal calcium-binding receptor. However, some protein breakdown products may facilitate or inhibit the uptake of calcium. This seems to be the case with basic amino acids, such as arginine or lysine, which have been shown to produce a marked enhancement in calcium absorption. This effect only plays a role with the non-mediated, bulk transport of the element since there were no differences between the D- and the L- stereoisomers of lysine. Solubility alone does not necessarily mandate the effectiveness of an amino acid as an enhancer of calcium absorption, since very soluble chelates, i.e. those with glycine, were not particularly effective. The hypothesis that single basic amino acids could neutralize organic acids, which may otherwise impair calcium absorption, has not been confirmed (Irving, 1973). The degree to which individual amino acids stimulate net water absorption in the small intestine may also play a role in the potential enhancement of calcium uptake by the gut. This property of individual amino acids may be linked to the identity of the specific mechanisms of amino acid transport, in particular, whether they are sodium-dependent or not (Johnstone, 1979). This situation stands in contrast with more convincing studies which documented the calcium absorption enhancing effects of lactose and fat, at least in milk and infant formulae (Allen, 1982).

We have tested experimentally the effect of a protein hydrolysate on the absorption of magnesium and calcium by rat jejunum (Table I). The results showed that the presence in the intestinal lumen of amino acids and oligopeptides with a mean molecular weight of 180 causes an increase in the absorption of both elements. The correlation between concentration of protein hydrolysate and mineral absorption is very significant for calcium, and to a lesser extent for magnesium. The enhancement of net water absorption is much less sensitive to the presence of protein breakdown products. The data also indicate that solvent drag plays only a limited role in the progressively greater calcium absorption associated with additional protein hydrolysate.

A similar effect to the one described with protein hydrolysate was demonstrated earlier, for magnesium, when variable amounts of protein (casein) were added to the diet of rats (Toothill, 1963). However, a doubling of the protein level only improved magnesium retention by about 50% (Table II). The combined amount of calcium and phosphorus in the diet of experimental animals has been shown to inversely correlate with the total amount of magnesium absorbed, and with the proportion of this element that is retained, even at constant levels of magnesium in the diet (Table III).

Table I. Absorption of magnesium, calcium and water fluxes in rat jejunum in the presence of a protein hydrolysate

Protein Hydrolysate (%)	Magnesium Absorption (nmol/min x cm)	Calcium Absorption (nmol/min x cm)	Net Water Absorption (μL/min x cm)
0.5	-0.36 ± 0.79	0.14 ± 0.12	1.29 ± 0.12
1.0	2.42 ± 1.24	0.40 ± 0.23	1.42 ± 0.08
2.0	2.98 ± 0.74	1.44 ± 0.14	1.50 ± 0.10
r versus Prot. Hydr.	0.426[a]	0.769[b]	0.290
r versus Net Water	0.425[a]	0.768[b]	—

N = 8 rats/group.
[a] $P < 0.05$.
[b] $P < 0.001$.

Table II. Effect of protein dietary content on magnesium absorption

Casein content (%)	Weight gain (g)	Mg intake (mg)	Mg retention (mg)	(%)
8	26.7	30.4	9.6	31.6
16	44.3	35.1	13.2	37.6

Adapted from Toothill, 1963.

Table III. Magnesium absorption: effect of calcium and phosphorus content

Ca in diet (g/kg)	P in diet (g/kg)	Ca + P (g/kg)	Mg intake (mg/day)	Mg absorption (mg)	(%)
3.35	3.92	7.27	25.8	17.2	66.7
3.23	7.91	11.14	26.5	12.4	46.8
6.82	3.89	10.71	26.9	11.6	43.1
6.52	7.84	14.36	24.5	7.0	28.6

r (Ca + P versus Mg absorption) = -0.990, $P < 0.01$.
Adapted from Toothill, 1963.

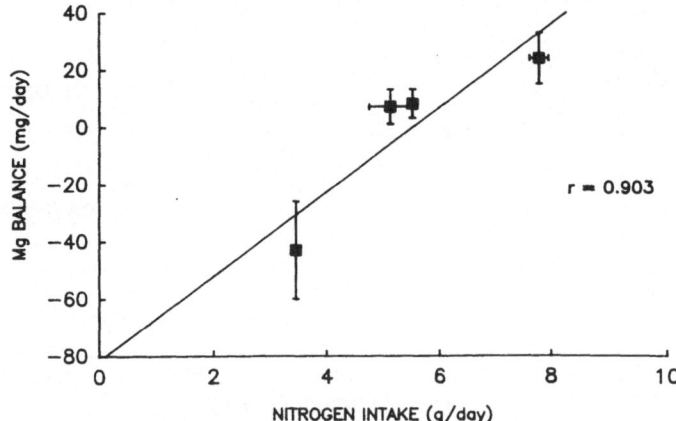

Figure 1. Correlation between mean daily nitrogen intake and magnesium utilization. Regression line between mean daily nitrogen intake, from protein, and magnesium balance in adult women who participated in a study with four types of diets. The correlation between both parameters was very significant: r = 0.903, P < 0.001, 16 d.f. (Adapted from Hunt & Schofield, 1969).

In human volunteers, when nitrogen intake and magnesium balance were considered, Hunt and Schofield (1969) demonstrated a direct correlation between both parameters. A restricted protein diet resulted in a negative magnesium balance. An intake greater than 5 g of nitrogen per day was necessary to achieve positive magnesium balance (Figure 1).

It has been shown repeatedly that increased losses of calcium occur when protein consumption is high (Johnson et al., 1970; Walker & Linkswiler, 1972; Margen et al., 1974; Allen et al., 1979a,b). It is now quite clear that the hypercalciuria is related to elevated urinary amino acid excretion and competition at the tubular resorption level. This renal amino acid effect was further demonstrated in patients receiving total parenteral nutrition. When amino acid infusion rates were boosted from 1 to 2 mg/kg per day, calcium excretion concomitantly increased from 287 to 455 mg per day (Bengoa et al., 1983).

In contrast to what was shown in experimental perfusions with amino acids (Table I), the negative effect of excess dietary protein on calcium balance does not seem to affect the intestinal absorptive stage. Nearly fifty years ago, McCance et al. (1942) presented data that showed a positive correlation between protein intake and calcium absorption, but not with magnesium absorption (Figure 2). Later on, Johnson et al. (1970) showed that, provided calcium and phosphorus were maintained at a fixed, elevated level (1,400 mg/day), a mean protein intake increase of 63 g/day, over a basal period at 48 g/day, did not result in changes in the absorption rate of calcium, although urinary excretion was proportionately increased. In other studies where nitrogen ingestion was the independent variable, calcium balance was negatively affected by an increase in nitrogen intake. In a group of middle age women ingesting self-selected diets, a 50% increment in dietary protein above the group mean resulted in a negative shift of 32 mg/day in mature women

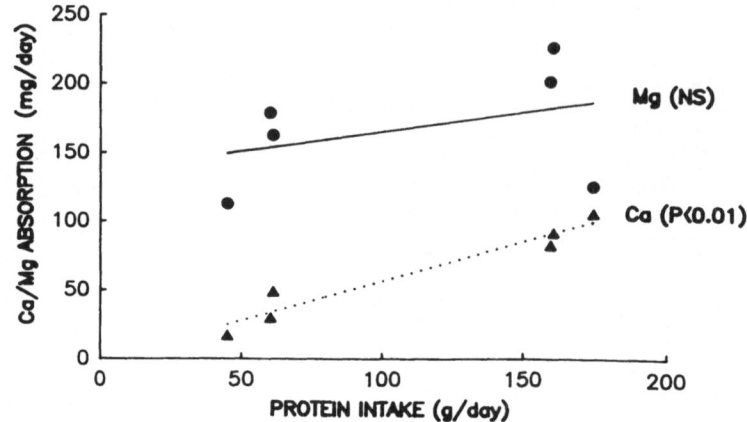

Figure 2. Correlation between protein intake and calcium and magnesium absorption. Scatter plot of magnesium and calcium absorption as a function of protein intake in five adults. The correlation was significant for calcium, but not for magnesium (Adapted from McCance et al., 1942).

who might be at risk for osteoporosis (Heaney & Recker, 1982). In contrast, evaluations of calcium and nitrogen balances in diets without and with additional meat intake, conducted by Spencer et al. (1978; 1983), lead to the conclusion that a greater intake of meat protein did not affect calcium balance or urinary losses, presumably due to the concurrent increase of phosphorus intake, which would effectively bind calcium. Thus, in a recent review, Spencer et al. (1988) severely criticized the notion that postmenopausal women and elderly persons, in general, should limit their protein intake in order to prevent calcium losses.

The hormonal component of calciuria was shown when changes in insulin and parathyroid hormone (PTH) levels were correlated with urinary calcium following the ingestions of meals with a low (15 g) or a high (45 g) protein content. An expected higher insulin peak occurred after high protein ingestion, and over a 31/2 h observation period there was a significant positive correlation between changes in percent calcium excretion and levels of serum insulin. The simultaneous changes of PTH were not affected by the amount of protein ingested (Allen et al., 1981).

Intestinal malabsorption of calcium can also occur as a consequence of protein losses, as in Crohn's disease, where enteric protein loss has been shown to be associated with calcium excretion. This finding could explain a specific nutritional handicap of these patients (Krawitt et al., 1976).

Some manifestations of renal impairment may lead to a negative calcium and magnesium balance. This was demonstrated in rats made diabetic with streptozotocin, which presented, in addition to glycosuria, significant calciuria and magnesuria (Fort et al., 1977). It is not clear whether concomitant aminoaciduria occurs in these animals, and if it plays a role in exacerbating mineral losses, or if this effect is purely osmotic.

Iron

This element and its absorption mechanisms have probably been more extensively studied than those of any other mineral of nutritional significance (Lynch, 1984). Hemoglobin and myoglobin account for 75% of the total iron adult human body content of 2.2-3.8 g (Hallberg, 1984; Dallman, 1986). Other heme and nonheme proteins play vital roles in energy, nucleic acid and amino acid metabolism. Dietary sources also correspond to heme and nonheme types. Heme-containing nutrients offer iron in the ferrous (divalent) oxidation state, in which it is more easily absorbed than in the ferric (trivalent) form. Stomach acidity contributes to the extraction of iron from foodstuffs and to the maintenance of the metal in the ferrous oxidation level. Iron in heme is taken up by the intestinal mucosa by an endocytotic process and, once in the enterocyte, it is incorporated into the intracellular pool which follows a common transport path with other sources of iron. Nonheme iron binds to specific high-affinity receptors in the small intestine and the translocation process occurs by an energy-dependent, mediated mechanism. Hemoglobin levels, however, cannot be taken as the only dependent variable in experimental nutritional studies. Serum ferritin, transferrin saturation and erythrocyte protoporphyrin have been postulated as useful indicators of iron sufficiency (Fairweather-Tait, 1987). Growth and total body iron are also among the better indicators of iron repletion.

Striated muscle dietary sources (meat) are both high-protein and high iron content nutrients. An inverse relationship between meat consumption and iron deficiency has been exhaustively proven (Layrisse et al., 1968; Takkunen & Seppanen, 1975; Bjorn-Rasmussen & Hallberg, 1979), although the total contribution of heme iron to the Western diet is much less than that of nonheme iron. The high bioavailability of iron from high protein content products of animal origin explains the disproportionate impact of this nutritional group in the maintenance of iron sufficiency. In normal, American style diets, heme iron is estimated to provide one third of adult requirements. However, chemically isolated hemoglobin is not as well absorbed (Bothwell et al., 1979). When ferritin, another high molecular weight source of iron was tested, the proportion absorbed sharply increased when veal was added (Table IV). In these studies, veal alone provided 13.2% bioavailable iron; therefore, the enhancement of iron absorption could only be attributed to hydrolytic products liberated from veal.

In experiments with rats, iron absorbability was shown to be directly proportional to casein concentration in the diet, independent of changes in carbohydrate and fat concentration (Conrad et al., 1967). A similar stimulation of iron absorption was reported during the *in vitro* uptake of iron in the presence of various potential chelators. While the uptake from ferrous sulfate produced a retention of 82 ppm, a crude protein chelate of vegetable origin raised it to 130 ppm and a fish meal preparation further enhanced uptake to 298 ppm (Ashmead et al., 1985).

All the preceding findings agree with the studies of Rao & Prabhavathi (1978), who postulated that iron bioavailability was related to the amount of iron that at pH 7.5 existed as freely diffusible ferrous ion, which, if from nonheme iron sources, was enhanced by the addition of meat extract and ascorbic acid. The addition of L-methionine as a complement to casein appears to be a key factor, beyond the simple protein concentration (Miller, 1983). Free amino acids have been postulated to be responsible for the enhancement of iron absorption, which

Table IV. Interaction of various foods with labeled ferritin and other iron salts on iron absorption

Ferritin +	Iron absorption from:		
	^{59}Fe-ferritin (%)	Other foods [55]Fe (%)	Fe 59:55
Soybean	0.5 ± 0.2	2.6 ± 0.9	0.19
Soybean + carrier liver	1.7 ± 0.7	5.0 ± 2.2	0.34
Ferric chloride	2.3 ± 0.5	11.7 ± 2.2	0.20
Ferric chloride + carrier liver	3.6 ± 0.6	19.7 ± 3.3	0.18
Veal muscle	11.7 ± 3.0	22.0 ± 2.1	0.53
Veal muscle (^{59}Fe in food)	6.6 ± 0.5	14.6 ± 1.8	0.45
Veal muscle (^{59}Fe in liquid)	11.1 ± 2.4	18.5 ± 1.9	0.60

Adapted from Layrisse et al. 1975.

adds a synergistic effect to the bioavailability of iron from grains and vegetables (Kroe et al., 1963; Martinez-Torres & Layrisse, 1970; Martinez-Torres et al., 1981). In spite of the conceptual attractiveness of the role of low molecular weight protein breakdown products, since egg albumin does not produce an enhancement of iron absorption capacity, the question is not totally answered (Hallberg, 1981). In addition, if phosphoproteins, which are present in significant amounts in eggs, are not excluded, the strong binding they exhibit for iron may reduce the bioavailability of the metal, even if during digestion an equivalent amount of low molecular weight oligopeptides and amino acids were generated (Callender et al., 1970; Monsen & Cook, 1979). A similar situation may exist in relation to soy protein isolates, resulting in a decreased iron absorption in man (Cook et al., 1981).

Infants exclusively fed breast milk fail to develop anemia, at least in the first six months of life, in spite of low iron intake levels (Saarinen, 1978). The well demonstrated high bioavailability of breast milk iron has been proposed to be due to the presence of certain free amino acids, such as cysteine and taurine, which are present in comparatively high concentrations in human breast milk (McMillan et al., 1976). However, additional intrinsic constituents of mammary gland secretions, including fat and various other low molecular weight fractions, could be among the yet not well characterized enhancers of iron absorption (Fransson & Lönnerdal, 1980). As will be described later, a similar phenomenon has been associated with zinc bioavailability.

Zinc

The interrelationships between zinc absorption, protein and amino acids are probably those that have been most intensively studied. The knowledge that many metalloproteins have one or more zinc atoms as constitutive elements of these molecules, and that zinc easily binds to serum proteins and amino acids *in vitro* and *in vivo* was the starting point for investigating the possible role of protein hydrolysis products on the luminal phase of zinc absorption (Prasad & Oberleas, 1970; Hallman et al., 1971; Giroux & Henkin, 1972; Henkin, 1974).

The association between protein and zinc nutrition has been demonstrated under many conditions. Certain tissues, such as testis, can accumulate zinc, even under conditions of limited protein intake (Oberleas & Prasad, 1969). Bone achieves a less efficient zinc storage and zinc requirements become more apparent (Figure 3). Animal protein sources provide a much greater zinc bioavailability than plant sources, and growth rates of the animals correlate well with mineral uptake only with feedings of proteins of animal origin (O'Dell et al., 1972). In addition, sampling of baby formulae in frequent use shows evidence of a significant correlation between protein and zinc content (Widdowson et al., 1974).

A group of intracellular proteins, first described by Kagi & Vallee (1960) in kidney and liver, and generically denominated metallothioneins (MT), exhibit great affinity for zinc and other divalent transition metals and have attracted the efforts of numerous investigators. MT unquestionably play a major regulatory role in the storage, homeostasis and release into the body of some essential trace elements, in particular zinc and copper, as well as in the handling of toxic metals, such as cadmium and mercury, among others (Richards & Cousins, 1976; Cousins, 1985; Hamer, 1986; Dunn et al., 1987).

Two components are considered to participate in the luminal phase of zinc absorption. One of these has been proposed to be membrane binding receptors that may be located either at the brush border or the basolateral membrane (Hahn & Evans, 1973; Schricker & Forbes, 1978). The molecular identity of these receptors has not yet been clarified. The processes by which the tightly bound zinc-MT in the enterocyte is delivered to membrane proteins and to extracellular albumin also need to be better defined.

The second component in the initial phase of intestinal zinc transport are the putative luminal factors which may allow or enhance zinc absorption. These potential transport vehicles have received possibly more attention than membrane receptors. This question arose from the initial demonstration that breast milk, but not cow's milk, was an effective therapy for acrodermatitis enteropathica. In fact, infants fed exclusively breast milk showed, as a group, higher plasma zinc levels than comparable infants fed a zinc-supplemented formula (Hambidge et al., 1979). Acrodermatitis enteropathica is an autosomal, recessively inherited disease characterized by an impairment in zinc absorption. It is generally manifested by skin lesions, diarrhea and hair loss, conditions which are consistent with a severe zinc deficiency state (Moynahan, 1974). In view of the successful treatment of acrodermatitis enteropathica by zinc and by agents capable of indirectly improving zinc absorption, questions remain about the nature of the luminal or dietary factors which may transform ingested zinc into a more bioavailable form.

One of the postulated low molecular weight (LMW) absorptive enhancers, picolinic acid, a minor metabolite of tryptophan, was suggested to be present in

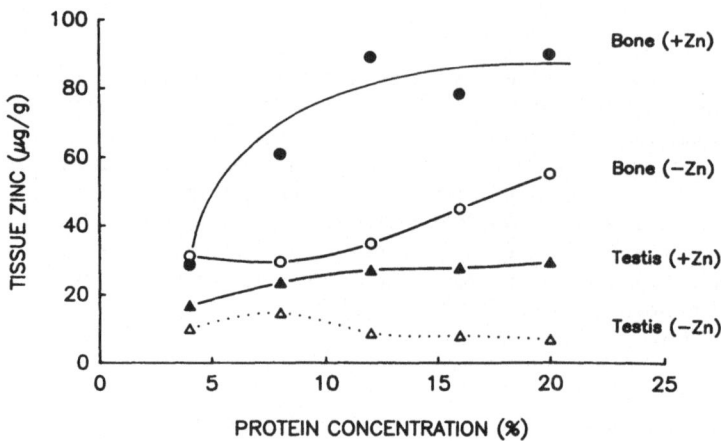

Figure 3. Tissue zinc levels as a function of dietary protein. Accumulation of zinc in tissues of rats fed variable concentrations of protein, without (–) or with (+) a zinc supplement (55 mg/kg). For each organ, the differences in zinc levels between the supplemented and the nonsupplemented animals were significant at the $P<0.005$ level (Adapted from Oberleas & Prasad, 1969).

pancreatic juice and in human breast milk, and to participate in the absorptive process for zinc (Evans, 1980; Evans & Johnson, 1980). Subsequently, Krieger et al. (1984) used picolinic acid in the treatment of acrodermatitis enteropathica. The results in alleviating the patients' symptomatology did not differ from those obtained with other LMW agents with high affinity for zinc. However, more recent experimental work, not only failed to validate an absorption enhancement of zinc by picolinate (Hill et al., 1987a), but even resulted in a depression of zinc absorption rates (Hill et al., 1987b).

The rationale for the role of LMW substances is that they could form complexes with very low dissociation constants which would successfully remove dietary zinc from semi-digested foodstuffs and be the vehicle delivering to the small intestinal mucosa soluble forms of the metal. Once at the brush border, zinc could be internalized by the paracellular route, that is, dragged by the normal water inflow, even in the absence of a specific carrier.

Other LMW ligands have been particularly studied. Closely following the first reports on picolinic acid, another group of investigators presented convincing evidence that the LMW ligand in human milk was citrate and not picolinate (Lönnerdal et al., 1980; Hurley & Lönnerdal, 1981). In addition, experiments on rats revealed that, at two levels of LMW ligand:zinc ratios, zinc was absorbed at higher rates in the presence of citrate or histidine, than with picolinate (Wapnir et al., 1981). It was also shown that ^{65}Zn was taken up by the pancreas in the presence of histidine at a rate twice that of picolinate (Johnson & Evans, 1982).

A likely role for amino acids in the luminal phase of zinc absorption has been accumulated from numerous reports of experimental and clinical work since the mid 1970's. An excess of histidine by either oral or parenteral route produced a sharp increase in urinary zinc excretion, in humans as well as in animals, without inducing deficiency symptoms (Henkin, 1972; Freeman & Taylor, 1977; Yunice et al., 1978). In work with dogs, an amino acid selectivity was demonstrated; cysteine, as well as histidine, increased zincuria, while an infusion of glycine was ineffective (Yunice et al., 1978).

Additional information supporting a significant role for amino acids and organic acids came from *in vivo* kinetic studies with rats, in our laboratory. We observed that the addition of increasing concentrations of certain putative LMW ligands, such as L-histidine, progressively reduced the ileal absorption of zinc, while with other amino acids, namely L-glutamate or L-tryptophan, or organic acids, such as D-galacturonate, the inhibition of zinc absorption was much less marked, or negligible. Further work with L-histidine yielded results compatible with a competitive inhibition of the amino acid on the L-histidine:zinc complex. This response to an amino acid excess was stereospecific for the L- isomer (Wapnir et al., 1983). Several amino acids reported to bind tightly to zinc were also shown to enhance zinc absorption in rat jejunum and ileum as compared to zinc perfused in the absence of LMW potential ligands. In addition, the small intestine, especially the ileum, recognized both the amino and the acidic functions of the amino acids as requirements for optimal zinc transport. This was shown when the amino acids were compared with homologues possessing similar structure, but lacking either the amino or the carboxylic moieties. Imidazole was most effective in mimicking the role played by the derived amino acid, L-histidine (Wapnir & Stiel, 1986).

Protein nutritional status can have an effect on zinc absorption, especially if oligopeptides are considered to be the major form in which digested protein is absorbed (Matthews, 1977). Thus, when zinc was presented to either rat jejunum, ileum or colon together with a hydrolysis-resistant dipeptide, glycylsarcosine, zinc absorption was sharply depressed in protein-energy malnourished animals, while the ligand absorption was not affected in the proximal and terminal regions of the gut. Only in the ileum were both glycylsarcosine and zinc absorption significantly decreased. These data may partially explain the hypozincemia of the malnourished rats, which were fed a diet with as much zinc as the controls (Wapnir et al., 1985).

Copper

At present, it is accepted that the intestinal absorption of copper is accomplished by mediated and nonmediated processes. The luminal phase of absorption is not as well understood as that of other components of copper homeostasis, namely, the enterohepatic circulation and body distribution of the element (Crampton et al., 1965; Evans, 1973). Inorganic copper salts are well absorbed, and the release by stomach acid of natural complexes with bound copper is physiologically compatible with a well developed absorptive mechanism in the duodenum (Marceau et al., 1970; Bronner & Yost, 1985). Although salivary and intestinal secretions may bind copper, this element remains available in easily dialyzable complexes (Gollan et al., 1971; Gollan, 1973). Most dietary copper in vegetables or plants is present as complexes with lectins or acidic glycoproteins which may be still available for extraction by gastric acid (Mills, 1956; Lo et al., 1984). Although high levels of organic phosphates, or phosphoproteins may reduce copper

bioavailability (Davis & Nightingale, 1975), phytate appears not to exerts a seques-
tering action on copper as strong as on zinc. Therefore, phytate may not be a serious interference on copper absorption (Lo et al. 1984), and may even enhance
copper availability by reducing the competition presented by zinc (Lee et al.,
1988).

The association of copper with amino acids has been well characterized, and,
based on dissociation constants of binary and ternary copper:amino acid complexes, the amino acid identity of the chelates in physiological fluids has been
predicted and found to agree with experimental findings (Berthon et al., 1986).
The affinity of copper for amino acids and oligopeptides is well known and is the
basis of the classical biuret reaction used for protein determination. Amino acids
have been postulated as the LMW ligands involved in the transmucosal uptake of
copper (Kirchgessner & Gassman, 1970). This concept was derived from data on
the enhancement of copper transport into liver and kidney slices or Ehrlich mouse
ascites cells by amino acids, which had been interpreted as indicative of active
transport. A copper transport alteration in the two well described inborn errors of
copper metabolism, Menkes' and Wilson's diseases, has been postulated as the
biochemical error responsible for either copper tissue accumulation or deficiency
(Neumann & Silverberg, 1966; Prohaska, 1986).

Data on the intestinal absorption of copper appear to agree with the findings
of those early studies in vitro. Apparently, the protein breakdown due to meat
cooking is sufficient to reverse copper deficiency produced in rats fed raw meat,
which apparently is not adequately digested by those animals (Moore et al., 1964).
Similar interpretation can be derived from experiments conducted with everted
intestinal sacs, where the addition of either fish or soybean meal enhanced inorganic copper absorption (Ashmead, 1970). Furthermore, it can be concluded that
only protein breakdown products, but not intact proteins, will improve copper
bioavailability and assist to its distribution throughout the body. This role is
shared by albumin and specific proteins, namely ceruloplasmin and transcuprein
(Solomons, 1985).

In man, an experimental increase in the protein content of the diet from 8.1
to 24.1 g of nitrogen per day by an enrichment of a special bread with extra
casein, lactalbumin, wheat gluten and dried egg white increased apparent copper
retention from a mean of 1.28 to 1.61 mg/day while reducing fecal losses from
1.80 to 1.54 mg/day (Greger & Snedeker, 1980). However, maintaining copper
sufficiency early in life may be threatened in high risk conditions, namely prema-
turity, prolonged intravenous alimentation and secondarily to malnutrition and
kwashiorkor (Ashkenazi et al., 1973; Graham & Cordano, 1976). Cow milk infant
formulae not appropriately enriched with minerals may pose the threat of copper
insufficiency, apparently because in cow's milk copper is evenly distributed
between casein and LMW protein fractions. In contrast, in human breast milk a
larger proportion of copper is associated with the whey fraction, and a smaller
percentage of this element is chelated by LMW ligands (Fransson & Lönnerdal,
1983). Nevertheless, trace mineral deficiency is also a risk factor for infants maintained largely on breast milk, due to the progressive concentration reduction of
copper and zinc through the postpartum period (Vuori & Kuitunen, 1979).

There is an apparent inconsistency between the concept of transport enhancement by amino acids and LMW oligopeptides, and the failure to do so by cow's
milk, a nutrient with a higher proportion of dialyzable copper than human breast

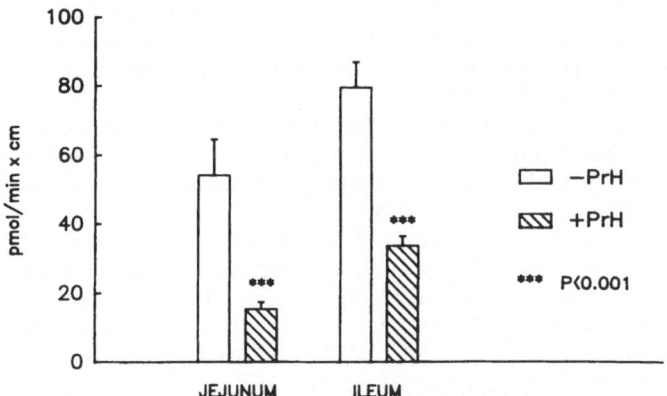

Figure 4. Copper absorption in the presence of a protein hydrolysate. Copper perfused at 31 μM concentration through rat jejunum in the absence and in the presence of a protein hydrolysate (PrH, mean m.w. 180 da.) added at a concentration of 60 mOsm/kg. The addition of PrH significantly reduced the rates of copper absorption (Adapted from Wapnir, 1985).

milk. This discrepancy can be better understood in the light of studies which have shown that an excess of amino acids with a great affinity for copper and zinc, such as histidine, can both enhance intestinal transport across the small intestinal mucosa as well as impair renal salvage of the amino acids. This may result in a net loss of amino acids and trace elements in the urine (Henkin et al., 1975; Harvey et al., 1981). Under experimental conditions, additional amounts of copper can compensate a large excess of an amino acid such as histidine (Harvey et al., 1981). However, more modest additions of either methionine, threonine or lysine to the diet did not affect copper balance of a group of adolescent girls (Price & Bunce, 1972). In studies conducted in our laboratory, with rats, we also observed a very sharp decline in copper absorption when this element was perfused in the presence of a large excess of amino acids and oligopeptides from a protein hydrolysate, present in a 2,000:1 proportion over the metal (Figure 4). This effect was noted both in the jejunum and in the ileum, and did not correlate with water transport from the lumen into the enterocyte, which was sharply stimulated in the presence of the protein hydrolysate (Wapnir, 1985).

These results are compatible with the concept that LMW ligands of proteinaceous origin are involved in the translocation of copper, and that excess potential chelators inhibit copper transport.

Manganese

Manganese, to a perhaps larger extent than other trace elements, has the dual characteristic of being both an essential nutrient and a toxic element. For this reason, the nature of the diet may play an important role in controlling the extent of the absorption of this mineral. This influence is well exemplified by the study of Murthy et al. (1981) in which they showed that feedings of a diet with only 10% casein could render rats more susceptible to the toxic effects of manganese than a protein sufficient diet with 21% casein.

Similarly, toxicity of manganese due to an excessive absorption of manganese from cow's milk has been presented as a potential source of concern. Cow's milk contains more casein and about five times more manganese (25.2 ± 2.6 μg/L) than human breast milk (4.9 ± 3.9 μg/L)(Stastny et al., 1984). What is more important is the difference in the proportion of manganese bound to ligands of various molecular weights in milk. In infant formulae and in cow's milk, manganese is 85-100% bound to LMW oligopeptides of less than 1,000 daltons. In contrast, when labeled manganese was added to human breast milk, none of the tagged metal was associated with LMW fractions. The label remained in its totality bound to proteins of 407,000 daltons (Lönnerdal et al., 1983). The greater absorbability of manganese associated with LMW protein breakdown products was demonstrated in animal experiments where cow's milk derived formulae were compared with breast milk (Bates et al., 1983). Moreover, the nature of the protein source in the formulations plays also a role in the absorbability of manganese. This was shown in a study using externally labeled manganese, where 80% of the metal was retained by a preparation based on cow's milk, while 60% of the manganese was absorbed from a product based on soy protein isolate (Keen et al., 1985). Under these conditions, bottled feedings may present the potential of allowing excessive absorption of manganese. This is a matter of concern since no well demonstrated manganese insufficiency has been demonstrated early in life. This and similar findings have prompted a considerable reduction in the metal content of manufactured infant feedings.

Rat jejunum appears to have mediated and nonmediated manganese transport mechanisms, with characteristics resembling those for zinc. However, the removal rate of manganese from the intestinal lumen is rapidly saturated and declines with time. LMW ligands, such as L-histidine or citrate, enhance the absorption rate of the metal and may act as "facilitators" of intestinal transport. This is best seen with the estimated initial uptake in the absence and in the presence of these chelators (Figure 5). The histidine:manganese absorption ratio, which is similar to the starting 2:1 stoichiometry rapidly increases, because the uptake of the amino acid remains unchanged but manganese removal from the lumen steadily falls off. In the nutritionally intact rat the enhancement of absorption by histidine is significant, and a mediated transport carrier with a $K_t = 56$ μM and a $V_{max} = 158$ pmol/min x cm can be characterized (Garcia-Aranda et al., 1983). The nutritional status of the animal also has an influence. In rats, growth retarded as a consequence of protein-energy deprivation, a greater uptake of the metal occurred in the absence of ligands. The addition of histidine did not affect the absorption rate (Garcia-Aranda et al., 1984).

Selenium

The interest in selenium nutrition has increased almost in a parallel fashion to the explosive expansion of research on zinc over the last thirty years. Selenium deficiency associated with areas of low soil selenium content resulted in a variety

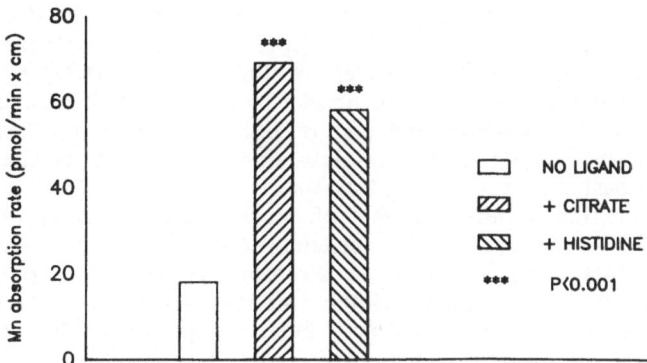

Figure 5. Effect of two low molecular weight ligands on the estimated maximum rat jejunal absorptive capacity for manganese. The absorption rates represent extrapolations to zero time for perfusions carried out at a 12.5 μM manganese concentration. The ligands were added at a 2:1 ratio to the metal. Both citrate and histidine significantly enhanced manganese absorption (Adapted from Garcia-Aranda et al., 1983).

of nutrient deficit diseases of fowls, pigs and sheep (Burk, 1983). In humans, the key role of selenium is its function as a component of the erythrocyte glutathione peroxidase (GSH-Px) molecule (Barbezat et al., 1984). In mammals, this is the one selenoprotein with biological significance. It reduces hydrogen peroxide, and can also reduce lipoperoxides. Bacteria have other selenium-dependent enzymes. Most organisms can utilize selenium in the form of selenites which, per se, have reducing properties and which potentiate the role of biologic antioxidants, namely, vitamin E. Thus, a constellation of possible nutritional deficiencies or disorders appear to be responsive to substances as diverse as chemical antioxidants, vitamin E and selenium.

The geochemistry of soils has also been linked to serum levels of selenium, with the lowest figures in certain populations groups being associated with Keshan disease, in China (Ge et al., 1983; Levander, 1987), and possibly, with Kashin-Beck disease, also described in several areas of the Far East (Sokoloff, 1988). Food analysis reveals a clear association between protein fractions and selenium content. Certain plants are good indicators of soil selenium levels, although this element may not play a biological role for vegetables. Animals are susceptible of exhibiting both selenium deficiency and selenium toxicity, according to the concentration of this element in their feeds (Oldfield, 1987). In contrast to divalent trace elements which are bound to proteins by covalent or coordinate covalent bonds, and alter the tertiary and quaternary structure of macromolecules, selenium can substitute directly for sulfur in sulfur-containing amino acids, cyst(e)ine and methionine, resulting in selenocyst(e)ine and selenomethionine, respectively. Therefore, selenoproteins may have a fraction of their cyst(e)ine and methionine residues replaced by selenium (Ganther, 1975).

In animal experiments, supplementation of selenium by selenomethionine is not effective in the absence of sufficient methionine. It appeared that selenomethionine was not directed to the target enzyme, GSH-Px, but to other proteins and, therefore, it may be inappropriate as a selenium supplement (Waschulewski & Sunde, 1988). In sheep, Wolffram et al. (1987) have shown that cysteine greatly enhances the mucosal uptake of selenite. This mechanism seems to be operating only at physiologic pH and is sodium-dependent. These findings are compatible with the view that seleno-dicysteine is absorbed by the same carriers that transport dibasic amino acids and cystine.

Inorganic selenide appears capable of incorporating directly into the protein matrix of GSH-Px and other selenoproteins, without necessitating an organoselenium intermediate (Sunde & Evenson, 1987). However, based on the chemical properties of selenium, protein homologues have been synthesized in which one or several sulfur atoms have been replaced by selenium. These substances, such as ribonuclease and heme iron proteins, if not of nutritional significance, may help to explain the mechanisms of selenium toxicity observed in animals feeding in high selenium pastures (Ganther, 1975).

An interesting aspect of selenium sufficiency and protein nutrition relates to the postulated association between kwashiorkor and selenium nutritional status. The work conducted by Schwarz (1961) on the nutritional rehabilitation of Jamaican children with kwashiorkor led to the proposal that the essential element selenium was also required for recuperation from the typical protein deficiency of kwashiorkor. Only by addition of selenium to the diet did two children undergoing a slow recovery improve markedly in weight gain. Several reports on marasmic children also support the contention that selenium deficiency is a notable component of protein-energy malnutrition. The evidence has been derived from studies in Jordan, Zaire, Guatemala and Thailand (Levander, 1987). The most significant results come from the latter country, where it was demonstrated that selenium deficiency is independent of serum protein levels and not only the resultant of the hypoproteinemia characteristic of children with marasmus and kwashiorkor (Levine & Olson, 1970). More recently, Golden et al. (1985) have postulated that one of the triggering causes of kwashiorkor may be the lack of antioxidant defenses in malnourished children, which could be linked to the levels of GSH-Px and, hence, to selenium nutriture. Golden's group considered that the measurement of erythrocyte GSH-Px could have a prognostic value in the eventual outcome of protein-energy malnutrition and kwashiorkor.

As described earlier for zinc and other trace elements, solutions for total parenteral nutrition lacking selenium can result in deficiency syndromes. In adults, insufficiency of this element has been reported to lead to cardiomyopathies, with possible fatal outcome (Van Rij et al., 1979; Johnson et al., 1981; Fleming et al., 1982). In addition, patients with congenital metabolic diseases such as phenylketonuria and maple syrup urine disease, placed on diets based on formulae low in certain essential amino acids, have been reported to develop selenium deficiency, either due to insufficient element intake, or to the presence of excess free amino acids (Lombeck & Bremer, 1977).

From another perspective, animal experiments have suggested the possibility that lactating mothers on a low selenium diet could induce a severe selenium deficiency in their offspring with concomitant side effects, such as anorexia and failure to grow (Ewan, 1976; Bunk & Combs, 1980).

Overview

The preceding review may serve to emphasize what, for some investigators, could be obvious — the connection between digestive processes involving protein and the absorption of many mineral elements essential for man and animals. This interaction includes the chemistry of proteins, the composition of macromolecules of biological significance and the source of foodstuffs. We are thus concerned with phenomena relating to the way minerals are bound to other nutrients and to the presence of chelating agents which can act as enhancers or inhibitors of the absorption of many elements.

The protein-mineral link has attracted the efforts of investigators in specialties as diverse as nutrition, physicochemistry, physiology and geochemistry. Governments and international agencies have been made aware of the importance of dietary factors, ethnic habits, and even international trade patterns which can alter sufficiency in essential metallic elements and result in symptoms of deficiency or toxicity. A more acute awareness of such relationships between nutrients, formally placed in very different categories may hopefully translate into a better utilization of food resources for man and animals and an eventual elimination of preventable disease conditions associated with protein and mineral nutrition.

Acknowledgement

This work was supported, in part, by NIH grant HD22585-02.

References

Adibi, S. A. (1971) *J. Clin. Invest.* 50, 2266-2275.
Allen, L. H., Oddoye, E. A., & Margen, S. (1979a) *Am. J. Clin. Nutr.* 32, 741-749.
Allen, L. H., Bartlett, R. S., & Block, G. D. (1979b) *J. Nutr.* 109, 1345-1350.
Allen, L. H., Block, G. D., Wood, R. J., & Bryce, G. F. (1981) *Nutr. Res.* 1, 3-11.
Allen, L. H. (1982) *Am. J. Clin. Nutr.* 35, 783-808.
Alpers, D. H., Lee, S. W., & Avioli, L. V. (1972) *Gastroenterology* 62, 559-565.
Ashkenazi, A., Levin, S., Djaldetti, M., Fishel, E., & Benvenisti, D. (1973) *Pediatrics* 52, 525-533.
Ashmead, H. (1970) *J. Appl. Nutr.* 22, 42-51.
Ashmead, H. D., Graff, D. J., & Ashmead, H. H. (1985) in *"Intestinal Absorption of Metal Ions and Chelates"*, pp 120-121, Charles C. Thomas, Springfield.
Barbezat, G. O., Casey, C. E., Reasbeck, P. G., Robinson, M. F., & Thomson, C. D. (1984) in *"Absorption and Malabsorption of Mineral Nutrients"* (Solomons, N. W., & Rosenberg, I. H., Eds.) pp 231-258, Alan R. Liss, New York.
Bates, J., Chan, W., Mahood, A., & Rennert, O. M. (1983) *Fed. Proc.* 42, 817.
Bengoa, J. M., Sitrin, M. D., Wood, R. J., & Rosenberg, I. H. (1983) *Am. J. Clin. Nutr.* 38, 264-269.

Berthon, G., Hacht, B., Blais, M. J., & May, P. M. (1986) *Inorg. Chim. Acta* 125, 219-227.

Birge, S. J. & Avioli, L. V. (1986) in *"Physiology of Membrane Disorders"* (Andreoli, T. E., Hoffman, J. F., Fanestil, D. D. & Schultz, S. G., Eds.) pp 887-906, Plenum, New York.

Bjorn-Rassmussen, E., & Hallberg, L. (1979) *Nutr. Metab.* 23, 192-198.

Block, G. D., Wood, R. J., & Allen, L. H. (1980) *Am. J. Clin. Nutr.* 33, 2128-2136.

Bothwell, T. H., Charlton, R. W., Cook, J. D., & Finch, C. A. (1979) *"Iron Metabolism in Man"*, Blackwell, Oxford.

Bronner, F., & Yost, J. H. (1985) *Am. J. Physiol.* 249, G108-G112.

Bunk, M. J., & Combs, G. F. (1980) *J. Nutr.* 110, 743-749.

Burk, R. F., Pearson, W. N., Wood, R. P., & Viteri, F. (1967) *Am. J. Clin. Nutr.* 20, 723-733.

Burk, R. F. (1983) *Ann. Rev. Nutr.* 3, 53-70.

Burston, D., Marrs, T. C., Sleisenger, M. H., Sopanen, T., & Matthews, D. M. (1977) *Ciba Fdn. Symp.* 50, 79-98.

Callender, S. T., Marney, S. R., & Warner, G. T. (1970) *Br. J. Haematol.* 19, 657-663.

Conrad, M. E., Foy, A. L., Williams, H. L., & Knospe, W. H. (1967) *Am. J. Physiol.* 213, 557-565.

Cook, J. D., Morck, T. A., & Lynch, S. R. (1981) *Am. J. Clin. Nutr.* 34, 2622-2629.

Cousins, R. J. (1985) *Physiol. Revs.* 65, 238-309.

Crampton, R. F., Matthews, D. M., & Poisner, R. (1965) *J. Physiol.* 178, 111-119.

Davis, N. T., & Nightingale, R. (1975) *Br. J. Nutr.* 34, 243-250.

Dallman, P. R. (1986) *Ann. Rev. Nutr.* 6, 13-40.

DeLuca, H. F., & Schones, H. K. (1976) *Ann. Rev. Biochem.* 45, 631-675.

Dunn, M. A., Blalock, T. L., & Cousins, R. J. (1987) *Proc. Soc. Exptl. Biol Med.* 185, 107-119.

Evans, G. W. (1973) *Physiol. Revs.* 53, 535-570.

Evans, G. W. (1980) *Nutr. Revs.* 38, 137-141.

Evans, G. W., & Johnson, E. C. (1980) *J. Nutr.* 110, 1076-1080.

Ewan, R. C. (1976) *J. Nutr.* 106, 702-709.

Fairweather-Tait, S. J. (1987) *Nutr. Res.* 7, 319-325.

Fleming, C. R., Lie, J. T., McCall, J. T., O'Brien, J. F., Baillie, E. E., & Thistle, J. L. (1982) *Gastroenterology* 83, 689-693.

Fort, P., Lifshitz, F., Wapnir, I. L., & Wapnir, R. A. (1977) *Diabetes* 26, 882-886.

Fransson, G.-B., & Lönnerdal, B. (1980) *J. Pediatr.* 96, 380-384.

Fransson, G.-B., & Lönnerdal, B. (1983) *Pediatr. Res.* 17, 912-915.

Freeman, R. M., & Taylor, P. R. (1977) *Am. J. Clin. Nutr.* 30, 523-527.

Ganther, H. E. (1975) *Chem. Scripta* (Sweden) 8A, 79-84.

Garcia-Aranda, J. A., Wapnir, R. A., & Lifshitz, F. (1983) *J. Nutr.* 113, 2601-2607.

Garcia-Aranda, J. A., Lifshitz, F., & Wapnir, R. A. (1984) *J. Pediatr. Gastro. Nutr.* 3, 602-607.

Garfinkel, L., & Garfinkel, D. (1985) *Magnesium* 4, 60-72.

Ge, K., Xue, A., & Bai, J. (1983) *Virchows Arch.* 401, 1-15.

Giroux, E. L., & Henkin, R. I. (1972) *Biochim. Biophys. Acta* 273, 64-74.

Giroux, E., & Prakash, N. K. (1977) *J. Pharm. Sci.* 66, 391-395.

Golden, M. H. N., Golden, B. E., & Bennett, F. I. (1985) in *"Trace Elements in Nutrition of Children"* (Chandra, R. K., Ed.) pp 185-207, Raven Press, New York.

Gollan, J. L., Davis, P. S., & Deller, D. J. (1971) *Am. J. Clin. Nutr.* 24, 1925-1935.

Gollan, J. L. (1973) *Clin. Sci.* 49, 237-244.

Graham, G. G., & Cordano, A. (1976) in *"Trace Elements in Human Health and Disease"* (Prasad, A. S., Ed.) pp 363-372, Academic Press, Inc. New York.

Greger, J. L., & Snedeker, S. M. (1980) *J. Nutr.* 110, 2243-2253.

Hahn, C., & Evans, G. W. (1973) *Proc. Soc. Exptl. Biol. Med.* 144, 793-795.

Hallberg, L. (1981) *Ann. Rev. Nutr.* 1, 123-147.

Hallberg, L. (1984) in *"Present Knowledge in Nutrition"* (Olson, R. E., Ed.) pp 459-478, The Nutrition Foundation, Washington, D. C.

Hallman, P. S., Perrin, D. D., & Watt, A. E. (1971) *Biochem. J.* 121, 549-555.

Hambidge, K. M., Walravens, P. A., Casey, C. E., Brown, R. M., & Bender, C. (1979) *J. Pediatr.* 94, 607-608.

Hamer, D. H. (1986) *Ann. Rev. Biochem.* 55, 913-951.

Harvey, P. W., Hunsaker, H. A., & Allen, K. G. D. (1981) *J. Nutr.* 111, 639-647.

Heaney, R. P., & Recker, R. R. (1982) *J. Lab. Clin. Med.* 99, 46-55.

Henkin, R. I., Keiser, H. R., & Bronzert, D. (1972) *J. Clin. Invest.* 51, 44a.

Henkin, R. I. (1974) *Adv. Exptl. Med. Biol.* 48, 297-327.

Henkin, R. I., Patten, B. M., Re, P. K., & Bronzert, D. A. (1975) *Arch. Neurol.* 32, 745-751.

Hill, D. A., Peo, E. R. Jr., & Lewis, A. J. (1987a) *Nutr. Rep. Intl.* 35, 1007-1014.

Hill, D. A., Peo, E. R. Jr., & Lewis, A. J. (1987b) *J. Nutr.* 117, 1704-1707.

Hunt, S. M., & Schofield, F. A. (1969) *Am. J. Clin. Nutr.* 22, 367-373.

Hurley, L. S., & Lönnerdal, B. (1981) *Pediatr. Res.* 15, 166-167.

Irving, J. T. (1973) *"Calcium and Phosphorus Metabolism"*, pp 25-26, Academic Press, New York.

Johnson, N. E., Alcantara, E. N. & Linkswiler, H. (1970) *J. Nutr.* 100, 1425-1430.

Johnson, W. T., & Evans, G. W. (1982) *J. Nutr.* 112, 914-919.

Johnson, R. A., Baker, S. S., Fallon, J. T., Maynard, E. P., Ruskin, J. N., Wen, Z., Ge, K., & Cohen, H. J. (1981) *N. Engl. J. Med.* 304, 1210-1212.

Johnstone, R. M. (1979) *Can. J. Physiol. Pharmacol.* 57, 1-15.

Kagi, J. H. R. & Vallee, B. L. (1960) *J. Biol. Chem.* 235, 3460-3465.

Keen, C. L., Bell, J. G., & Lönnerdal, B. (1985) *Fed. Proc.* 44, 1850.

Kirchgessner, M. & Grassman, E. (1970) in *"Proceedings of WAAP/IBP International Symposium on Trace Element Metabolism in Animals"* (Mills, C. F., Ed.) pp 277-287, E. & S. Livingstone, Edinburgh.

Krawitt, E. L., Beeken, W. L., & Janney, C. D. (1976) *Gastroenterology* 71, 251-254.

Krieger, I., Cash, R., & Evans, G. W. (1984) *J. Pediatr. Gastro. Nutr.* 3, 62-68.

Kroe, D., Kinney, T. D., Kaufman, N., & Klavins, J. V. (1963) *Blood* 21, 546-551.

Layrisse, M., Martinez-Torres, C., & Roche, M. (1968) *Am. J. Clin. Nutr.* 21, 1175-1183.

Layrisse, M., Martinez-Torres, C., Renzi, M., & Leets, I. (1975) *Blood* 45, 688-696.

Lee, D.-Y., Schroeder, J. III, & Gordon, D. T. (1988) *J. Nutr.* 118, 712-717.

Levander, O. A. (1987) *Ann. Rev. Nutr.* 7, 227-250.

Levine, R. J., & Olson, R. E. (1970) *Proc. Soc. Exptl. Biol. Med.* 134, 1030-1034.

Lo, G. S., Settle, S. L., & Steinke, F. H. (1984) *J. Nutr.* 114, 332-340.

Lombeck, I., & Bremer, H. J. (1977) *Nutr. Metab.* 21, 49-64.

Lönnerdal, B., Stanislowski, A. G., & Hurley, L. S. (1980) *J. Inorg. Biochem.* 12, 71-78.

Lönnerdal, B., Keen, C. L., Ohtake, M., & Tamura, T. (1983) *Am. J. Dis. Child.* 137, 433-439.

Lynch, S. R. (1984) in *"Absorption and Malabsorption of Mineral Nutrients"* (Solomons, N. W. & Rosenberg, I. H., Eds.), Alan R. Liss, New York.

Marceau, N., Aspin, N., & Sass-Kortsak, A. (1970) *Am. J. Physiol.* 218, 377-384.

Martinez-Torres, C., & Layrisse, M. (1970) *Blood* 35, 669-675.

Martinez-Torres, C., Romano, E., & Layrisse, M. (1981) *Am. J. Clin. Nutr.* 34, 322-327.

Matthews, D. M. (1977) *Gastroenterology* 73, 1267-1279.

McCance, R. A., Widdowson, E. M., & Lehmann, H. (1942) *Biochem. J.* 36, 686-691.

McMillan, J. A., Landaw, S. A., & Oski, F. (1976) *Pediatrics* 38, 686-693.

Miller, J. (1983) *Nutr. Rep. Intl.* 27, 1187-1197.

Mills, C. F. (1956) *Biochem J.* 63, 190-193.

Monsen, E. R., & Cook, J. D. (1979) *Am. J. Clin. Nutr.* 32, 804-810.

Moore, T., Constable, B. J., Day, K. C., Impey, S. G., & Symonds, K. R. (1964) *Br. J. Nutr.* 18, 135-142.

Moynahan, E. J. (1974) *Lancet* 2, 399-400.

Murthy, R. C., Lal, S., Saxena, D. K., Shukla, G. S., Ali, M. M., & Chandra, S. V. (1981) *Chem. Biol. Inter.* 37, 299-304.

Neumann, P. Z., & Silverberg, M. (1966) *Nature* 210, 414-416.

Newey, H., & Smyth, D. H. (1962) *J. Physiol.* (London), 164, 527-561.

Nixon, S. E., & Mawer, G. E. (1970) *Brit. J. Nutr.* 24, 241-258.

Oberleas, D., & Prasad, A. S. (1969) *Am. J. Clin. Nutr.* 22, 1304-1314.

O'Dell, B. L., Burpo, C. E., & Savage, J. E. (1972) *J. Nutr.* 102, 653-660.

Oldfield, J. E. (1987) *J. Nutr.* 117, 2002-2008.

Prasad, A. S., & Oberleas, D. (1970) *J. Lab. Clin. Med.* 3, 416-425.

Price, N. O., & Bunce, G. E. (1972) *Nutr. Rep. Intl.* 5, 275-284.

Prohaska, J. R. (1986) *Clin. Physiol. Biochem.* 4, 87-93.

Rao, B. S. N., & Prabhavathi, T. (1978) *Am. J. Clin. Nutr.* 31, 169-175.

Richards, M. P., & Cousins, R. J. (1976) *J. Nutr.* 106, 1591-1599.

Saarinen, U. M. (1978) *J. Pediatr.* 93, 177-180.

Schuette, S. A., & Linkswiler, H. M. (1984) in *"Present Knowledge in Nutrition"* (Olson, R. E., Ed.) pp 400-412, The Nutrition Foundation, Washington, D.C.

Schricker, B. R., & Forbes, R. M. (1978) *Nutr. Rep. Intl.* 18, 159-166.

Schwarz, K. (1961) *Fed. Proc.* 20, 666-673.

Silk, D. B. A., Marrs, T. C., Addison, J. M., Burston, D., Clark, M. L., & Matthews, D. M. (1973) *Clin. Sci. Mol. Med.* 45, 715-719.

Sokoloff, L. (1988) *Nutr. Revs.* 46, 113-119.

Solomons, N. W. (1985) *J. Amer. Coll. Nutr.* 4, 83-105.

Spencer, H., Kramer, L., & Osis, D. (1978) *Am. J. Clin. Nutr.* 31, 2167-2180.

Spencer, H., Kramer, L., DeBartolo, M., Norris, C., & Osis, D. (1983) *Am. J. Clin. Nutr.* 37, 924-929.

Spencer, H., Kramer, L., & Osis, D. (1988) *J. Nutr.* 118, 657-660.

Stastny, D., Vogel, R. S., & Picciano, M. F. (1984) *Am. J. Clin. Nutr.* 39, 872-878.

Sunde, R. A., & Evenson, J. K. (1987) *J. Biol. Chem.* 262, 933-937.

Takkunen, H., & Seppanen, R. (1975) *Am. J. Clin. Nutr.* 28, 1141-1148.

Toothill, J. (1963) *Brit. J. Nutr.* 17, 125-134.

Van Rij, A. M., Thomson, C. D., McKenzie, J. M., & Robinson, M. F. (1979) *Biol. Reprod.* 8, 625-629.

Van Slyke, D. D., & Meyer, G. M. (1912) *J. Biol. Chem.* 12, 399-410.

Vuori, E., & Kuitunen, P. (1979) *Acta Paediatr. Scand.* 68, 33-37.

Walker, R. M., & Linkswiler, H. (1972) *J. Nutr.* 102, 1297-130 .

Wapnir, R. A ., Wang, J., Exeni, R. A., & McVicar, M. (1981) *Am. J. Clin. Nutr.* 34, 651.

Wapnir, R. A., Khani, D. E., Bayne, M. A., & Lifshitz, F. (1983) *J. Nutr.* 113, 1346-1354.

Wapnir, R. A. (1985) in *"Nutrition for Special Needs of Infancy - Protein Hydrolysates"* (Lifshitz, F., Ed.) pp 37-57, Marcel Dekker, Inc., New York.

Wapnir, R. A., & Stiel, L. (1986) *J. Nutr.* 116, 2171-2179.

Waschulewski, I. H., & Sunde, R. A. (1988) *J. Nutr.* 118, 367-374.

Widdowson, E. M., Southgate, D. A. T., & Schutz, Y. (1974) *Arch. Dis. Child.* 49, 867-873.

Wolffram, S., Wurmli, R., & Scharrer, E. (1987) in *"TEMA 6"*, Conference Abs. p 61, Pacific Grove, CA.

Yunice, A. A., King, R. W. Jr., Kraikitpanitch, S., Haygood, C. C., & Lindeman, R. D. (1978) *Am. J. Physiol.* 235, F40-F45.

8

The Effect of Dietary Proteins on Iron Bioavailability in Man[1]

Sean R. Lynch, Richard F. Hurrell, Sandra A. Dassenko, and James D. Cook

Normal iron nutriture in human beings depends on an adequate supply of bioavailable dietary iron. The quantity of food iron absorbed from any meal is determined not only by the amount, but also the form of iron present, and the composition of the meal (Monsen et al., 1978). The complex diets of adults living in Western countries generally contain relatively large amounts of animal tissue and ensure both a stable iron supply and adequate absorption. Factors affecting bioavailability may be a much more important determinant of adequate iron nutrition in the relatively monotonous vegetable diets of developing countries (Bothwell et al., 1979). Unfortunately, even in Western nations, the diets of infants and children (infant formulas, infant cereals, and weaning foods) tend to be less varied. They contain little animal tissue and do not always include foods that naturally promote iron absorption. An adequate supply of bioavailable iron is essential during this period of life because of the iron demands of growth (Stekel, 1984) and because iron stores have not yet been accumulated. Therefore, careful attention must be paid to iron content and its bioavailability in foods prepared for infants and children.

Current trends in nutritional counseling and product development may make the effect of proteins on iron bioavailability more important to other segments of the population in the future. Our increasing use of processed food as well as the replacement of some of the protein in our diets that was traditionally derived from meat with protein from other sources will make an accurate knowledge of protein iron interactions affecting iron bioavailability important to individuals of all ages.

Measurement of Iron Absorption in Man

In vitro testing to determine the solubility or dialyzability of iron is a satisfactory method for screening compounds as well as food items to determine whether

---

1 Supported in part by NIH grant #DK39246

the iron is potentially bioavailable to human beings. Miller et al. (1981) found particularly good agreement between relative availability determined by a method involving simulated gastrointestinal digestion and actual food iron absorption. Although this method is useful for identifying enhancers and inhibitors of nonheme iron absorption, the magnitude of the effect tends to be exaggerated (Hurrell et al., 1988a,b).

Animal models, particularly the rat hemoglobin repletion method have also been used extensively for evaluating iron bioavailability (Fritz et al., 1970, 1972). A recent study demonstrated that the rat hemoglobin repletion method is valuable for screening compounds that could be used for iron fortification (Forbes et al., 1988). However, it appears to be unsatisfactory for predicting the bioavailability of food iron for human beings (Hurrell & Brown, unpublished observations). Precise information about bioavailability in man ultimately necessitates that iron absorption be measured in human beings.

Radioisotopic Methods

Classical chemical balance studies of iron absorption are unsatisfactory for studying human iron absorption because the fraction of dietary iron assimilated normally represents only a small difference between iron intake and fecal loss. Most of the present knowledge about iron nutrition is based on radioisotopic measurements of iron absorption (Bothwell et al., 1979). While several theoretical criticisms of these studies have been made through the years, the body of evidence that has been accumulated from several different laboratories is surprisingly consistent. Moreover, the information is supported by our understanding of the physiology of iron balance based on other information such as rates of iron excretion (Green et al., 1968).

In the early studies of food iron absorption an intrinsic tag technique was used. Test meals consisted of single foods that had been labeled biosynthetically with radioiron (Moore & Dubach, 1951). Marked variations in iron absorption were noted. Iron derived from animal tissue was more available than that of vegetable origin (Layrisse et al., 1969). However, when two different food items were separately labeled with ^{59}Fe and ^{55}Fe and then eaten in the same meal, it became apparent that absorption from each was affected by the other. For example, when maize and meat were eaten together, absorption from maize was markedly enhanced while a smaller percentage of the meat iron was assimilated (Martinez-Torres & Layrisse, 1971), indicating that absorption was a property of overall meal composition.

Extrinsic tag technique. The complexity of Western diets precluded biosynthetic labeling of all foods in a meal and limited the application of this method. The large body of information about human food iron absorption that has been accumulated in the last two decades was made possible by a crucial observation reported in the early 1970s. When a small quantity of inorganic radioiron is mixed with a vegetable food before it is eaten, percentage absorption from this extrinsic tag is virtually identical to that of the biosynthetically incorporated label (Cook et al., 1972; Bjorn-Rasmussen et al., 1972). These and subsequent similar observations have demonstrated that when several foods are eaten in the same meal, the nonheme iron destined for absorption behaves as though it is derived from a common pool. Iron absorption can be measured by determining the size of the pool and the percentage absorption of a radioiron tracer (extrinsic tag) mixed with the pool. To ensure adequate labeling of the pool, it is usually necessary to mix the tracer with a major component of the meal (Hallberg, 1980). The bioavailability of iron in the common nonheme pool is determined by the balance of factors in the meal that either enhance or inhibit absorption.

Numerous studies from many different laboratories have revealed only a few situations in which absorption of the extrinsic tag may be misleading. It may not exchange completely with intrinsic iron in whole grain rice presumably because it fails to permeate the rice kernel (Bjorn-Rasmussen et al., 1973). Meat iron in the form of ferritin or hemosiderin may also not equilibrate fully with the common pool (Layrisse et al., 1975; Martinez-Torres et al., 1976; Martinez-Torres et al., 1986). It has been suggested that the protein shell inhibits exchange between the common iron pool and iron contained within the central core of ferritin. Insoluble iron salts used for fortification and contaminant inorganic iron also fail to exchange completely with the common nonheme iron pool (Cook et al., 1973; Derman et al., 1977; Hallberg & Bjorn-Rasmussen, 1981).

A similar but separate common absorption pool exists for heme iron derived principally from hemoglobin and myoglobin in meat. Iron in this pool is particularly well absorbed and enters the mucosal cell while still within the porphyrin ring (Weintraub et al., 1968). The principle of extrinsic tagging described for the nonheme pool is equally applicable to the heme pool if biosynthetically labeled hemoglobin is added to the meat in the meal (Layrisse & Martinez-Torres, 1972). The availability of two separate iron radioisotopes (^{55}Fe and ^{59}Fe) that have energy levels sufficiently different to allow their quantitation in the same sample makes it possible to tag the two major dietary iron pools independently and measure total iron absorption from mixed meat containing meals. Bjorn-Rasmussen et al. (1974) used double extrinsic tags to measure absorption from a complete day's diet which was designed to be representative of normal eating habits in 32 young, Swedish men. The result illustrates the importance of the small, highly bioavailable heme iron pool in ensuring an adequate dietary iron supply; 0.37 mg iron was absorbed from the 1.0 mg heme iron in the day's diet (37.3%) while only 0.88 mg was absorbed from the 16.4 mg nonheme pool (5.3%).

Quantitation of radioiron absorption. Appropriately radiolabeled test meals are usually administered after an overnight fast. Radioiron absorption may be quantitated by one of several methods including fecal radioiron balance, plasma radioiron tolerance curves, measurements of incorporated red cell radioactivity and, in the case of ^{59}Fe, whole body counting. Only the latter two are used extensively. For normal individuals values based on measured red-cell radioactivity and a calculated blood volume are sufficiently accurate. Moreover, the availability of both ^{59}Fe and ^{55}Fe permits direct comparisons between different meals in a single individual. Whole body counting is more cumbersome and is generally reserved for clinical conditions in which red cell radioiron incorporation is unpredictable (Bothwell et al., 1979).

Unfortunately, food iron absorption varies markedly in normal individuals. The primary factor responsible for the wide range of "normal" values is differences in iron status. For this reason it was necessary to devise a method for comparing measurements in subjects with differing iron needs. The use of a "reference dose" consisting of a freshly prepared solution of 3 mg iron as $FeSO_4$ and sufficient ascorbic acid to provide a 2:1 molar ratio (ascorbate:Fe) made intersubject comparisons possible (Layrisse et al., 1968). Iron in this form is essentially all bioavailable and differences in absorption are a reflection only of the physiological factors that control its assimilation in the individual being studied (Hallberg, 1980). The reference dose is administered in the fasting state on a different day using the other iron isotope and test meal absorption values are "corrected" to the same reference dose value, usually 40%, or expressed as a fraction of the reference dose. More recently it has become apparent from comparisons between serum ferritin concentrations and reference dose absorption that similar calculations can be based on serum ferritin values (Bezwoda et al., 1979).

Applicability of single meal studies to dietary iron absorption. Most radioisotopic studies of human iron absorption have been based on single meals. The practical relevance of these single meal studies to "real-life" iron nutrition may be questioned. Some support for the validity of single meal observations is provided by complementary information based on world-wide patterns of food consumption and the prevalence of nutritional iron deficiency (Bothwell et al., 1979; Hallberg, 1981). Cereal- and legume-based diets are associated with a high prevalence of iron deficiency despite adequate quantities of iron in the diet. Iron deficiency is uncommon in countries where meat is readily available. Moreover, Takkunen and Seppanen (1976) found a significant correlation between the intake of meat products and iron status in a study of 7000 people in Finland.

We recently obtained additional preliminary experimental evidence supporting the validity of single meal studies (Cook, Dassenko, & Lynch, unpublished observations). A direct comparison was made between radioiron absorption from a single meal considered typical of the diet of the subject being studied which was administered in the laboratory and average absorption from 28 meals eaten over a period of 2 weeks in the individual's usual surroundings. Almost identical mean absorption values were obtained for the single meal and the 14-day diet. Similar findings were obtained when diets were designed to include factors known to reduce or increase iron absorption respectively. These observations provide direct evidence that single meal studies are representative of dietary iron availability in free living individuals over an extended period.

Protein Rich Foods and Iron Bioavailability

Animals proteins. Animal tissues have the common property of enhancing iron absorption by both providing highly bioavailable heme iron and enhancing the absorption from the nonheme pool derived from the meat as well as other components of the meal. The enhancing effect of animal tissues on nonheme iron absorption has been demonstrated in studies using either biosynthetically labeled foods or the extrinsic tag technique. The results are very similar. Several representative studies summarized in Table I demonstrate that percentage absorption was increased an average of 2.6-fold when animal tissues were incorporated into a vegetable meal. The dose effect of increasing the quantity of animal tissue in vegetable meals has not been studied rigorously, but a modest further

Table I. Effect of animal tissues on nonheme iron bioavailability

| Meal | Animal Tissue | Nonheme Iron Absorption (%) | | Ratio (B:A) |
		Alone (A)	With Animal Tissue (B)	
Maize[a]	Veal muscle	4.1	7.6	1.87
Black beans[a]	Veal muscle	4.8	10.7	2.21
Maize[b]	Veal liver	4.9	10.9	2.22
Maize[b]	Veal liver	2.2	7.0	3.17
Maize[c]	Fish	4.2	7.5	1.78
Black beans[c]	Fish	1.0	1.7	1.70
Maize[d]	Beef muscle	2.2	7.2	3.80
Maize[d]	Chicken muscle	2.4	5.7	3.24
Maize[d]	Fish	0.4	1.3	4.37
Maize[d]	Calf thymus	0.9	2.26	2.97
Maize[e]	Beef	0.5	1.6	3.22
Wheat bread[e]	Beef	3.0	3.2	1.07

[a] Martinez-Torres & Layrisse, 1971.
[b] Martinez-Torres et al., 1974.
[c] Layrisse et al., 1968.
[d] Bjorn-Rasmussen & Hallberg, 1979.
[e] Hurrell et al., 1988.

improvement in bioavailability appears to occur when the quantity is increased (Table II).

A carefully controlled study conducted by Cook & Monsen (1976) using two standardized meals provides the most detailed information on the relative effects of different animal tissues as well as other animal proteins on nonheme iron bioavailability. They used the extrinsic tag technique to examine absorption from a standard mixed meal (STM) chosen to be representative of the typical American diet. It consisted of ground beef, potatoes, cornbread, margarine, ice milk, and peaches. Other protein sources were then substituted for the beef on an equiprotein basis in different studies. Although it was not possible to match the nutrient composition or iron content of the substituted meals exactly, a much better level of standardization was achieved than had been the case in earlier studies. The results demonstrated that there was no statistical difference in percentage nonheme iron absorption from meals containing beef, pork, lamb, liver, chicken, or fish.

An even more precise characterization of the effect of animal proteins on the bioavailability of iron was achieved by designing a meal comprising three semipurified ingredients (SPM), hydrolyzed maize starch, corn oil, and sprayed dried egg white, which were blended together with dibasic calcium phosphate and potassium phosphate as well as sufficient ferric chloride to adjust the meal iron content to 4.1 mg. The ingredients were chosen to provide the same quantities of the major dietary nutrients as were present in the STM described above. When

Table II.   Effect of quality of animal tissues on bioavailability

| Meal | Animal Tissue | Amount (g) | Nonheme Iron Absorption (%) | | Ratio (B:A) |
			Alone (A)	Tissue (B)	
Maize[a]	Fish	10	2.2	3.7	1.52
		20	0.4	1.3	4.37
Wheat[b]	Beef	40	2.0	2.5	1.25
		80	2.0	3.9	1.95
		160	2.0	4.2	2.10

[a] Bjorn-Rasmussen & Hallberg, 1979.
[b] Lynch, Cook, & Dassenko, unpublished observations.

other proteins were substituted for the egg white in this meal, the remaining ingredients could be adjusted to maintain a relatively constant chemical composition. Iron absorption from the SPM containing egg white was much lower than from the STM. Mean absorption values in 9 different groups of normal volunteers studied ranged from 0.7% and 2.0% (STM 3.8% to 14.8%). The substitution of animal tissue led to a marked improvement in absorption (2.05 to 3.86-fold, Table III).

The enhancing effect of animal tissues does not appear to be a general property of animal proteins. Early studies of other important dietary sources of animal protein demonstrated an inhibitory effect on iron absorption. Iron was poorly absorbed from a meal containing eggs unless orange juice was added (Callender et al., 1970) and the addition of an egg to a breakfast meal containing bread prepared from wheat that had been labeled biosynthetically with radioiron markedly reduced absorption (Elwood et al., 1968). The inhibitory effect of powdered egg which was comparable to that of egg white was confirmed by Cook & Monsen (1976).

Most of the published reports on the effect of milk or milk- products on iron absorption have suggested an inhibitory effect (Abernathy et al., 1965; Cook & Monsen, 1976) although Hallberg & Rossander (1982b) reported that the substitution of milk for water in a hamburger meal did not influence iron absorption. In the carefully controlled studies of Cook and Monsen, the substitution of milk or cheese for meat in the STM reduced absorption from 5.5% to 1.6% and 9.4% to 3.6% respectively. Absorption from the SPM was not significantly different when these proteins were substituted for egg white (Table III).

Vegetable proteins. Iron derived from vegetable sources is generally less well absorbed than that derived from animal foods (Layrisse et al., 1969), although a high content of ascorbic acid and possibly other organic acids may sometimes render the nonheme iron as bioavailable as it is in meat containing meals (Hallberg & Rossander, 1982a; Gillooly et al., 1983). Poorer bioavailability has been attributed to several factors including fiber (Cook et al., 1983), polyphenols (Disler et al., 1975a; Disler et al., 1975b; Gillooly et al., 1983), phytates (Widdowson &

Table III. Relative effect of different protein sources on nonheme iron absorption from SPM

| Substitute | Mean Iron Absorption (%) | | Absorption Ratio (A:B) |
	Substitute (A)	Egg White Control (B)	
No Protein[a]	10.6	3.0	3.53
Animal Tissues			
Beef muscle[b]	5.1	1.7	3.00
Pork[b]	5.2	1.6	3.25
Lamb[b]	5.2	1.6	3.25
Liver[b]	5.4	1.4	3.86
Chicken[b]	3.4	1.4	2.43
Fish[b]	3.9	1.9	2.05
Animal Protein Foods			
Milk[b]	0.9	0.7	1.29
Cheese[b]	2.4	2.0	1.20
Whole egg[b]	0.7	0.5	0.88
Vegetable Protein Foods			
Full fat soy flour[c]	1.0	5.5	0.18
Textured soy flour[c]	1.9	5.5	0.35
Semi-purified & purified protein fractions			
Bovine serum albumin[a]	5.7	3.0	1.90
Casein[c]	2.7	2.5	1.08
Casein[d]	3.7	6.7	0.55
Whey protein[d]	1.0	2.5	0.40
Wheat gluten[d]	2.1	3.0	0.70
Soy protein isolate[c]	0.5	2.5	0.20
Soy protein isolate[c]	0.4	5.5	0.08

[a] Hurrell et al., 1988a.
[b] Cook & Monsen, 1976.
[c] Cook et al., 1981.
[d] Hurrel et al., 1988b.

McCance, 1942; Hallberg et al., 1987) and inorganic calcium and phosphates (Monsen & Cook, 1976). Evaluation of a possible role for the protein component of vegetable foods has been limited to a few observations using soybean products rich in protein. When full fat soy flour or defatted textured soy flour were substituted for egg white in the SPM absorption was significantly reduced (Cook et al., 1981; Table III).

Effects of Purified and Semi-purified Proteins on Bioavailability

While the studies described above provide circumstantial evidence that the bioavailability of food iron is affected both by the quantity and the nature of dietary protein, definitive proof depends on studies of purified protein fractions. Only a few such studies have been carried out, and in most cases it was only possible to evaluate products that consisted predominantly of the major food protein in a semi-purified form. Unfortunately, the preparations varied in their content of factors such as calcium, phosphate, and phytate that are known to affect iron absorption. Nevertheless, the highest absorption ratio (test meal:control meal containing egg white) was observed in the protein free meal (Table 3). Thus, all protein sources tested in the SPM reduced absorption when compared with the protein free meal (Table III). Inhibition was least marked with bovine serum albumin. Percentage absorption fell from 10.6 to 5.7 ($P < 0.05$), but remained significantly higher than the same meal with egg white (3.0%, Hurrell et al., 1988). Soy protein isolate was the most inhibitory. Mean percentage nonheme iron absorption in two studies was 0.5 and 0.4 (only 20% and 10% of the value for the meal with egg white, Cook et al., 1981).

Additional evidence that specifically implicates the protein component in some of these purified protein-rich products has been obtained from the study of hydrolyzed preparations. Once again, it is important to inject a note of caution into the interpretation of the results, since other factors known to affect iron bioavailability could not be controlled completely. Nevertheless, it is apparent that absorption improved when the protein was hydrolyzed prior to consumption (Table IV). The improvement in absorption appeared to be partly dependent on the extent of hydrolysis and perhaps on the enzyme used. The milk protein hydrolyzates were prepared with trypsin and pancreatin. Papain was used for the soy protein products.

Mechanism by which Proteins Affect Iron Bioavailability

The enhancing effect of meat on nonheme iron absorption has been studied in the greatest detail. It appears to exert its influence on the intraluminal milieu and does not seem to act indirectly by stimulating gastric secretion of hydrochloric acid. In one study, meat increased absorption from maize from 0.7% to 2.1% in patients with histamine-fast achlorhydria (Bjorn-Rasmussen & Hallberg, 1979). The three-fold greater absorption with meat is similar to that observed in other studies with normal individuals (Table I). Further evidence for an intraluminal effect was provided by the observation that meat did not increase absorption from a solution of ferrous sulfate, but nevertheless, reduced the inhibitory effect of sodium phytate on absorption from both ferrous sulfate and ferric chloride (Bjorn-Rasmussen & Hallberg, 1979). The possibility that the effect of meat might be due to it's nucleoprotein content was considered by Bjorn-Rasmussen and Hallberg, but calf thymus which is particularly rich in nucleoproteins had a promoting effect that was no greater than that of other meat products. This series of studies also demonstrated that when minced beef was boiled in water the enhancing factor was found in the meat residue rather than the broth.

Table IV. Effect of enzymatic hydrolysis on inhibitory effect of proteins on nonheme iron absorption

Protein	Extent of Hydrolysis (%)	Percentage Absorption	Ratio (Hydr:Intact)
Whey protein (WP)[a]	0	1.0	
Hydrolyzed WP	16	1.1	1.08
Hydrolyzed WP	36	1.7	1.74
Casein	0	3.7	
Hydrolyzed Casein	84	7.7	2.10*
Soy protein isolate (SPI)[b]	0	0.3	
Hydrolyzed soybean grits	24[+]	1.9	8.29**
Hydrolyzed SPI	52	5.3	22.70**

[a] Hurrell et al., 1988.
[b] Lynch et al., 1986.
* $P < 0.05$; ** $P < 0.01$; + approximate values.

The possibility that protein digestion products may merely act as nonspecific ligands that increase iron solubility has been considered by several groups of investigators. Pepsin digestion products in chicken muscle with molecular weights less than 10,000 increase the solubility of inorganic iron (Slatkavitz & Clydesdale, 1988). Kane and Miller (1984) quantitated the fraction of iron that became dialyzable under simulated gastrointestinal conditions. Various animal tissues and vegetable proteins were digested *in vitro* at 37°C with pepsin and then pancreatin under careful pH control. Low molecular weight digestion products of beef and bovine serum albumin enhanced iron dialyzability. On the other hand, digestion products of gelatin, casein, defatted soy flour, gluten and soy protein isolate reduced percentage dialyzability. They postulated that the influence of proteins on iron bioavailability is related to the affinity of undigested or partially digested protein for iron. Hurrell et al. (1988a), using the same *in vitro* test, demonstrated that bovine serum albumin also increased the dialyzable iron in cornmeal, bread, rice flour, and rice and wheat based infant cereals. However, the improvement in dialyzability was not associated with improved absorption in most of the meals, suggesting that some peptide digestion products may render nonheme food iron soluble, but nevertheless not enhance its absorption.

In 1970 Martinez-Torres and Layrisse proposed that the enhancing effect of meat on nonheme iron absorption is a more specific property of its amino acid composition. They based their postulate on the observation that the percentage absorption of iron from black beans increased two-fold when the food was eaten either with 100 g fish or a quantitatively equivalent amino acid mixture. Studies with specific amino acids demonstrated that the effect was due to the presence of cysteine or cysteine plus methionine. In these studies cysteine was administered in a capsule in the middle of the meal. No effect was seen when the amino acid was mixed with vegetable foods before the final cooking (Martinez-Torres et al., 1981) or even mixed with maize porridge immediately before serving (Bjorn-Rasmussen

& Hallberg, 1979). While the explanation for this discrepancy is uncertain, oxidation of cysteine to cystine is rapid at neutral or basic pH, with loss of the thiol groups that are postulated to be responsible for facilitating iron absorption.

It is unlikely that free cysteine is an important enhancer of iron bioavailability, but Taylor et al. (1986) have proposed recently that cysteine-containing peptides produced during peptic digestion of beef increase nonheme iron bioavailability. Myosin and actin are the major myofibrillary proteins of meat. Both contain a relatively high number of free sulfhydryl groups. Myosin (MW 475,000) has 40-42 cysteine residues per molecule and actin (MW 42,000) five. Bovine serum albumin (MW 69,000) has only one. It is therefore possible that the different effects of beef and serum albumin could result from digestion products generated in the upper small intestine that differ in the level of cysteine-containing peptides.

There are several reasons to suspect that the mechanisms by which proteins modify nonheme bioavailability may be quite complex. Phytates (Hallberg et al., 1987); polyphenols (Disler et al., 1975a; Disler et al., 1975b; Gillooly et al., 1983) and inorganic calcium and phosphate salts (Monsen & Cook, 1976) have been established as important inhibitors of iron absorption in vegetable-based meals. Proteins could bind iron directly or have an indirect effect by modifying other factors that affect bioavailability. The following are possible examples. At low pH phytic acid forms electrostatic linkages with the basic lysine, arginine and histidine residues of proteins resulting in insoluble complexes that dissolve only below pH 3. At neutral and basic pH, phytate and most proteins dissociate because both have a net negative charge. However, in the presence of multivalent cations soluble protein-cation-phytate complexes occur (Graf, 1986). Vegetable proteins and phytates could both be components of an intraluminal inhibitory effect on nonheme iron absorption.

Tannin in tea is a powerful inhibitor of iron absorption (Disler et al., 1975). Gillooly et al. (1983) found a strong inverse correlation between total polyphenol content and nonheme iron absorption from vegetable meals. Torrance et al. (1982) suggested that the enhancing effect of meat in vegetable and cereal meals may merely result from a reduction in the inhibitory influence of polyphenols. Like phytate, polyphenols form strong complexes with proteins. Meat digestion products could sequester inhibitory polyphenol ligands and thus facilitate nonheme iron absorption.

Ascorbic acid is a major enhancer of nonheme iron absorption. The degree of enhancement is dose dependent (Lynch & Cook, 1980), but the relative improvement in bioavailability may be affected by other factors in the meal. Protein may be one of them. Ascorbic acid is relatively less effective in meals containing meat. Cook & Monsen (1977) examined the effect of 100 mg ascorbic acid on their SPM. The mean absorption ratio for iron from the meal with ascorbic acid to that without was 3.19. However, when the same amount of ascorbic acid was studied in the STM the absorption ratio was only 1.67. Meat appears to reduce the relative effect of ascorbic acid. At concentrations of ascorbic acid (40 mg/100 g) used for commercial fortification, a soy-based and a milk-based infant formula with similar protein contents was tested (Gillooly et al., 1984) and iron absorption was significantly better from the milk formula. The addition of 40 mg ascorbic acid to 100 g soy-based infant formula (14% protein, iron content 6 mg/100 g) did not increase iron absorption significantly (mean values 1.87 and 3.3%). Absorption did rise significantly to 6.9% with 80 mg, but the further increase with 160 mg was minimal and not statistically significant (7.7%). A direct comparison between the soy based product and a milk based formula (16% protein, iron content 6 mg/100 g) demonstrated a much greater enhancement of absorption with the latter. All of these observations point to the existence of more complex interactions between iron, protein and other iron binding ligands.

Effects of Specific Iron Storage and Transport Proteins

Iron is essential to almost all living organisms, but free ionic iron is highly toxic. Consequently, elaborate biological systems have been developed for the procurement of iron from the environment, its distribution within organisms, and storage. Proteins are an important component, particularly in animal systems. Since these proteins have high affinities for iron under certain conditions they merit special attention as factors that could modify bioavailability if resistant to digestion in the upper gastrointestinal tract of human beings.

Ferritin and hemosiderin. From a quantitative point of view the major storage proteins, ferritin and hemosiderin, are the most important. In animal tissues, 20-60% of the iron is in this form. Ferritin similar to that found in mammalian systems is also present in plants (Crichton et al., 1978; Sczekan & Joshi, 1987) and may account for a significant fraction of the iron in some soy flours (Lynch & Covell, 1987). The absorption of iron from animal ferritin has been studied in human beings using purified material biosynthetically labelled with radioiron (Hussain et al., 1965; Layrisse et al., 1975). In the latter investigation the geometric mean value for iron absorption from purified ferritin administered in a solution to fasting subjects with normal iron status was 0.9%. Values of 2.5% and 5.7% were obtained in individuals with moderate and marked iron deficiency. Mean absorption for the whole group was 1.9%, a value similar to that reported for vegetable foods and much lower than that for meat. However, these very low bioavailability values may be of little practical significance since meat enhanced absorption markedly. The mean absorption of 2 mg ferritin iron given alone was 1.3%. When given with veal muscle, absorption rose to 12%. A similar increase from 1.7% to 6.6% was seen with the addition of the liver.

Ferritin iron absorption is also modified by other factors known to affect the common nonheme pool. Vegetable foods such as maize, wheat, and soybean reduce absorption even in the presence of meat, while ascorbic acid has a marked enhancing effect (Layrisse et al., 1975; Derman et al., 1982). Iron absorption from hemosiderin, the insoluble fraction of storage iron in animal foods, is also limited when administered alone (Martinez-Torres et al., 1976). As with ferritin, it is enhanced by meat or ascorbic acid.

Although iron absorption from ferritin and hemosiderin is affected by ligands that determine common nonheme pool iron bioavailability, equilibration with the common pool may be incomplete (Layrisse et al., 1975; Martinez-Torres et al., 1976; Martinez-Torres et al., 1986). Initial studies with meat demonstrated significantly lower absorption from a trace label incorporated into purified ferritin than from biosynthetically tagged meat. In this case, the difference appeared to result from absorption of the radioiron tag in the highly available heme fraction of the meat. When dehemoglobinized meat was used, values were almost identical

(Martinez-Torres et al., 1976). However, in the case of meals containing vegetable foods, iron entering the common pool is significantly better absorbed than ferritin iron added to the same meal even in the presence of meat (Layrisse et al., 1975; Martinez-Torres et al., 1986). The nature and extent of the exchange between iron and ferritin and the common nonheme pool remains incompletely characterized.

Transferrin and lactoferrin. The effect of two other iron binding proteins on its bioavailability has been studied in human beings. Bezwoda et al. (1986) compared absorption from diferric human transferrin and ferric chloride in subjects with histamine fast achlorhydria. The geometric mean absorption values of 1.4% and 1.9% respectively were not significantly different. They concluded that transferrin does not play a significant role in human iron absorption.

Lactoferrin, a protein with several properties that are similar to those of transferrin, is present in many body fluids and is found in relatively high concentrations in human milk. Its functions in milk are uncertain. *In vitro* studies have demonstrated a bacteriostatic effect (Bullen et al., 1972; Arnold et al., 1977). Lonnerdal (1984) suggested that it might also act as a promoter of iron absorption. The marked difference in iron bioavailability between human milk and cows milk could be explained by the difference in lactoferrin concentration which is found only in low concentrations in cow's milk (Lonnerdal, 1984; Lonnerdal, 1985). Evidence for the presence of a lactoferrin receptor in the human jejunum provides some support for this postulate (Cox et al., 1979). However, lactoferrin does not enhance the absorption of iron in adult human beings (McMillan et al., 1977). The low concentration of lactoferrin in cows milk and the rapid loss of its iron binding properties on heating (Ford et al., 1977) make any important effect on nonheme bioavailability in nonbreast fed infants, older children, and adults unlikely.

Nutritional Significance of Bioavailability Studies in the Context of the Western Diet

The observations described above demonstrate that many important sources of dietary protein have a significant effect on the bioavailability of nonheme food iron when tested in single meals under experimental conditions. However, this information should be used with caution in attempts to predict the impact of changes in protein source on human iron nutrition in the context of the complex Western diet. One study involving the replacement of a portion of the meat protein in a mixed meal, with soy protein provides a good illustration of this point (Lynch et al., 1985). Table V demonstrates that the inclusion of soy protein in meat meals markedly reduced nonheme bioavailability. However, the composite effect on overall absolute iron absorption was much less. Study II is the most representative of the use of soy protein as a substitute for meat in the United States. Percentage nonheme iron absorption in the soy flour containing meal was decreased 5% to 2%, but the size of the pool was increased by the relatively high iron content of the soy flour. Although there was less heme in the substituted meal, percentage heme iron absorption was better. The net result of these different effects was a modest (28%) decrease in absolute iron absorption. Similar conclusions have been drawn by Hallberg & Rossander (1982c) using different complex meals.

Table V. Quantities of nonheme (NH), heme (H), and total (T) iron absorbed from beef and mixed beef and soy flour meals[a]

Meal[b] Studied	Form of Iron	Iron Content		Iron Absorption		Changes in Absorption
		A	B	A	B	
		mg		mg (%)		mg
I	NH	1.50	4.50	0.37 (25)	0.04 (1)	-0.33
	H	1.20	0.84	0.20 (17)	0.23 (27)	+0.03
	T	2.70	5.34	0.57 (21)	0.27 (5)	-0.30
II	NH	3.20	4.15	0.16 (5)	0.08 (2)	-0.08
	H	1.20	0.84	0.40 (33)	0.35 (42)	-0.05
	T	4.20	4.99	0.56 (13)	0.43 (9)	-0.13
III	NH	4.70	4.70	0.27 (6)	0.15 (3)	-0.12
	H	1.20	1.20	0.21 (18)	0.34 (29)	+0.13
	T	5.90	5.90	0.48 (8)	0.49 (8)	+0.01

[a] Data from Lynch et al., 1985.
[b] Meals:
   I.   A - 100 g beef patty.
        B - 70 g beef + 75 g hydrated textured soy flour.
   II. A - 100 g beef, bun, french fries, milk shake.
        B - 70 g, 30 g hydrated soy flour, bun, french fries, milk shake.
   III. A - 100 g beef, bun, french fries, milk shake, with 2.0 mg iron supplement.
        B - 100 g beef, 30 g hydrated textured soy flour, bun, french fries, milk shake.

Until we understand the factors in protein foods that are responsible for modifying the bioavailability of food iron, it will be difficult to make any general predictions about the consequences of substituting one protein source for another in the Western diet. Moreover, other enhancers of iron absorption are plentiful in Western diets. The iron status of menstruating, predominantly vegetarian women was as good as that of omnivorous women in one recent study (Bindra & Gibson, 1986), presumably because of a sufficiency of promoters of absorption other than animal tissue.

On the other hand, there is adequate justification for applying some experimental information on bioavailability directly to the design of infant formulas, infant cereals, and vegetable based food supplements. Ascorbic acid supplementation of milk based infant formulas is an effective method of improving iron bioavailability (Derman et al., 1980; Stekel et al., 1986). Similar results may be obtained with soy-based formulas, but larger quantities of ascorbic acid are required (Gillooly et al., 1984).

References

Abernathy, R. P., Miller, J., Wentworth, J., & Spiers, M. (1965) *J. Nutr.* 85, 265-270.

Arnold, R. R., Cole, M. F., & McGhee, J. R. (1977) *Science* 197, 263-265.

Bezwoda, W. R., Bothwell, T. H., Torrance, J. D., MacPhail, A. P., Charlton, R. W., Kay, G., & Levin, J. (1979) *Scand. J. Hematol.* 22, 113-120.

Bezwoda, W. R., MacPhail, A. P., Bothwell, T. H., Baynes, R. D., Derman, D. P., & Torrance, J. D. (1986) *Brit. J. Haematol.* 63, 749-752.

Bindra, G. S., & Gibson, R. S. (1986) *Am. J. Clin. Nutr.* 44, 643-652.

Bjorn-Rasmussen, E., & Hallberg, L. (1979) *Nutr. Metab.* 23, 192-202.

Bjorn-Rasmussen, E., Hallberg, L., Isaksson, B., & Arvidsson, B. (1974) *J. Clin. Invest.* 53, 247-255.

Bjorn-Rasmussen, E., Hallberg, L., & Walker, R. B. (1972) *Am. J. Clin. Nutr.* 25, 317-323.

Bjorn-Rasumssen, E., Hallberg, L., & Walker, R. B. (1973) *Am. J. Clin. Nutr.* 26, 1311-1319.

Bothwell, T. H., Charlton, R. W., Cook, J. D., & Finch, C. A. (1979) in *Iron Metabolism in Man*, Blackwell Scientific Publications, Oxford.

Bullen, J. J., Rogers, H. J., & Leigh, L. (1972) *Brit. Med. J.* 1, 69-75.

Callender, S. T., Marney, Jr., S. R., & Warner, G. T. (1970) *Brit. J. Haematol.* 19, 657-665.

Cook, J. D., Layrisse, M., Martinez-Torres, C., Walker, R., Monsen, E., & Finch, C. A. (1972) *J. Clin. Invest.* 51, 805-815.

Cook, J. D., Minnich, V., Moore, C. V., Rasmussen, A., Bradley, W. B., & Finch, C. A. (1973) *Am. J. Clin. Nutr.* 26, 861-872.

Cook, J. D., & Monsen, E. R. (1977) *Am. J. Clin. Nutr.* 30, 235-241.

Cook, J. D., Morck, T. A., & Lynch, S. R. (1981) *Am. J. Clin. Nutr.* 34, 2622-2629.

Cook, J. D., Noble, N. L., Morck, T. A., Lynch, S. R., & Petersburg, S. J. (1983) *Gastroenterology* 85, 1354-1358.

Cook, J. D., Watson, S. S., Simpson, K. M., Lipschitz, D. A., & Skikne, B. S. (1984) *Blood* 64, 721-726.

Cox, T. M., Mazurier, J., Spik, G., Montreuil, J., & Peters, T. J. (1979) *Biochim. Biophys. Acta* 588, 120-128.

Crichton, R. R., Ponce-Ortiz, Y., Koch, M. H. J., Parfait, R., & Stuhrmann, H. B. (1978) *Biochem. J.* 171, 349-356.

Derman, D. P., Bothwell, T. H., MacPhail, A. P., Torrance, J. D., Bezwoda, W. R., Charlton, R. W., & Mayet, F. G. (1980) *Scand. J. Haematol.* 25, 193-201.

Derman, D. P., Bothwell, T. H., Torrance, J. D., MacPhail, A. P., Bezwoda, W. R., Charlton, R. W., & Mayet, F. G. H. (1982) *Scand. J. Haematol.* 29, 18-24.

Derman, D., Sayers, M., Lynch, S. R., Charlton, R. W., Bothwell, T. H., & Mayet, F. (1977) *Brit. J. Nutr.* 38, 261-269.

Disler, P. B., Lynch, S. R., Charlton, R. W., Torrance, J. D., Bothwell, T. H., Walker, R. B., & Mayet, F. (1975a) *Gut* 16, 193-200.

Disler, P. B., Lynch, S. R., Torrance, J. D., Sayers, M. H., Bothwell, T. H., & Charlton, R. W. (1975b) *S. Afr. J. Sci.* 40, 109-116

Elwood, P. C., Newton, D., Eakins, J. D., & Brown, D. A. (1968) *Am. J. Clin. Nutr.* 21, 1162-1169.

Forbes, A. L., Adams, C. E., Arnaud, M. J., Chichester, C. O., Cook, J. D., Harrison, B. N., Hurrell, R. F., Kahn, S. G., Morris, E. R., Tanner, J. T., & Whittaker, P. (1988) *Am. J. Clin. Nutr.* (In press).

Ford, J. E., Law, B. A., Marshall, V. M. E., & Reiter, B. (1977) *J. Pediatr.* 90, 29-35.

Fritz, J. C., & Pla, G. W. (1972) *J. Assoc. Off. Anal. Chem.* 55, 1128-1132.

Fritz, J. C., Pla, G. W., Roberts, T., Boehne, J. W., & Hove, E. L. (1970) *J. Agric. Food. Chem.* 18, 647-651.

Gillooly, M., Bothwell, T. H., Torrance, J. D., MacPhail, A. P., Derman, D. P., Bezwoda, W. R., Mills, W., & Charlton, R. W. (1983) *Brit. J. Nutr.* 49, 331-342.

Gillooly, M, Torrance, J. D., Bothwell, T. H., MacPhail, A. P., Derman, D., Mills, W., & Mayet, F. (1984) *Am. J. Clin. Nutr.* 40, 522-527.

Graf, E. (1986) in *Phytic Acid Chemistry and Application* (Graf, E., Ed.) pp 1-21, Pilatus Press, Minneapolis, USA.

Green, R., Charlton, R. W., Seftel, H., Bothwell, T., Mayet, F., Adams, B., Finch, C., & Layrisse, M., (1968) *Am. J. Med.* 45, 336-353.

Hallberg, L. (1980) in *Iron* (Cook, J. D., Ed.) pp 116-133, Churchill Livingstone, New York, U.S.A

Hallberg, L. (1981) *Ann. Rev. Nutr.* 1, 123-147.

Hallberg, L., & Bjorn-Rasmussen, E. (1981) *Am. J. Clin. Nutr.* 34, 2808-2815.

Hallberg, L., & Rossander, L. (1982a) *Am. J. Clin. Nutr.* 35, 502-509.

Hallberg, L., & Rossander, L. (1982b) *Hum. Nutr. Appl. Nutr.* 36, 116-123.

Hallberg, L., & Rossander, L. (1982c) *Am. J. Clin. Nutr.* 36, 514-520.

Hallberg, L., Rossander, L., & Skanberg, A-B. (1987) *Am. J. Clin. Nutr.* 45, 988-996.

Hurrell, R. F., Lynch, S. R., Trinidad, T. P., Dassenko, S. A., & Cook, J. D. (1988a) *Am. J. Clin. Nutr.* 47, 102-107.

Hurrell, R. F., Lynch, S. R., Trinidad, T. P., Dassenko, S. A., & Cook, J. D. (1988b) *Am. J. Clin. Nutr.* In press.

Hussain, R., Walker, R. B., Layrisse, M., Clark, P., & Finch, C. A. (1965) *Am. J. Clin. Nutr.* 16, 464-471.

Kane, A. P., & Miller, D. M. (1984) *Am. J. Clin. Nutr.* 39, 393-401.

Layrisse, M., Cook, J. D., Martinez, C., Roche, M., Kuhn, I. N., Walker, R. B., & Finch, C. A. (1969) *Blood* 33, 430-443.

Layrisse, M., & Martinez-Torres, C. (1972) *Am. J. Clin. Nutr.* 25, 401-411.

Layrisse, M., Martinez-Torres, C., Renzi, M., & Leets, I. (1975) *Blood* 45, 689-698.

Layrisse, M., Martinez-Torres, C., & Roche, M. (1968) *Am. J. Clin. Nutr.* 21, 1175-1183.

Lönnerdal, B. (1984) in *Iron Nutrition in Infancy and Childhood*, Nestle Nutrition Workshop Series, Vol 4. (Stekel, A., Ed.) pp 95-118, Raven Press, New York, U.S.A.

Lönnerdal, B. (1985) *Am. J. Clin. Nutr.* 42, 1299-1317.

Lynch, S. R., & Cook, J. D. (1980) *Ann. N.Y. Acad. Sci.* 355, 32-44.

Lynch, S. R., & Covell, A. M., (1987) *Clin. Res.* 35, 775A

Lynch, S. R., Dassenko, S. A., Morck, T. A., Beard, J. L., & Cook, J. D. (1985) *Am. J. Clin. Nutr.* 41, 13-20.

Lynch, S. R., Hurrell, R., Dassenko, S. A., & Cook, J. D. (1986) *Clin. Res.* 34, 800A.

McMillan, J. A., Oski, F. A., Lourie, G., Tomarelli, R. M., & Landaw, S. A. (1977) *Pediatrics* 60, 896-900.

Martinez-Torres, C., & Layrisse, M. (1970) *Blood* 35, 669-682.

Martinez-Torres, C., & Layrisse, M. (1971) *Am. J. Clin. Nutr.* 24, 531-540.

Martinez-Torres, C., & Layrisse, M. (1973) in *Clinics in Haematology*, Vol. 2 (Callender, S. T., Ed.) pp 339-352, W. B. Saunders & Co., London, U.K.

Martinez-Torres, C., Leets, I., Renzi, M., & Layrisse, M. (1974) *J. Nutr.* 104, 983-993.

Martinez-Torres, C., Leets, I., Taylor, P., Ramirez, J., Camacho, M. dV., & Layrisse, M. (1986) *J. Nutr.* 116, 1720-1725.

Martinez-Torres, C., Renzi, M., & Layrisse, M. (1976) *J. Nutr.* 106, 128-135.

Martinez-Torres, C., Romano, E., & Layrisse, M. (1981) *Am. J. Clin. Nutr.* 34, 322-327.

Miller, D. D., Schricker, B. R., Rasmussen, R. R., & Van Campen, D. (1981) *Am. J. Clin. Nutr.* 34, 2248-2256.

Monsen, E. R., & Cook, J. D. (1976) *Am. J. Clin. Nutr.* 29, 1142-1148.

Monsen, E. R., Hallberg, L., Layrisse, M., Hegsted, D. M., Cook, J. D., Mertz, W., & Finch, C. A. (1978) *Am. J. Clin. Nutr.* 31, 134-141.

Moore, C. V., & Dubach, R. (1951) *Trans. Assoc. Am. Physicians* 64, 245-256.

Reddy, N. S., & Kumak, R. L. (1988) *Nutr. Reports Internat.* 37, 77-81.

Sczekan, S. R., & Joshi, J. G. (1987) *J. Biol. Chem.* 262, 13780-13788.

Slatkavitz, C. A., & Clydesdale, F. M. (1988) *Am. J. Clin. Nutr.* 47, 487-495.

Stekel, A. (1984) in *Iron Nutrition in Infancy and Childhood* (Stekel, A., Ed.) pp 1-10, Raven Press, New York, U.S.A.

Stekel, A., Olivares, M., Pizarro, F., Chadud, P., Lopez, I., & Amar, M. (1986) *Am. J. Clin. Nutr.* 43, 917-922.

Takkunen, H., & Seppanen, R. (1976) *Am. J. Clin. Nutr.* 28, 1141-1147.

Taylor, P. G., Martinez-Torres, C., Romano, E. L., & Layrisse, M. (1986) *Am. J. Clin. Nutr.* 43, 68-71.

Torrance, J. D., Gillooly, M., Mills, W., Mayet, F., & Bothwell, T. H. (1982) in *The Biochemistry and Physiology of Iron* (Saltman, P., & Hegenauer, J., Eds.) pp 819-820, Elsevier Biomedical, New York, U.S.A.

Weintraub, L. R., Weinstein, M. B., Huser, H-J., & Rafal, S. (1968) *J. Clin. Invest.* 47, 531-539.

Widdowson, E. M., & McCance, R. A. (1942) *Lancet* 1, 588-591.

9

Effect of Gastrointestinal Conditions on the Mineral–Binding Properties of Dietary Fibers[1,2]

Joseph A. Laszlo

Investigations into the relationship between dietary fiber content and mineral-nutrient bioavailability of diets have generally shown an inverse relationship (Munoz, 1986). The inhibitory effect of fiber on mineral absorption, although perhaps more appropriately attributed to phytic acid in some studies, thus seems well established. The process by which fiber exerts its inhibitory effect is less well characterized. Three modes of inhibition have been hypothesized (Kelsay, 1981): 1) fiber greatly increases fecal bulk and motility, thus reducing the time available for absorption or access to transport mechanisms; 2) fiber directly or indirectly alters luminal-to-serosal transport mechanisms in the mucosa (such as the ferritin system); 3) the formation of stable, unabsorbable mineral-fiber complexes reduces the pool of available minerals. The latter hypothesis, utilized by most investigators, as well as in this work, posits that minerals bound to large macromolecules can not be absorbed directly nor transfer to mineral-transporter moieties. Thus, within the context of the subject matter of these proceedings, the present work addresses the issue of "To what extent might a plant-derived macromolecular complex (i.e., plant cell walls) impede mineral absorption?"

Dietary fiber may be simply characterized as being the undigestible fraction of plant cell walls, although more exact definitions are available (Trowell, 1974; Trowell, 1976). Cell walls are comprised of assorted polysaccharides (cellulose, pectins and hemi-celluloses), polyphenols (lignin and tannin), and proteins (Selvendran, 1984). The amount and type of each of these polymers in the cell wall varies considerably with the plant source. Thus, the relationship between mineral bioavailability and dietary fiber may vary substantially depending on the source of the fiber.

---

1   The mention of firm names or trade products does not imply that they are endorsed or recommended by the U.S. Department of Agriculture over other firms or similar products not mentioned.

2   This article is not copyrighted, therefore is in the public domain.

Two disparate sources of dietary fiber, corn bran (pericarp) and soybean hull (seed coat), were examined in this study. The cell walls of corn, a monocot, and soybean, a dicot, differ substantially, particularly in their acidic polysaccharide content (Darvill et al., 1980). This difference should be reflected in the mineral-binding properties of the two tissues. The *in vivo* behavior of corn bran (Dintzis et al., 1985, 1989) and soybean hull (Dintzis et al., 1985; Ward & Reichert, 1986; Lykken et al., 1987; Moore & Kornegay, 1987) have been examined in relationship to mineral bioavailability, and various aspects of their mineral-binding attributes have been explored *in vitro* (Rasper, 1979; Thompson & Weber, 1979; Laszlo, 1987, 1988a,b). Both tissues are employed as ingredients in human and animal diets.

In this work, the mineral-binding properties of corn bran and soybean hull were compared under simulated monogastric gastrointestinal conditions. Although soluble pectins present in such tissues have demonstrable effects on mineral absorption (Monnier et al., 1980), only the insoluble fraction is treated here.

Experimental Procedures

Fiber sources. Dry-milled corn bran (18-30 mesh) was provided by Lauhoff Grain Co. (Danville, IL). Soybean seeds (cultivar Century) were obtained locally. Seeds were passed through a cracking mill. The hulls were collected by hand and ground to a coarse powder with a coffee mill.

Fiber preparation. For experiments in which the endogenous minerals of the fiber sources were examined, the fibers were washed extensively with 70% ethanol and then with acetone. The washed material was collected by filtration on a coarse glass filter, air dried, then stored under vacuum. The ethanol-washed corn bran and soybean hull fibers were suspended in 1.0 mM 4-morpholinepropane-sulfonic acid (Mops) buffer, pH 7.2, at a concentration of 4 g fiber/L. The fibers were stirred for 2 h at room temperature. The buffer was decanted and the process repeated. The buffer-washed fibers were washed with acetone, collected by filtration, air dried, and stored under vacuum. For experiments concerned with the binding of added minerals, buffer-washed fibers were treated with 0.05 N HCl (25 g fiber/L) and washed extensively with water. The acid-extracted fibers were collected, dried and stored as above.

Analysis of endogenous-mineral content. Buffer-washed fibers were subjected to solutions of various ionic composition to observe the extent of mineral retention by the fibers. Buffer-washed fiber (0.2 g) was suspended in a 100-mL solution. For experiments in which only the effect of pH was studied, the solution/fiber mixture was pH adjusted with dilute HCl or KOH. For studies of the effect of ionic strength, the KCl concentration of 1.0 mM Mops buffered solutions were varied. In either case, fiber was equilibrated with solution for 2 h while stirring at 25°C. The treated fiber was collected by filtration, washed with acetone, and dried under vacuum overnight. The recovered fiber samples were wet ashed by a microwave digestion procedure. Digestion was performed in a Microwave Digestion System model MDS-81D (CEM Corp., Indian Trail, NC) operated in closed-vessel mode. Samples were contained in 20-mL scintillation vials placed within 100-mL capacity Teflon digestion vessels. Trace-metal-grade nitric acid (6 mL) was added to the scintillation vials, then the samples were heated in three stages at 5, 15 and 25% power for 10 min at each stage. After cooling, the digestion vials were unsealed. Samples were taken to dryness (open-vessel mode) with a heating regime of 60, 80 and 100% power, 10 min each. The sample ash residue was suspended in 1 mL of 0.2 N HCl containing 0.5 mM ascorbic acid, then filtered through a Centrifree micropartition unit (Amicon Corp.), and stored frozen until analyzed.

Mineral analysis was performed with a Dionex 2010i series ion chromatography system. Transition metals were detected colorimetrically after post-column reaction with 4-(2-pyridylazo)resorcinol. Calcium and magnesium were detected by conductivity. The signal from either detector was fed to a Spectra-Physics 4270 reporting integrator for quantitation.

Analysis of added-mineral binding. The acid-extracted fibers were tested for their mineral-binding affinity and capacity in solutions of varying ionic composition. Acid-extracted fiber (0.1 g) was suspended in 100-mL buffered solutions. Buffered solutions were composed of 2.0 mM 4-morpholineethanesulfonic acid (Mes), and were adjusted to pH 6.0 with KOH. The use of Good's buffers (Mes or Mops) to control solution pH is justified because they don't bind cations (Good et al., 1966), nor should the zwitterionic or anionic forms of these buffers compete with cations for binding to the fibers. Solution ionic strength was adjusted by the addition of KCL. Indicated solution ionic strengths are based solely on the total K concentration, ignoring the contributions of other added ions (i.e., calcium or Mes). Calcium was added to the solutions to give total calcium concentrations of 0.05-2.5 mM. The solutions were stirred for 2 h, except where noted, and then the fiber was collected by filtration and washed sequentially with small aliquots of water and acetone. The collected fiber was dried, weighed, and extracted with 10 mL of 0.2 N HCL. The acid extract was filtered, and analyzed for calcium and potassium content by ion chromatography. Calculation of the solution free-calcium concentrations at equilibrium with the fiber was performed as described previously (Laszlo, 1987).

Results

The endogenous magnesium, calcium, iron and zinc contents of the corn-bran and soybean-hull fiber preparations are given in Table I. Soybean hull contained 10- to 20-fold greater quantities of calcium and iron. Thus, soybean hull represents a potentially richer source of nutritionally important minerals. However, the availability of minerals from these fibers for absorption may be limited by the extent to which the minerals are extracted from the matrix of the fiber under the conditions present in the gastrointestinal tract.

Simulation of stomach pH conditions. To examine the amount of minerals that may be extracted in the stomach, the fibers were subjected to treatment over a range of pH values expected to be encountered. The ionic strengths of these test solutions were not adjusted, thus were quite low. A more realistic simulation of stomach ionic conditions would include a supporting ionic strength of ~0.075 (Alexander, 1962), but this approach was not elected so that the individual effects

Table I. Mineral contents of corn bran and soy hull

Element	Mineral contents (μg/g dry wt)	
	corn bran	soy hull
Mg	400	1,360
Ca	150	3,870
Fe	15	200
Zn	10	20

of pH and ionic strength could be evaluated. The data depicted in Figure 1 demonstrate that little calcium or magnesium was removed from the fibers over the pH range 4.5-6.0. Below pH 4.5, calcium and magnesium were substantially extracted, with little or none remaining below pH 3.0. The behavior of zinc and iron in these tissues is strikingly different (Figure 2). At or above pH 4.0, zinc and iron were not extracted. Over the pH range 3.2-0.7, zinc in both tissues and iron in corn bran were progressively extracted. Much higher acid concentrations were required to remove iron from soybean hull. These results imply that the fibers bind zinc and iron more tightly than calcium or magnesium.

The acid extractability of soybean-hull iron was examined more closely. The cultivar of soybean utilized in this study contained approximately equal proportions of Fe(II) and Fe(III) in the hull (Laszlo, 1988a). Figure 3 shows the extent of extraction of each of these ions at various HCl concentrations. At HCl concentrations approaching the lower achievable physiological stomach pH range (~pH 1.0), Fe(II) was readily extracted, substantially more so than Fe(III). Only 2.0 N HCl was able to quantitatively remove Fe(III) from the soybean hull. More than 90% of the corn-bran iron was found to be in the Fe(II) oxidation state. This suggests that the difference between soybean-hull and corn-bran iron extractability (Figure 2) is due to the presence of the more tightly bound Fe(III) in soybean hull.

Simulation of small intestine ionic conditions. As food passes from the stomach to the intestinal tract, it mixes with secretions from the pancreas resulting in a nearly-neutral pH, high ionic strength solution. The mineral-binding behavior of corn-bran and soybean-hull fibers was examined under simulated small intestine ionic conditions.

It is presumed in these simulations that ingested fibers are in contact with digesta media sufficiently long to allow complete equilibrium of fiber and digesta ionic constituents to be achieved. The adequacy of this assumption was tested. Figure 4 demonstrates the time required for two samples of hydrated, acid-extracted corn bran to equilibrate with a solution containing calcium. Corn-bran fiber bound its maximum amount of calcium (i.e., reached equilibrium) within 30 min. Ninety-five percent of the equilibrium value was reached in about 15 min. This implies that ingested fiber should have little difficulty in equilibrating with digesta ions during transit, at least when fully hydrated and not enveloped in food boluses or fecal matter. Therefore, fiber-solution ion exchanges examined at equilibrium adequately reflect the *in vivo* state.

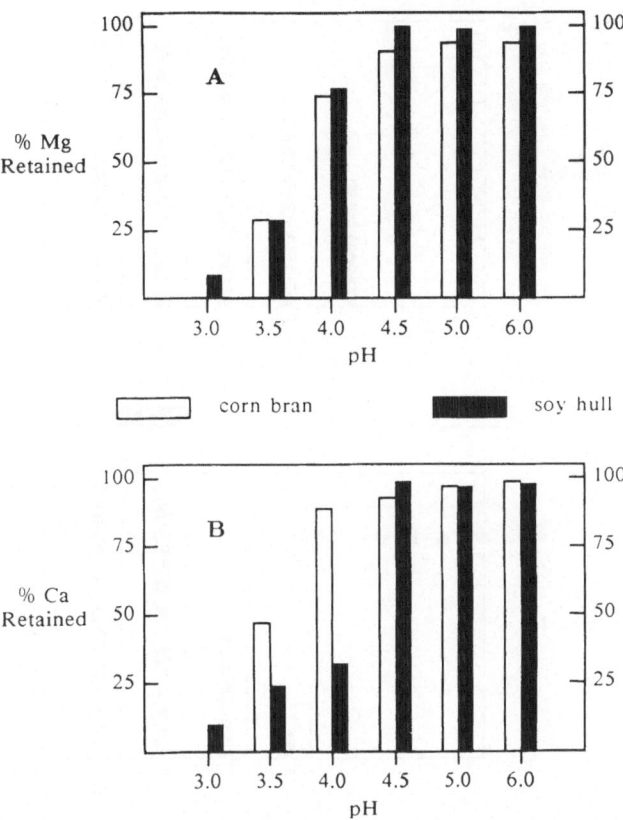

Figure 1. Effect of simulated gastric pH on Ca and Mg contents of fibers. Buffer-washed corn-bran and soybean-hull fibers were treated with solutions at indicated pH values, then examined for amounts of endogenous (A) magnesium and (B) calcium remaining in the fibers. See Table I for mineral contents of untreated samples.

Depending on the acidity of the stomach, the minerals in soybean hull and corn bran may be only partially extracted, as indicated by the results given above, before passing into the small intestine. Figure 5 shows that the calcium and magnesium present in these fibers are progressively more extracted in higher ionic strength media. Thus, the high salt conditions of the intestine should facilitate removal of calcium and magnesium. Note, however, that soybean hull retained a greater proportion of these ions than corn bran at any given ionic strength. This suggests that soybean hull binds calcium and magnesium more tightly. Also, at any given ionic strength, more calcium was retained than magnesium (percentage basis) in either fiber. Solutions with KCl concentrations as high as 150 mM released less than 10% of the iron and zinc from these samples (data not shown). Therefore, while any residual quantities of calcium or magnesium in the fibers leaving the stomach would be extracted in the small intestine, iron and zinc would remain bound.

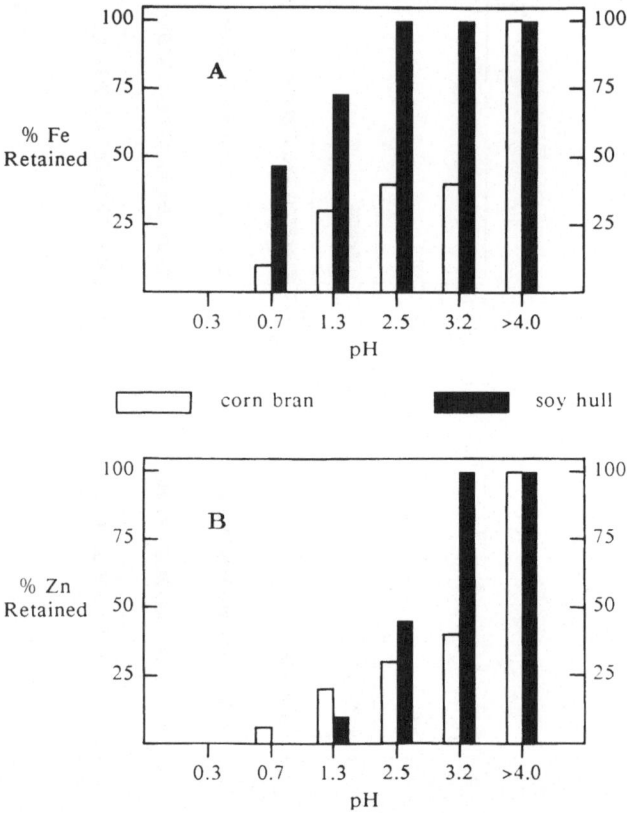

Figure 2. Effect of simulated gastric pH on Fe and Zn contents of fibers. Buffer-washed corn bran and soybean hull were examined for amount of (A) Fe (total) and (B) Zn retained after treatment in various pH solutions. The control (100%) values are given in Table I.

To test whether demineralized fiber emptying from the stomach may re-bind nutritionally important minerals in the small intestine, the mineral-binding capacity and affinity of corn bran and soybean hull were investigated. The total ion-binding capacity of the corn-bran fiber was 195 ± 5 μeq/g dry wt. Figure 6 demonstrates the relationship between solution calcium concentration and the amount of calcium bound by acid-extracted corn bran in various ionic strength media. As expected, the extent of calcium bound was proportional (but not linearly so) to solution free-calcium concentration, and inversely proportional to solution monovalent cation concentration. In 100 mM KCl, calcium filled less than 25% of the corn-bran ion-exchange sites at solution calcium concentrations exceeding the likely physiological level (< 2.5 mM) of free calcium. This is in agreement with the observed effects of ionic strength on endogenous-calcium binding in corn bran (Figure 5).

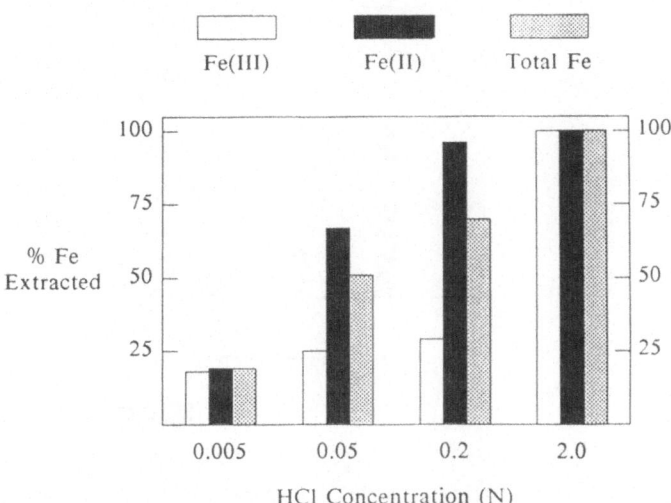

Figure 3. Effect of HCl concentration on iron contents of buffer-washed soybean hulls.

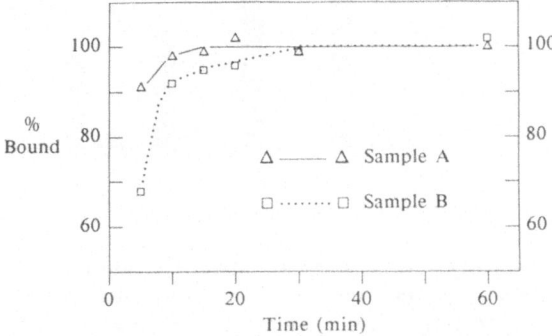

Figure 4. Time required for corn bran to equilibrate with calcium. Two identical samples (A and B) of acid-extracted corn bran (0.2 g) were suspended in 100-mL 2.0 mM Mes buffer, pH 6.0, containing 10 mM potassium. After rehydrating the corn bran for 1 h, Ca was added to a final concentration of 0.25 mM. At time intervals, aliquots (0.75 mL) were sampled to measure free Ca. Bound Ca values were calculated by subtraction of free values from the total (initial) value, and expressed as a percentage of the values found after 24 h.

In similar fashion, the relative affinities of acid-extracted soybean-hull and corn-bran fibers for calcium were compared. At any given solution concentration of calcium and monovalent cations, soybean hull bound a greater total amount of calcium (not shown) and filled a higher percentage of its available binding sites with calcium (Figure 7). This behavior is consistent with the indication of a

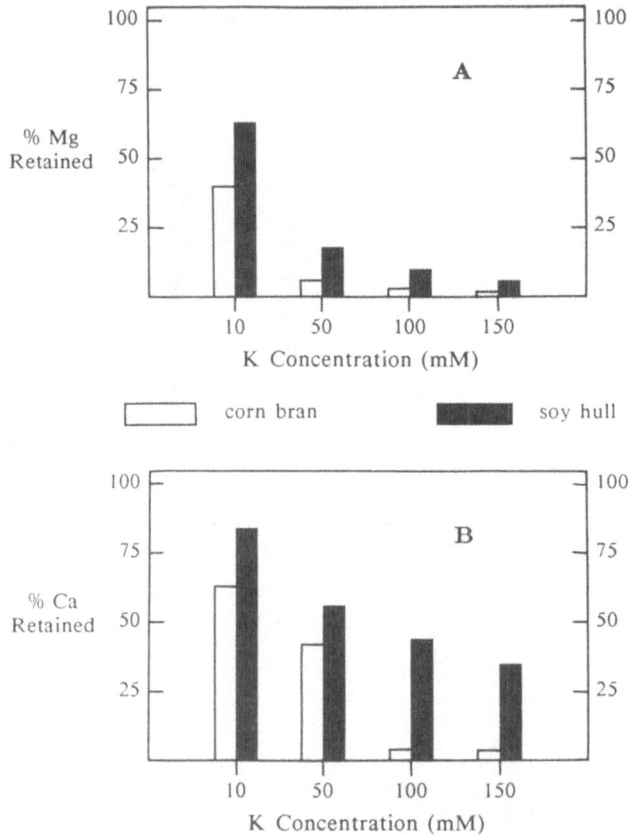

Figure 5. Effect of simulated small intestinal ionic conditions on Mg and Ca in fibers. Buffer-washed corn bran and soybean hulls were treated in 1.0 mM Mops buffer, pH 7.2, with KCl added to adjust the final solution K concentration to the indicated values. (A) Magnesium and (B) calcium contents were measured on the treated fibers and compared to the mineral values given in Table I.

greater binding affinity of soybean hull for calcium suggested by the data in Figure 5. The total ion-exchange capacity of acid-washed soybean hull was approximately twice that of corn bran.

Discussion

The vast majority of ion-exchange (i.e., cation binding) sites in dietary fiber are contributed by acidic polysaccharides present in the plant cell wall. Since dicot cell walls usually contain far more acidic polysaccharides than monocot cell walls, it is not surprising that the soybean hull tissue was found to have a higher cation-binding capacity, and a concomitantly higher level of endogenous minerals

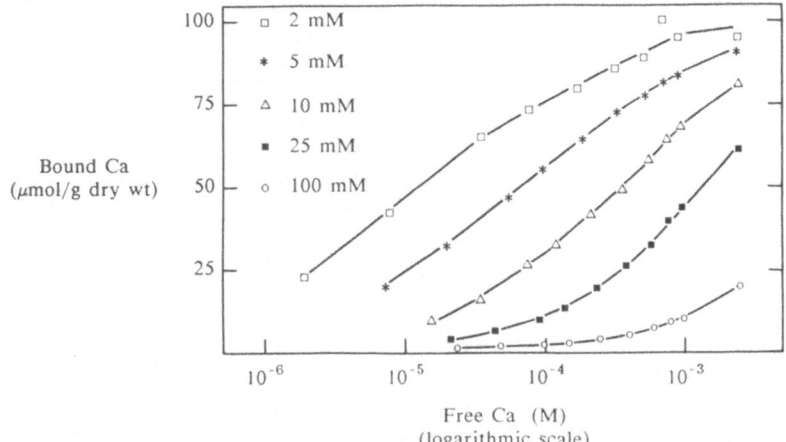

Figure 6. Relationship between calcium concentration, ionic strength, and calcium bound to corn bran. Acid-extracted corn bran was equilibrated with solutions of varying ionic strength (K concentration) and Ca, then examined for Ca content. (See Experimental Procedures for details.)

than corn bran tissue (Table I). In fact, much of the binding capacity of soybean hull is lost by the removal of pectins during the buffer-wash step (Aspinall et al., 1966, 1967; Schweizer & Würsch, 1979; Laszlo, 1987). Rasper (1979) found similar cation-exchange capacities of dietary fibers prepared by several different methods from corn bran to that reported here. Thus, while soybean hull may serve as a greater source of minerals than corn bran, it may potentially act as a greater sink for nutritionally important minerals under physiological conditions.

In addition to defining the total mineral binding capacity of a fiber (James et al., 1978), the uronic acid groups of the constituent acidic polysaccharides determine ion selectivity as well. Typically, plant cell walls display a relative binding affinity for divalent cations of: Cu > Fe, Zn > Ca > Mg (Van Cutsem & Gillet, 1982, 1983; Amory & Dufey, 1984). Previous work on acid-extracted soybean hulls demonstrated they too exhibit this trend (Laszlo, 1987). The extraction behavior of calcium and magnesium in soybean-hull and corn-bran fiber by protons (Figure 1) or salts (Figure 5) was entirely consistent with the notion that these ions are bound to uronic acid groups. However, it is unclear why soybean hull bound calcium more tightly than did corn bran under similar solution ionic conditions (Figures 5 and 7). Two causes can be suggested. The type of uronic acid comprising the acidic polysaccharide fraction of each tissue might be different, with different intrinsic affinities for calcium (and maybe magnesium). Alternatively, the concentration of uronic acid groups may differ, giving rise to different Donnan potentials between the fibers and test solutions (Dainty & Hope, 1961; Sentenac & Grignon, 1981). Resolution of this question will require further compositional and physical studies.

The properties of the endogenous iron and zinc, particularly iron in soybean hull, strongly suggest that these ions are bound to the fibers other than by uronic

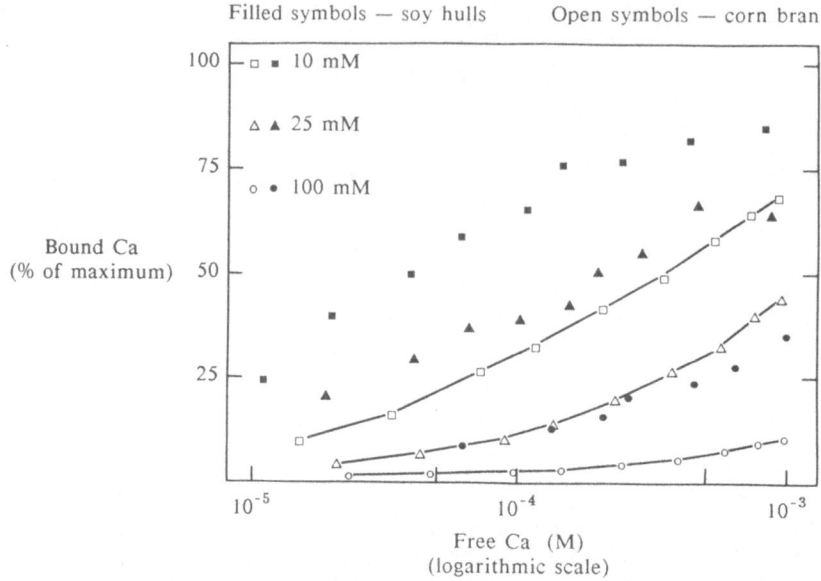

Figure 7. Comparison of calcium binding to corn bran and soybean hull. Acid-extracted corn bran and soybean hull were treated as in Figure 6.

acid groups. Both the very low pH required for extraction (Figures 2 and 3) and ineffectiveness of high salt concentrations are indicative of the presence of other types of mineral-binding sites in these fibers. The inability of low pH to extract iron from the soybean-hull tissue has been noted by others (Thompson & Weber, 1979). The unusual oxidation-reduction properties of the soybean-hull iron also suggests a unique binding site environment (Laszlo, 1988b). Phytic acid, a metal chelator commonly found in dietary fiber preparations, is not present in these tissues (Graf & Dintzis, 1982). Lignin, a potential iron-binding polymer (Fernandez & Phillips, 1982; Platt & Clydesdale, 1987), is present in these tissues at low levels (Rasper, 1979). However, the phenolic groups in lignin have such a high pKa that ferrous iron binding occurs only near neutrality (Reinhold et al., 1981). The tenacity with which soybean hull retains its iron at low pH seems to rule out a role for lignin in the binding of endogenous minerals. In fact, the release of the very tightly held iron at low pH may reflect a pH-induced structural change of the iron-binding site, rather than a simple proton-iron exchange reaction.

The applicability of the results reported herein are dependent on how well the *in vitro* conditions employed mimic *in vivo* states. *In situ* measurements of human stomach acidity suggest that pH 2.0 is an appropriate value to utilize when modeling normal (i.e., healthy) gastric conditions (Ovesen et al., 1986). Ingestion of food causes a transient pH rise, but the original gastric pH value is restored within about an hour (Ovesen et al., 1986). Therefore, it would be expected that all minerals except iron would be completely extracted, or nearly so, from the studied fibers in the human stomach. However, the certainty of such an assertion may be questioned. Tadesse (1986) has recently demonstrated that the buffering capacity of ingested fiber is sufficient to significantly raise the pH (> 3.0) of the gastric contents. Thus the minerals may be less than completely solubilized.

The poor extractability of soybean-hull iron seems to be at odds with reports of its high bioavailability (Jacob et al., 1980; Lykken et al., 1987). Part of this apparent disparity may be due to the fact that the soybean-hull samples examined in this work were depleted of a soluble fraction representing 10-25% of the hull iron (Laszlo, unpublished observation). This iron may be associated with the solubilized pectins, and may be the source of bioavailable iron. Other components of the gastrointestinal tract (i.e., free amino acids, bile salts, etc), while effective in increasing iron solubility in certain food systems (Slatkavitz & Clydesdale, 1988), are not expected to increase the extractability of soybean-hull iron because strong iron-chelating agents such as EDTA are ineffective (Laszlo, unpublished observation). The one exception, ascorbic acid, has been shown to solubilize a substantial portion of soybean-hull iron (Laszlo, 1988a,b).

The mineral content of corn bran during passage through the swine gastrointestinal tract has been recently examined by Dintzis and co-workers (Dintzis et al., 1989). Their work indicated that the calcium content of corn bran actually increased in the stomach, contradicting the *in vitro* studies described here. One plausible explanation for this apparent discrepancy rests on the observation of Alexander (1962) that the pig stomach pH falls in the range of 4.2-5.1, substantially higher than human gastric pH and more nearly in the region where corn bran can bind significant quantities of calcium. This fact, coupled with the very high mineral supplementation of swine feed and the relatively low amount of calcium initially in corn bran, may produce conditions wherein calcium loading of bran proceeds in accordance with the *in vitro* model.

Although two diverse sources of dietary fiber were examined in this study, several potential mineral-binding components commonly found associated with other dietary fibers were not included. Lignins, tannins, phytic acid and silica all may significantly alter the mineral-binding properties of fiber, changing both its ion-exchange capacity and ion selectivity (or rather, providing multiple ion selectivities).

A critical question left unanswered by this research is whether fiber from corn bran or soybean hull, or dietary fiber in general, diminishes mineral bioavailability. If it does, then the present study suggests that fiber affects mineral absorption by a process other than by virtue of its inherent ion-exchange properties. Future research may well lead us to find that fiber, in-of-itself, has no significant adverse impact on human mineral nutrition. Such a conclusion, as yet unproven, will not negate the value of current investigations into fiber-mineral interactions. Work in this field has broader significance in terms of understanding the mechanisms of mineral absorption in the human gastrointestinal tract.

References

Alexander, F. (1962) *Res. Vet. Sci.* 3, 78-84.
Amory, D. L., & Dufey, J. E. (1984) *Plant Soil* 80, 181-190.

Aspinall, G. O., Hunt, K., & Morrison, I. M. (1966) *J. Chem. Soc.* 1966, 1945-1949.

Aspinall, G. O., Hunt, K., & Morrison, I. M. (1967) *J. Chem. Soc.* 1967c, 1080-1086.

Dainty, J., & Hope, A. B. (1961) *Aust. J. Biol. Sci.* 14, 541-551.

Darvill, A., McNeil, M., Albersheim, P., & Delmer, D. P. (1980) in *The Biochemistry of Plants* (Tolbert, N. E., Ed.) Vol 1, pp 91-162, Academic Press, New York.

Dintzis, F. R., Baker, F. L., & Calvert, C. (1989) *Biol. Trace Elem. Res.* 19, in press.

Dintzis, F. R., Watson, P. R., & Sandstead, H. H. (1985) *Am. J. Clin. Nutr.* 41, 901-908.

Fernandez, R., & Phillips, S. F. (1982) *Amer. J. Clin. Nutr.* 35, 100-106.

Good, N. E., Winget, G. E., Winter, W., Connolly, T. N., Izawa, S., & Singh, R. M. M. (1966) *Biochemistry* 5, 467-477.

Graf, E., & Dintzis, F. R. (1982) *Anal. Biochem.* 119, 413-417.

Jacob, R. A., Sandstead, H. H., Klevay, L. M., & Johnson, L. K. (1980) *Blood*, 56, 786-791.

James, W. P. T., Branch, W. J., & Southgate, D. A. T. (1978) *Lancet* 1, 638-639.

Kelsay, J. L. (1981) *Cereal Chem.* 58, 2-5.

Laszlo, J. A. (1987) *J. Agric. Food Chem.* 35, 593-600.

Laszlo, J. A. (1988a) *Cereal Chem.* 65, 20-23.

Laszlo, J. A. (1988b) in *Soybean Utilization Alternatives* (McCann, L., Ed.) pp 333-341, University of Minnesota Press, St. Paul.

Lykken, G. I., Mahalko, J. R., Nielsen, E. J., & Dintzis, F. R. (1987) *J. Food Sci.* 52, 1545-1548.

Monnier, l., Colette, C., Aguirre, L., & Mirouze, J. (1980) *Am. J. Clin. Nutr.* 33, 1225-1232.

Moore, R. J., & Kornegay, E. T. (1987) *Nutr. Rep. Int.* 36, 1237-1249.

Munoz, J. M. (1986) in *CRC Handbook of Dietary Fiber in Human Nutrition* (Spiller, G. A., Ed.) pp 193-200, CRC Press, Boca Raton.

Ovesen, L., Bendtsen, F., Tage-Jensen, U., Pedersen, N. T., Gram, B. R., & Rune, S. J. (1986) *Gastroenterology* 90, 958-962.

Platt, S. R., & Clydesdale, F. M. (1987) *J. Food Sci.* 52, 1414-1419.

Rasper, V. F. (1979) in *Dietary Fibers: Chemistry and Nutrition* (Inglett G. E., & Falkehag S. I., Eds.) pp 93-115, Academic Press, New York.

Reinhold, J. G., Garcia L, J. S., & Garzon, P. (1981) *Am. J. Clin. Nutr.* 34, 1384-1391.

Schweizer, T. F., & Würsch, P. (1979) *J. Sci. Food Agric.* 30, 613-619.

Selvendran, R. R. (1984) *Amer. J. Clin. Nutr.* 39, 320-337.

Sentenac, H., & Grignon, C. (1981) *Plant Physiol.* 68, 415-419.

Slatkavitz, C. A., & Clydesdale, F. M. (1988) *Am. J. Clin. Nutr.* 47, 487-495.

Spiller, G. A. (1986) in *CRC Handbook of Dietary Fiber in Human Nutrition* (Spiller, G. A., Ed.) pp 15-18, CRC Press, Boca Raton.

Tadesse, K. (1986) *Brit. J. Nutr.* 55, 507-513.

Thompson, S. A., & Weber, C. W. (1979) *J. Food Sci.* 44, 752-754.

Trowell, H. (1974) *Lancet* 1, 503.

Trowell, H., Southgate, D. A. T., Wolever, T. M. S., Leeds, A. R., Gassull, M. A., & Jenkins, D. J. A. (1976) *Lancet* 1, 967.

Van Cutsem, P., & Gillet, C. (1982) *J. Exp. Bot.* 33, 847-853.

Van Cutsem, P., & Gillet, C. (1983) *Plant Physiol.* 73, 865-867.

Ward, A. T., & Reichert, R. D. (1986) *J. Nutr.* 116, 233-241.

10

In Vivo Mineral Contents of Dietary Fiber Determined by EDX Analysis[1,2]

Frederick R. Dintzis[3], Frederick L. Baker and Tim S. Stahly

In the past fifteen years there has been extensive research into relationships between the dietary fiber content of human and animal diets and health and nutrition. A continuing concern is that binding of minerals to dietary fiber may impair mineral bioavailability (Kies, 1985; Sandstrom et al., 1987). The *in vitro* binding of elements such as Ca, Fe, Mg, and Zn to various fiber substrates has been reported (Camire & Clydesdale, 1981; Reinhold et al., 1981). Numerous feeding studies in recent literature (reviewed by Kelsay, 1986) also address questions of effects on mineral bioavailability of dietary fiber in human and animal diets. An interesting question is whether or not the plant cell walls of the dietary fiber source impede mineral absorption by acting as mineral sinks that remove significant amounts of cations from the intestinal lumen. However, there are relatively few studies that examine changes in the mineral content of such tissues to directly measure *in vivo* mineral binding.

The feasibility of directly measuring *in vivo* binding of minerals to dietary fiber by energy-dispersive X-ray (EDX) analysis was demonstrated in an earlier study (Dintzis et al., in press). Mineral content of corn pericarp (corn bran or the hull of the maize kernel) retrieved from the stomach, ileum, and rectum of killed pigs was examined by EDX analysis. We have now applied and extended techniques of EDX analysis to examine the mineral content of oat hulls as a function of location during passage through the pig gastrointestinal (GI) tract. The pig was chosen as a model animal because of similarities of digestive physiology with humans (Cummings, 1981; Miller & Ullrey, 1987). Oat hull (husk) was chosen as a tissue because its initial mineral content differs significantly from corn bran and,

---

1 The mention of firm names or trade products does not imply that they are endorsed or recommended by the U.S. Department of Agriculture over other firms or similar products not mentioned.

2 This article is not copyrighted, therefore is in the public domain.

3 Author to whom correspondence should be addressed.

like corn bran, is relatively indigestible. Hence, it is a substrate of approximately constant composition and morphology and, therefore, suitable for testing the general applicability of EDX analysis and for determining *in vivo* mineral binding characteristics.

The principles and techniques of EDX analysis have been presented by Goldstein et al. (1981). In EDX analysis, a specimen is bombarded with electrons and a portion of the characteristic X-rays generated during the collisions with elements in the sample are collected by an energy-sensitive detector. The numbers of X-rays characteristic of a given element that are generated and counted depend upon many factors, some of which are: electron beam energy and current, number of atoms of the element excited by the electron beam in the target micro-volume, atomic number of the element, and average atomic number and density of the target. Two basic assumptions, on which this study is based, are: 1) that X-ray counts measured over three areas of a specimen cross-section adequately represent an average within the specimen, and 2) that such averages are proportional to element concentrations within the specimen.

Experimental

Four pigs, Hampshire × Yorkshire barrows, were fed a diet consisting of ground corn and dehulled soybean meal, 68% and 19% respectively, 10% oat hulls, and usual mineral and vitamin supplements. Purchased oat hulls were ground through a 1/4-inch screen before they were added to the diet. Whole oat hulls (donated by the Quaker Oats Co., Cedar Rapids, IA) were used for *in vitro* mineral loading studies. The animals were housed in concrete-floored pens, bedded with straw, in an open-front building and were permitted to feed *ad libitum*. At the start of this 92-day feeding experiment the average age of the pigs was 105 days. Average initial and final weights, respectively, were 47 kg and 119 kg. To ensure that the GI tract contained normal amounts of digesta, neither feed nor water was withdrawn prior to slaughter. At the termination of the experiment the pigs were removed from their pens, loaded on a common truck, shipped four miles to the University Meat Laboratory, and killed approximately 2 h after removal from their pens. Digesta were collected immediately after each animal was electrically stunned and bled. The samples were removed from the stomach, terminal ileum, proximal colon (15 to 30 cm post-cecal), distal colon, and the rectum and placed directly into plastic cups, frozen and freeze-dried. The freeze-dried samples were then shipped to Peoria where they were stored initially at 0-4°C. These hygroscopic samples were later transferred to glass jars and stored at room temperature until needed.

The oat hull fragments, which were easily identifiable, were first separated from digesta by sieving over a 20 mesh screen (U.S.S.-A.S.T.M., 0.86 mm openings). Individual hull fragments were then picked out with tweezers while the sieved material was viewed with the aid of a 10× binocular microscope. Hull fragments were also picked directly from unsieved digesta. Particles of corn pericarp, while present in much lower quantities than oat hull fragments, also were identified and were of sufficient size to provide suitable specimens. Thus, particles of oat hull (glume and lemma) and corn pericarp were available from the same sample of intestinal contents retrieved from a specific part of the GI tract.

Details of specimen preparation have been given previously and therefore will be summarized only briefly (Dintzis et al., in press). After oat hull fragments had been embedded directly in effapoxy resin (Ernest F. Fullam, Inc. Latham, NY), transverse sections were sawed perpendicular to the longitudinal axis of the hull. Embedded specimens were dry-cut by a glass knife on a Porter-Blum microtome and mounted on 3/8" diameter × 1/16" thick, spectroscopic-grade, carbon planchets so that the longitudinal axis of the hull was perpendicular to the planchet surface. These bulk specimens were about 1.0 mm thick. The microtomed areas varied with the size of the hull fragment cross-section and could be quite large, perhaps up to 1.0 mm × 0.5 mm. X-ray counts were taken on carbon-coated specimens.

X-ray measurements were made with an ISI-SS130 scanning electron microscope equipped with a microprobe detector with a 12 mm^2 beryllium window. Count data were processed with a Princeton Gamma Tech System 4. An electron beam voltage of 15 kV, a beam current of 1.0 nA, an angle of 47 deg (take-off angle) between planchet surface and detector, a working distance of 20 mm from sample to detector and a 5 min counting period, were used for all measurements.

A scanning electron micrograph of a sectioned oat hull is presented in Figure 1. The surrounding embedding resin, top left and bottom right, has pulled away from the plant tissue. In addition to the existence of voids, the heterogeneity of substrate morphology is evident as indicated by the folded and compressed cell walls. Oat hull and corn pericarp sections were scanned with the electron beam so as to include most of the width dimension, but not the embedding resin at the edges. This was done to minimize the risk of generating X-rays from extraneous digesta that might adhere to the hulls' exterior. Such materials were presumed to contain high mineral concentrations typical of digesta. X-ray counts, designated "resin blank," were taken on areas of the microtomed, carbon-coated, embedding resin to serve as a control for spurious counts that might occur from interactions within the specimen chamber/resin.

An average of about 1100 total counts per second was obtained from the oat hull specimens. X-ray count values presented for elements in the table and figures were background corrected. The background-corrected count for an element was a small fraction of the total count from the specimen. Thus, the mean background-corrected count from oat hulls loaded with 3160 ppm calcium was 3180 counts per 5 minutes (Figure 2). Counts for calcium were corrected by subtracting overlapping counts from potassium k-beta X-rays. Powdered KCl was used as a calibration standard to determine that in our system the overlapping potassium k-beta counts were 7% of the potassium k-alpha signal.

Oat hulls were loaded *in vitro* to prepare batches of tissues containing known concentrations of elements. This was done to establish a relationship between the mineral content of the hulls and the X-ray count values (Figure 2). The hulls, 5–10 g, were immersed overnight at room temperature in 1.0 L of appropriate salt solutions (KCl, CaCl$_2$, KH$_2$PO$_4$). Concentrations of salts up to 1.0 M were used to obtain maximum loading. After the hulls had been in contact with these high salt concentrations, they were aspirated dry on filter paper, rinsed for 30 s in a 0.1 M solution of the salt, aspirated dry, then rinsed in 95% ethanol, aspirated dry, and finally dried in a vacuum oven at room temperature and stored in glass jars. This procedure was helpful in preventing formation of salt residues on the hull exterior. If such residues were observed during routine observation with a 60×

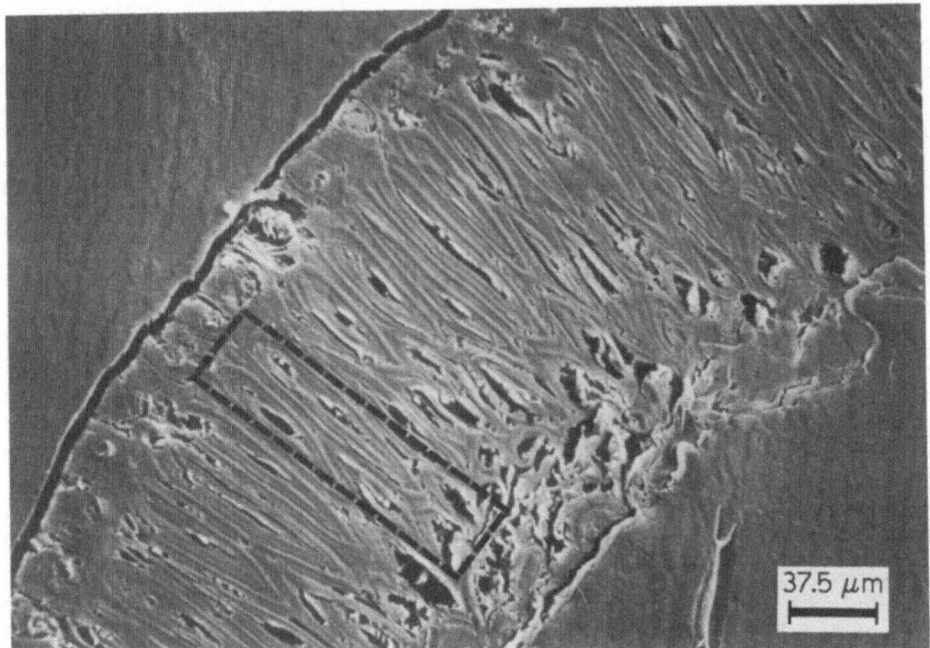

Figure 1. Scanning electron micrograph of Au-Pd shadowed oat hull specimen, original magnification approximately 400×. The rectangle enclosed by the dashed lines represents a hypothetical area scanned by the electron beam during a five-minute counting period. Three different, non-contiguous, areas were scanned within each specimen cross-section.

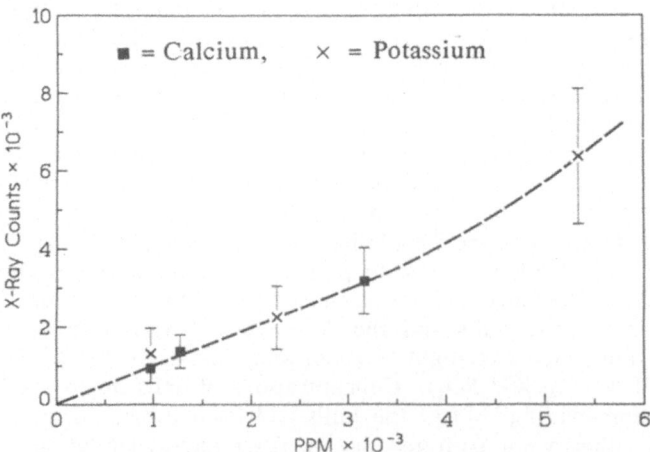

Figure 2. Relationship between concentrations of Ca and K in oat hulls loaded *in vitro* (as determined by atomic absorption) and X-ray counts taken from specimen cross-sections. Each mean represents 18 observations: 6 specimens × 3 different areas within each cross-section.

microscope, an additional washing of these dried tissues, for 1 min or less, with 50 mL distilled water or with a salt solution, 0.01-0.05 M, was needed to remove the salt residues.

From each 5-10 g batch of loaded oat hulls, six different hull fragments were selected to be sources of specimens, one from each fragment, to be examined with the electron beam. X-ray count averages obtained from the six specimens were considered to be representative of the specific batch of *in vitro* loaded tissue. Our assumption was that the organic composition and morphology of these hulls would be sufficiently similar to hulls retrieved from the pigs that the *in vitro* loaded specimens could serve as calibration sources for the *in vivo* loaded tissues.

Concentrations of minerals in the hulls and digesta were determined by atomic absorption measurements (Garcia et al., 1972). Samples of mineral-loaded oat hulls or digesta, 0.5-1.0 g, were wet-ashed and prepared as 25.0 mL solutions. Mineral contents of digesta refer to total mineral contents of the freeze-dried solids and do not indicate the amounts of mineral available as ionic species during GI tract residence. The oat hull and corn pericarp had the desirable properties of remaining intact and relatively rigid, both prior to and after passage through the pig GI tract and after *in vitro* mineral loading.

Digesta from four pigs were examined. For three of the pigs samples were available from each location (stomach, ileum, proximal colon, distal colon and rectum); in the remaining pig sufficient amounts of GI tract contents were available only from the proximal and distal colon. The mineral content of digesta at each location in each pig was measured at least once, and frequently in duplicate. Three oat hull specimens were prepared from three randomly chosen particles obtained from digesta retrieved at a specific location from each pig. X-ray counts were obtained from three randomly chosen and separated areas within the cross-section of each specimen. In like manner, X-ray counts were made on corn bran specimens obtained from the stomach, ileum, and rectum of two pigs.

Results

The relationship between X-ray counts measured from oat hull specimens loaded with potassium or calcium and concentrations of these elements determined by atomic absorption is displayed in Figure 2. Within the experimental error of comparing X-ray counts from relatively few particles with the macro-concentration in 0.5 g distributions of a large number of particles, the relationship is linear within the 0-4000 ppm concentration range and the same for both elements. However, at higher concentrations (data not shown), X-ray counts are greater than would be predicted from count values at lower mineral concentrations.

Histograms in Figures 3 through 6 present pooled data from the pigs. For greater clarity, only the upper half of the standard deviation (error bar) is shown. X-ray counts of Na, K, and Ca from initial oat hulls and hulls retrieved from a given GI tract location are in the left portion of each figure and concentrations (ppm, obtained by atomic absorption) in initial oat hulls and in digesta are in the right part of the figures. Thus, the left and right ordinates are different. It is appropriate to compare quantitatively the magnitude of the bars in either the right or left set of a specific figure and the overall symmetry of the envelopes of the two sets of histograms, but not the heights of bars in one set with the heights of the bars in the other. The X-ray count values of sodium include a significant "resin blank" contribution, 2630 ± 350 counts/5 min, from either the embedding resin or specimen chamber interactions, or from both of these sources. Significant X-ray counts were not detected for K, Ca, P, or S when the embedding resin was examined.

The patterns of pooled measurements on sodium, Figure 3, demonstrated the greatest symmetry between magnitude of X-ray counts in oat hull specimens and concentration of an element in digesta. In general, coefficients of variation (CV) in X-ray counts were lowest for sodium. The X-ray count pattern showed that sodium was: 1) loaded onto oat hull in the stomach; 2) greatly increased in the hulls in the ileum, 3) unloaded as the hulls passed through the large intestine. Sodium concentrations in digesta exhibited a pattern similar to X-ray counts in retrieved oat hulls. The higher values of sodium X-ray counts from oat hulls at various GI tract locations versus initial oat hulls were all significant at a level of $P < 0.001$, where P, the probability of no difference between means, was determined by analysis of variance. Higher sodium contents of digesta from the ileum versus stomach, distal colon and rectum digesta samples, respectively, were significant, $P < 0.001$. Sodium content of proximal colon digesta was different from that of other locations, $P < 0.01$; there was no significant difference between sodium content of digesta from distal colon and rectum. Initial oat hull contained less sodium than all digesta samples, $P < 0.0001$. The amount of sodium in the initial hulls, approximately 100 ppm, was too low to provide counts above the "resin blank" background.

The behavior of potassium, Figure 4, was different than that of sodium. Note that the X-ray counts show potassium was unloaded from the oat hull in the stomach, $P < 0.01$. The X-ray counts then increased to a relatively constant level in hulls retrieved from ileum, proximal colon and distal colon such that differences were non-significant, $P > 0.05$. Potassium counts from rectum oat hulls were higher than from hulls retrieved at other locations, $P < 0.001$. Concentrations of potassium in digesta from the stomach were lower than in digesta from the proximal colon, distal colon, rectum, and in the initial oat hulls, $P < 0.01$. Concentrations of potassium were not significantly different between initial oat hulls and digesta from ileum, proximal colon and distal colon. Digesta from the rectum had greater potassium concentrations than from the stomach, $P < 0.01$, or distal colon, $P < 0.05$, or in initial oat hulls, $P < 0.01$.

The pattern of calcium X-ray counts in oat hulls from the GI tract, Figure 5, is quite different from that of calcium concentrations in the digesta. Except for a higher mean count from oat hulls retrieved from the proximal colon, the trend is that of decreasing calcium counts as the hulls traveled through the GI tract. Counts from the initial hulls were significantly lower than counts from hulls retrieved from locations other than the rectum: for initial hulls versus hulls from stomach, $P < 0.001$. While concentrations of calcium in digesta were not significantly different between stomach and ileum, the general trend was that of an increase in concentration from ileum to rectum.

The X-ray counts of phosphorus and sulfur, Figure 6, were low and therefore subject to greater variation. Phosphorus counts were significantly lower from initial hulls versus hulls from the GI tract. Sulfur counts from hulls from the ileum were significantly higher than in hulls from all other locations, $P < 0.001$. Sulfur

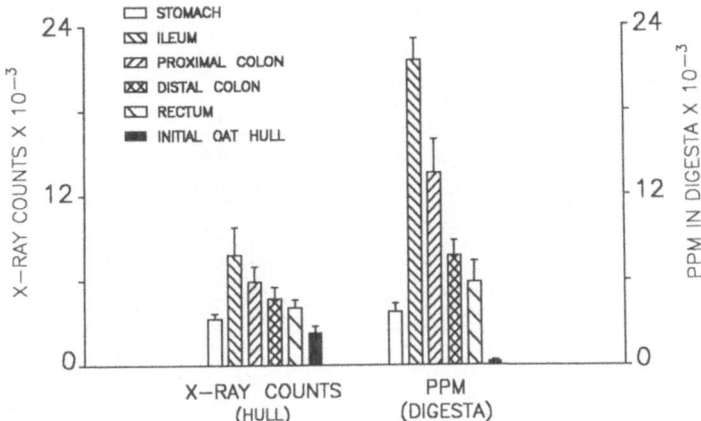

Figure 3. Comparisons of sodium X-ray counts from initial oat hulls and oat hulls retrieved from pigs, and sodium content of digesta (pooled values) and initial hulls.

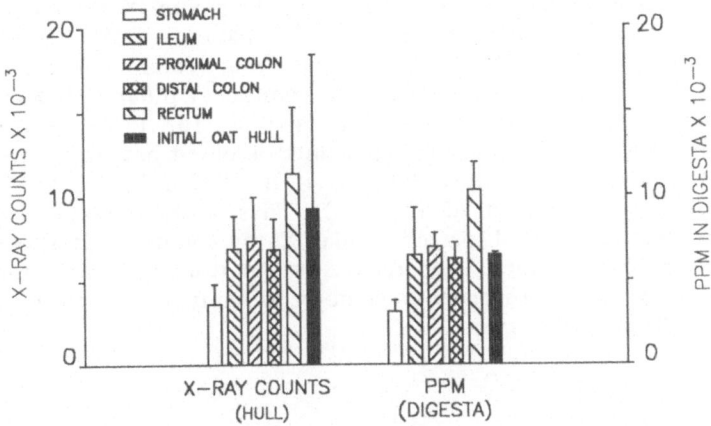

Figure 4. Comparisons of potassium X-ray counts from initial oat hulls and oat hulls retrieved from pigs, and potassium content of digesta (pooled values) and initial hulls.

counts were not significantly different for stomach vs initial hulls. Sulfur counts from hulls from proximal colon, vs distal colon vs rectum were not significantly different from each other, but were higher than counts from stomach and initial hulls, $P < 0.001$. There was no apparent general correlation between concentrations of phosphorus in digesta samples and X-ray counts of phosphorus in retrieved oat hulls (data not shown). Sulfur contents of digesta were not measured.

Values are given in Table I of pooled X-ray counts for corn bran and oat hulls retrieved from the same digesta sample obtained from specific locations in two pigs. Thus, the two types of tissues are presumed to have been exposed to

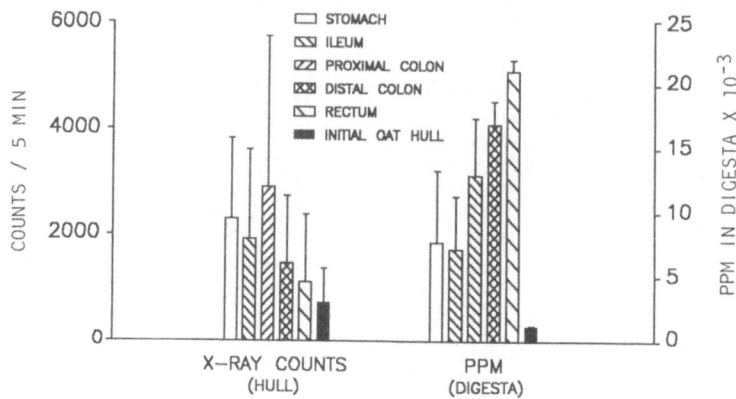

Figure 5. Comparisons of calcium X-ray counts from initial oat hulls and oat hulls retrieved from pigs, and calcium contents of digesta (pooled values) and initial hulls.

essentially the same conditions. The trend of X-ray count values for Na, P and S was to peak in tissues retrieved from the ileum. Potassium X-ray counts increased as the tissues traveled through the GI tract. The pattern of calcium X-ray counts from oat hulls listed in the table, i.e., counts from rectum samples significantly lower than from stomach and ileum and no significant difference between counts from stomach and ileum hulls, was the same as for three pigs (Figure 5). Although the high variation in calcium counts obscured any trend for oat hulls, calcium counts decreased in corn bran as it traveled through the GI tract, as reported previously (Dintzis et al., in press). Thus, a major point of the table is that the two types of tissue displayed similar X-ray count trends as a function of passage through the GI tract. For reasons to be discussed later, the reader is warned that it is **not** appropriate to compare directly the magnitude of counts between oat hulls and corn bran.

Discussion

The data in Figure 2 show the expected relationship that mean X-ray counts are proportional to macro-concentrations of an element (Ca and K). The high variation in counts may be explained by at least two mechanisms: 1) the six specimens chosen for X-ray measurements may have contained a different average amount of an element than the larger distribution of particles and 2) the distribution of an element within the plant tissue cross-section was heterogeneous. A major conclusion from Figure 2 (and Table I) is that the methods used in this study offer a precision limited to a coefficient of variation of not less than 10%. A realistic minimum CV would be of the order of 20%. Corn bran samples loaded *in vitro* had minimum CV's of about 25% (Dintzis et al., in press).

We infer from Figure 3 that because the loading of sodium onto the oat hull was proportional to the concentration in digesta, the sodium ion was able to diffuse into and out of the oat hull in a manner proportional to the sodium concentration

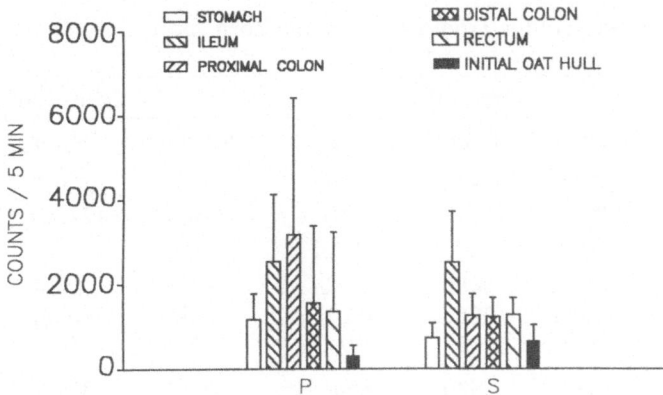

Figure 6. Comparisons of phosphorus and sulfur X-ray counts from oat hulls retrieved from pigs (pooled data) with initial hulls.

gradient between the hulls and chyme. The large increase of sodium in digesta retrieved from the ileum was caused mainly by pancreatic secretions into the small intestine. Daily throughputs of 21.6 g of Na in the duodenum (Partridge, 1978), a daily output of 18.4 g of Na in pancreatic juice (Partridge et al., 1982), and Na outputs of 6.5 to 15.3 g/day in pancreatic juices of pigs (Zebrowska, 1985), have been reported.

X-ray count values of potassium in retrieved oat hulls, Figure 4, generally follow the pattern of concentrations in digesta. Thus, the amount of potassium in the oat hull was proportional to the concentration in the digesta. From this we infer that potassium, like sodium, was able to diffuse into and out of the oat hull during passage through the GI tract. Comparisons involving counts of potassium in initial oat hull were confounded by high variation. We infer from this that the distribution of potassium in oat hulls was significantly more heterogeneous than the distribution of sodium.

Our conclusion from data shown in Figure 5 is that oat hulls in the stomach were loaded with calcium and then unloaded to approximately initial values during completion of passage through the GI tract. Examination of data from individual pigs indicates that in the stomach the loading of calcium onto oat hulls was proportional to the calcium concentration in the digesta.

X-ray data in Figure 6 leads us to conclude that both phosphorus and sulfur were loaded onto oat hulls during GI tract residence and that the hulls leave the pig containing more phosphorus, but not more sulfur, than prior to ingestion. The sudden increase in sulfur counts from oat hulls retrieved from the ileum might be explained by the presence of sulfur containing bile constituents, such as taurocholic acid or taurine. Products of digestion, such as phosphorus and sulfur-containing amino acids or small peptides, might also contribute to counts of these elements.

In metabolism trials with young pigs (39 kg) fed diets containing 10% oat hulls, Moser et al. (1982) found that the presence of oat hulls; 1) did not affect

Table I. X-ray counts from oat hulls and corn bran

Element	Oat hulls			Corn bran		
	Stomach	Ileum	Rectum	Stomach	Ileum	Rectum
Na	3270	8800	4180	4740	17700	6260
	(390)[a]	(1510)	(550)	(1070)	(2220)	(1410)
	12[b]	17	13	23	13	23
K	3640	6480	11700	9320	11560	21400
	(1210)	(2060)	(4520)	(3640)	(1630)	(4700)
	33	32	39	39	14	22
Ca	1920	2480	850	7550	3590	1880
	(1260)	(1781)	(1170)	(5040)	(770)	(570)
	66	72	140	67	21	30
P	1100	2720	1300	3140	3820	1880
	(580)	(1620)	(1900)	(1350)	(1010)	(1980)
	53	60	150	43	26	83
S	820	1940	1330	1460	2650	1340
	(360)	(570)	(450)	(400)	(680)	(380)
	44	29	34	27	26	28

Pooled data from tissues retrieved from digesta of two pigs,
n = 6 for each count mean, three from each pig.
[a] Standard deviation.
[b] Coefficient of variation, units of percent.

excretion of Ca, 2) increased ($P < 0.1$) fecal excretion of P, 3) did not affect retention of Ca or P. In balance studies involving growing pigs (30 or 50 kg) fed diets containing 10% oat hulls, Moore et al. (1986) found that the presence of oat hulls; 1) decreased Ca ($P < 0.06$) and P ($P < 0.10$) balance, 2) depressed ($P < 0.01$) absorptions of Na and K, but did not significantly affect balance of these minerals. Moore et al. (1986) concluded that oat hulls decreased mineral balance in pigs. X-ray count patterns of Na, K, Ca, and P in oat hulls during passage through the GI tract seem compatible with results of these feeding studies, but our data base is too small to permit us to form conclusions with respect to effects of oat hulls on mineral nutriture in pigs. Therefore, correlations between the flows of minerals into and out of oat hulls (and corn bran) during GI tract passage and the effects of oat hulls (and corn bran) on mineral bioavailability to the pig are yet to be determined.

The first major point of Table I is that the X-ray count patterns of the two plant tissues were similar, except for calcium. The relatively high initial X-ray counts of calcium from corn bran in the pig stomach, which then decreased substantially during the remainder of GI tract passage, was observed previously (Dintzis et al., in press). It is possible that a similarity between calcium X-ray counts from oat hulls and corn pericarp was obscured by the high variation in counts from oat hulls.

Variations in X-ray counts could arise from a variety of sources. Two sources would be differences between times of feed ingestion and metabolic differences between pigs. Thus, the free ion concentrations experienced by plant tissues within the chyme are expected to vary significantly from pig to pig. Stomach samples (Table I) were generated from tissues exposed to digesta containing either 13200 ± 460 or 1910 ± 90 ppm Ca. This difference in calcium content of stomach digesta likely was caused by different times of feed ingestion. While the relationship between content of an element in the digesta and concentration of the diffusible ion is unknown, these values suggest the likelihood of significant differences in Ca concentrations in the stomachs of the two pigs. The high CV's in the table are caused by low signals and a very small data base, and, for calcium in the stomach contents, by different times of feed ingestion. The exceptionally low CV's of <20% probably represent artifacts arising from a very small data base.

From the presence of voids in the sample interior (Figure 1) we infer that penetration of embedding resin into the specimens was limited. This belief seems verified by the relatively low values of chlorine X-ray counts (data not shown) measured in sample cross-sections compared with counts in the resin blank (the resin contained significant amounts of chlorine). We also believe that residues of chyme did not penetrate into the oat hull (or corn bran) specimens because of the presence of "empty" voids and because such materials would have generated X-ray counts significantly higher than the measured averages. In principle, the use of EDX analysis to examine specimens obtained directly from digesta should avoid altering concentrations of labile cations within the tissue. Concentrations of sodium and potassium in oat hulls and corn pericarp would be significantly decreased by use of aqueous solutions intended to remove extraneous matter adhering to the tissue exterior.

Heterogeneity in specimen morphology, and therefore specimen density, has been demonstrated for oat hull (Figure 1) and this sort of heterogeneity is also present in corn pericarp (Dintzis et al., in press). Since X-ray count values also depend upon average atomic number of the target micro-volume (Goldstein et al., 1981) variations in this average, caused by differences in target density, might explain some of the variation in counts. Heterogeneity of mineral distribution within a specimen cross-section, caused by asymmetric distribution of binding sites, also would contribute to variation in X-ray counts. Thus, we believe a significant component of the total variation in X-ray counts is related to heterogeneities intrinsic to the relatively large areas scanned within the two types of plant tissues.

Significant differences have been observed in X-ray count values between *in vitro* loaded oat hulls and corn bran. While it is not within the scope of this paper to investigate further such differences, we consider the effect might be caused by a strong asymmetry of mineral binding within the oat hull, by a significant difference in average atomic number of the tissue matrix associated with minerals in the two tissues, or both of these factors (such matters will be the subject of a future publication). The point for this study is that the relationship between concentration of an element and X-ray count values was different for oat hulls and for corn pericarp. Therefore, on the basis of X-ray counts, one should not directly compare concentrations of an element in one tissue with that in the other. Thus, the potassium and calcium "calibration" graph, Figure 2, for oat hulls should not be used for corn pericarp.

Summary

EDX measurements of the mineral content of oat hulls in the pig GI tract revealed that the hulls from the rectum contained more Na, P and S than prior to ingestion; while contents of K and Ca were not significantly different than in initial hulls. X-ray measurements indicated that potassium was the only element of the five examined which was unloaded from the initial oat hulls during passage through the GI tract. During this passage, the flows of Na and K into and out of oat hulls were proportional to concentrations of these elements in digesta. Although Ca was loaded onto oat hulls in the stomach, it was unloaded during subsequent passage, even though the concentration of Ca in digesta increased significantly in the large intestine. The behavior of corn pericarp generally was similar to that of oat hulls. We consider it unwise to attempt quantitative comparisons of corn pericarp behavior in our previous work (Dintzis et al., in press) with results in this study. The data bases are very small and feeding situations and diets were not equivalent. However, results from both studies show similar behavior in loading and unloading of Na, Ca, and S from the plant tissues, and possible differences with K and P.

The finding that X-ray count values were different for oat hulls and corn pericarp when the tissues were loaded with equal amounts of calcium or potassium serves as a stark warning that additional work is required before measurements of this sort can provide quantitative results and a basis for comparisons between different plant tissues. Nevertheless, EDX analysis has provided information about the loading of Na, K, Ca, S, and P onto plant tissues during passage in the GI tract of growing pigs. The techniques used in this study appear worthy of further effort, for we believe they have the potential to provide significant information about *in vivo* interactions between plant tissues and minerals in the diet.

Acknowledgement

The assistance of Cecil Harris in expeditiously and competently measuring mineral contents by atomic absorption analysis is gratefully acknowledged.

References

Camire, A. L., & Clydesdale, F. M. (1981) *J. Food Sci.* 46, 548-551.
Cummings, J. H. (1981) *Br. Med. Bull.* 37, 65-70.
Dintzis, F. R., Baker, F. L. & Calvert, C. C. (1989) *J. Biol. Trace Element Res.* 19, in press.
Garcia, W. J., Blessin, C. W., Inglett, G. E., & Carlson, R. O. (1972) *Cereal Chem.* 49, 158-167.
Goldstein, J. I., Newbury, D. E., Echlin, P., Joy, D. C., Fiori, C., & Lifchin, E. (1981) *Scanning Electron Microscopy and X-ray Microanalysis*, Plenum Press, New York.

Kelsay, J. L. (1986) in *Dietary Fiber Basic and Clinical Aspects*, (Vahouny, G. V., & Kritchevsky, D., Eds.) pp 361-372, Plenum Press, New York.

Kies, C. (1985) in *Nutritional Bioavailability of Calcium*, (Kies, C., Ed.) p 175-187, ACS Symposium Series 275, American Chemical Society, Washington, DC.

Miller, E. R., & Ullrey, D.E. (1987) *Ann. Rev. Nutr.* 7, 361-382.

Moore, R. J., Kornegay, E. T., & Lindemann, M. D. (1986) *Can. J. Anim. Sci.* 66, 267-276.

Moser, R. L., Peo, Jr., E. R., Moser, B. D., & Lewis, A. J. (1982) *J. Anim. Sci.* 54, 800-805.

Partridge, I. G. (1978) *Br. J. Nutr.* 39, 527-537.

Partridge, I. G., Low, A. G., Sambrook, I. E., & Corring, T. (1982) *Br. J. Nutr.* 48, 137-145.

Reinhold, J. G., Salvador Garcia J., & Garzon, P. (1981) *Am. J. Clin. Nutr.* 4, 1384-1391.

Sandstrom, B., Almgren, A., Kivisto, B., & Cederblad, A. (1987) *J. Nutr.* 117, 898-1902.

Zebrowska, T. (1985) in *Proceedings of the 3rd International Seminar on Digestive Physiology in the Pig* (Just, S., Jorgensen, H., & Fernandez, J. A., Eds.) pp 152-154, Copenhagen, Denmark.

11

Phytic Acid Interactions with Divalent Cations in Foods and in the Gastrointestinal Tract

John W. Erdman, Jr. and Angela Poneros-Schneier

The proper chemical designation for phytic acid is myoinositol 1,2,3,4,5,6-hexa kis (dihydrogen phosphate). Phytic acid and/or its salt (phytate) are found in all plant seeds and in low concentrations in some roots and tubers (Table I). Phytates are considered to be the chief storage form of phosphate and inositol in almost all seeds (Cosgrove, 1966). During the ripening process of cereal grains, active transport of phosphorus from the leaves and roots to the seeds occurs. Up to 60-80% of the total phosphorus in seeds is accumulated in the form of phytic acid. During germination, the phytic acid molecule can be rapidly hydrolyzed to inositol and phosphate to supply the nutritional needs of the plant.

Phytic acid was isolated from plant seeds over a century ago (Oberleas, 1983), yet the exact conformational structure of this chelating agent is still controversial (Erdman, 1979). Moreover, the extent to which phytic acid interacts with other components of seeds *in situ* is still unclear. While these uncertainties remain unresolved, the mineral chelation potential of phytic acid has been more clearly defined. Phytic acid has tremendous affinity for divalent cations or for other plant components with positive charge(s). Phytic acid forms salts or complexes with most heavy metals. The relative stability and solubility of the complex depends not only on pH, but also on the presence of other cations (Oberleas, 1983).

Table I shows the concentration of phytic acid in a variety of seeds, legumes, and flours. An expanded list of phytic acid content of foods has been published by Oberleas & Harland (1981). Whole grain cereals contain about 1 percent of this chelator (dry basis), while oilseeds contain about 1.5 percent or higher. Phytic acid distribution within various morphological portions of seeds varies greatly. The endosperm of wheat and rice kernels are almost devoid of phytate. The majority of phytate is concentrated in the germ portion and the aleurone layer cells of the kernel and in the bran or hull. However, corn is unique from most cereals since almost 90% of the phytic acid is concentrated in the germ portion of the kernel (O'Dell et al., 1972; Erdman, 1979). Oilseeds contain little or no endosperm and the phytate tends to be more equally distributed throughout the seed. Often phytate in oilseeds is localized within subcellular inclusions called aleurone grains or protein bodies (Martinez, 1977). In some oilseeds, such as cottonseed,

Table I. Phytic acid concentrations in components
or products of cereals, legumes and oilseeds[a]

Sample	Phytic acid (%)[b]
Corn, Hybrid	0.89
Germ	6.38
Endosperm	0.04
Aleurone	4.11
Hull	0.07
Wheat, Soft	1.13
Germ	3.90
Endosperm	0.01
Hull	N.D.[c]
Rice, Brown	0.89
Germ	3.48
Endosperm	0.01
Pericarp	3.37
Rice, polished, long grain	0.34
Cottonseed globoids	60.00
Rapeseed protein concentrate	5.3-7.5
Soybean, whole, meal or flour	1.4-1.6
Soy protein isolate or concentrate	1.6-2.4
Peanuts	0.80
Peanut meal, defatted and dehulled	5.20
Sesame meal, dehulled	3.60
Sesame meal, defatted and dehulled	5.20
Beans, red kidney	1.9-2.1
Beans, black eyed	1.2-1.6
Beans, pigeon	1.9-2.0
Beans, white	1.8-2.0
Peas, field	0.85

[a] Sources: Beal et al., 1984; Erdman, 1979; Lathia et al., 1987; O'Dell et al., 1972; Pons et al., 1953; Reddy & Salunkhe, 1980.
[b] On a dry basis assuming 28.2% phosphorus in phytic acid.
[c] None detectable.

sunflower and peanuts, the phytic acid is further concentrated in substructures of protein bodies called crystalloids or globoids. In cottonseed the globoids can be isolated intact and have been found to contain 60% phytic acid and 10% non-phosphorus elements (Lui & Altshul, 1967). Globoid-type structures have also been reported in wheat bran (Fulcher & Wong, 1980) and oat bran (Yui & Mongeau, 1987).

Thus, in different seed types phytic acid is associated with different seed components and it may be preferentially extracted with those components. Some natural association of phytic acid with minerals and protein (primarily storage proteins) occurs. Although phytate from seeds was generally thought to be a significant mineral storage chelate of a variety of elements, such as calcium and trace elements, modern analytic procedures applied to a variety of species have shown that potassium and magnesium are the most common cationic constituents associated with phytate. Calcium, manganese, iron and zinc may be present in low concentrations depending upon the species, the tissue region and the soil conditions (Lott & Ockenden, 1986). The phytate chelate in seeds does not serve as a reservoir for the majority of seed cations.

Effects of Food Processing upon Phytic Acid Interactions within Food

Phytic acid is far from inert in food systems, especially when seeds, grains or kernels are ground and water is added prior to or during processing. At neutral pH, phytic acid is very negatively charged and the phosphate groups are free to associate loosely or bind chemically with a variety of food components. As foods are modified during various food processing procedures, the chemical environment is altered and new interactions may take place. Of a variety of different common food processing procedures, those involving heat; fermentation; the addition or removal of moisture; and the addition of certain food additives, such as EDTA, acids, bases, enzymes or mineral supplements are most likely to affect mineral binding to phytic acid (Erdman et al., 1987). Several excellent reviews of the chemistry of binding of phytic acid to minerals and/or proteins have been published (Cheryan, 1980; Reddy et al., 1982; Cosgrove, 1966).

Foods containing phytate are rarely consumed raw. Cereals and legumes require heating and further processing to increase the palatability, to increase the digestibility of the protein and other food components and to reduce heat-labile antinutritional factors (for example, trypsin inhibitors in legumes). Phytic acid is very stable during heating: for example, autoclaving of soybean flakes for 60 minutes (an extensive amount of heat treatment) only reduced phytate content by about 15% (de Boland et al., 1976).

Tempering or soaking of certain beans and seeds is a common practice in many cultures since many beans are difficult to hydrate and require soaking for many hours. Additionally, soaking (a process also used as the first step in germination) is a common practice prior to or concurrent with fermentation. During this soaking period, the phytase enzyme, if present, can hydrolyze phosphate groups from phytic acid thus reducing its mineral chelation potential. During germination of cereals and legumes phytase activity rises rapidly, resulting in a decrease in phytate content (Nayini & Markakis, 1986). Phytases in plants and microorganisms generally completely remove all phosphate groups from myoinositol, negating the binding potential of phytic acid. While not present in significant quantities in plants, mono- through pentaphosphate inositols are known to be present in measurable quantities in processed foods (Phillippy et al., 1986). Their chelation potential has not been carefully studied.

Ranhotra et al. (1974) reported that all or most of the phytate in wheat and other variety breads was hydrolyzed during the process of bread making. Both the wheat and the yeast used to leaven bread are rich sources of phytase. When chemical leavening instead of yeast leavening is used in baked products, phytic

Table II. Losses of phytic acid phosphorus during fermentation and baking of bread

Nature of Product	Phytic acid phosphorus present originally in flour (mg/100 g)	Phytic acid phosphorus hydrolyzed (%)
Bread made from 92% extraction wheat meal with yeast	214	31.0
Bread made from 92% extraction wheat meal with baking power	214	5.0

Source: Reddy et al. (1982), calculated from the data of Widdowson (1941).

acid hydrolysis is much lower (Table II). During the fermentation of soybeans to produce tempeh, a 33% reduction in phytic acid occurred. This was attributed to the phytase production by the inoculated mold (Sudarmadji & Markakis, 1977). Phytate reduction can have positive effect on zinc bioavailability. Morris & Ellis (1980a) showed that phytate reduction with phytase enzyme improved zinc (but not iron) bioavailability from wheat bran for rats. Lönnerdal et al. (1986) also reported that phytase reduction of phytate in soy formula improved zinc bioavailability for the Rhesus monkey.

Other food processes such as milling or grinding, which break cell walls, can also affect phytic acid interactions in processed foods. Upon disruption of plant cells, phytic acid can react with protein and/or minerals depending upon pH, ionic strength, mineral profile, moisture content and other conditions. The role of pH on protein-phytic acid interactions has been studied by several workers (Fontaine et al., 1946; de Rham & Jost, 1979). Of significance in food systems is the observation that protein and phytic acid tend to interact strongly near neutral pH. For example, de Rham & Jost (1979) found that in soybean extracts, 40% of the phytic acid was protein bound (nondialyzable) at 7.5. These researchers suggested that calcium and other cations are probably involved as a salt bridge between phytic acid and protein at neutral pH.

Our laboratory has extensively studied the bioavailability of zinc and other minerals from a variety of soybean protein products (Erdman & Forbes, 1981; Erdman et al., 1980; Ketelsen et al., 1984). In the soy concentrate and soy isolate systems, we have demonstrated that neutralized, as compared to acid-precipitated, soy products exhibit reduced zinc bioavailability in rats. For example, Ketelsen et al. (1984) produced a defatted soy flour, an acid precipitated and dried, and a neutralized and dried soy concentrate from a single lot of ^{65}Zn, intrinsically labeled soybeans. Retention of ^{65}Zn in bone or in the whole body 12 days after a test meal (see Table III), revealed that neutralization of soy, prior to drying, depressed zinc bioavailability.

Table III. Retention of ^{65}Zn by rats fed meals containing soy flour, acid-precipitated or neutralized soy concentrate

Diet Description	% of initial activity retained in two tibias after 12 days	Whole body ^{65}Zn retention	
		Day 1	Day 2
		% dose	
Soy flour	0.17 ± 0.01[a]	83.1 ± 1.5[a]	74.5 ± 1.5[a]
Acid-precipitated soy concentrate	0.15 ± 0.01[a]	75.9 ± 2.2[b]	68.0 ± 2.0[b]
Neutralized soy concentrate	0.12 ± 0.01[b]	64.7 ± 1.8[c]	52.3 ± 1.8[c]

Source: Ketelsen et al. (1984). Differing superscript letters within a column indicate significant differences (P < 0.05).

The reduction of zinc bioavailability at neutral pH may be a result of the formation of stable protein-phytic acid-zinc complexes in the dried neutral product. Since protein-phytic acid-mineral associations occur in solution at a neutral pH (de Rham & Jost, 1979), these associations may well form more tightly-bound complexes during the drying of the soy protein. The exclusion of water from the protein-phytic acid-mineral system could lead to complexes that are much more thermodynamically stable than the associations occurring in solution. In the digestive tract, these stable complexes may inhibit the complete digestion of protein to free amino acids. Short peptides or amino acid residues bound to zinc and phytic acid may result. These would be resistant to digestion with consequent inefficient absorption of zinc or other minerals (Erdman et al., 1980).

Cheryan (1980) suggested that the imidazole group of histidine is a probable binding site for phytic acid through a divalent mineral bridge. Other amino acids likely for such involvement are glutamate and aspartate. These are found in large quantities in soya protein and, at neutral pH, their free carboxyl groups could easily complex with phytic acid through a Zn(II) bridge. Alternatively, it is possible that basic amino acids at neutral pH might bind directly with a free phosphate group of a phytic acid-zinc chelate. Then, upon drying, a conformational change of protein could trap the zinc or other cation and reduce its availability (Erdman & Forbes, 1981).

Elevated levels of dietary calcium accentuate the negative effect of phytate on zinc bioavailability (Oberleas et al., 1966a; Morris & Ellis, 1980b; Forbes et al., 1984). The formation of zinc-calcium-phytate complexes or other zinc phytate complexes in foods or in the upper GI tract of monogastric animals may be a major mechanism by which phytic acid reduces dietary zinc bioavailability (Fordyce et al., 1987). Controlled studies with rats (Morris & Ellis, 1980b or Forbes et al., 1984) have demonstrated such a clear interrelationship of dietary levels of phytic acid and calcium with zinc bioavailability, that several groups have suggested the use of a phytate x calcium/zinc [(P)(C)/(Z)] molar ratio to predict zinc bioavailability. Bindra et al., (1986) evaluated diets and zinc status of several groups of Punjabi Sikh Canadian immigrants. One lacto-ovo vegetarian group frequently consumed milk and milk products as well has high levels of phytate. This group with the highest (P)(C)/(Z) molar ratio (~250 mM/1000 Kcal) also had low serum zinc status (32% were below 70 μg/dL zinc). Morris & Ellis (1988) and our laboratory (Fordyce et al., 1987) have suggested that (P)(C)/(Z) ratios of 150-200 mM/1000 Kcal in human diets may result in low zinc status.

Phytic acid interactions in food systems are also affected by extrusion cooking, a high temperature and pressure procedure commonly utilized to produce most breakfast cereals and snack items. Recently Sandberg & coworkers (1987) investigated the digestion of dietary phytic acid from unprocessed and extruded wheat bran products (30% bran) in human subjects with an established ileostomy (surgical passage through the abdominal wall into the ileum allowing for collection of digesta from the lower small intestine). In unprocessed bran 58% of the phytic acid was hydrolyzed to penta-, tetra- and triphosphates during passage through the small intestine. When bran was extrusion-cooked, phytase activity of the bran ceased and only 25% of the inositol hexaphosphate was hydrolyzed. The authors speculated that the reduced digestibility of phytic acid may have been due to the lost phytase activity or to formation of undigestible complexes during extrusion cooking. These same workers (Kivistö et al., 1986) further showed that extrusion cooking of the bran product resulted in reduced absorption of zinc, magnesium and phosphorus from the product in these subjects with an ileostomy.

Phytic Acid Interactions with Minerals in the Gastrointestinal Tract

As foods are ingested and the digesta travels through the GI tract, phytic acid may continue to maintain associations that developed during ripening or during the processing of foods. On the other hand, phytic acid interactions may be altered during digestion. In a dilute, hydrated environment, first at low pH in the stomach and then about neutral pH in the upper intestine, phytate complexes may dissociate and other chelates may form. Binding of the phytic acid with minerals depends upon the pH of the element. For example, *in vitro* studies at pH 7.4 indicate that phytic acid complexes with single, nutritionally important ions in the following decreasing order: Cu(II) > Zn(II) > Co(II) > Mn(II) > Fe(III) > Ca(II) (Maddariah et al., 1964; Vohra et al., 1965; Oberleas, 1983).

Phytic acid complexes may be fully or partially hydrolyzed by intestinal phytase(s) or other enzymes. Sandberg & Andersson (1988) recently reported that mucosal phytase, if present in the human small intestine, does not seem to play a significant role in phytate digestion in humans. The hydrolysis of phytate that does occur in the GI tract is probably due to microbial phytases or due to non-enzymatic cleavage (Reddy et al., 1982).

Predicting the specific interactions of phytic acid in the GI tract and the nutritional implications of these interactions is very difficult with the current state of knowledge. A great deal of interactive factors confound such predictions. These include: type and solubility of phytic acid/phytate complexes entering and formed within the GI tract, level of phytic acid/phytate complexes present, level and type of minerals in GI tract (from food and endogenous origin), levels of other chelators in the GI tract (such as EDTA, oxalates or fiber from food or secreted ligands from GI tract), and mineral status of the individual (with low status, active transport systems in mucosal cells may be turned on, for example). The solubility of phytate complexes is a critical and perhaps overriding issue because complexes that are insoluble in the upper small intestine are highly unlikely to provide absorbable essential elements. Once these insoluble complexes are formed, presence of enzymes or other ligands may not reverse phytic acid's negative affects on mineral absorption.

The mineral binding capacity in the small intestine is in a constant state of flux as meals, snacks and beverages move through it. The mucosal cells are normally respondent to changing body needs. Therefore, the efficiency of mucosal cells to absorb chelates and their ability to compete with chelates for minerals is also in flux.

In the stomach, phytate is very negatively charged. Six of the 12 dissociable protons of phytic acid are strongly dissociated with a pKa of about 1.8 or at a pH of about 2.0. (Crean & Haisman, 1963; Reddy et al., 1982). Since proteins are strongly positively charged at pH 2.0, formation of new phytate-protein complexes is very probable in the stomach. The concurrent action of the protease pepsin in the stomach will also affect such complex formation. Rizk & Clydesdale (1985) studied the solubility of iron in various soy-based foods systems with and without pepsin treatment. They noted improvements of iron solubility after pepsin digestion, especially when ascorbic acid and other enhancers of iron solubility were added. More studies of this type are needed to better understand the complexity of mineral interactions in the GI tract.

In the upper GI tract, where maximum mineral absorption normally occurs, chemical interactions of phytic acid with minerals are of particular concern. At pH 6, the approximate pH of the upper duodenum, there is maximum precipitation (insolubility) of zinc phytate and zinc-calcium-phytate complexes (Oberleas, 1983; Reddy et al., 1982). Phytate complexation with other cations such as iron under these conditions is also of concern.

A number of endogenous or exogenous chelating agents may successfully compete with mineral-phytate complexes for essential minerals. To be nutritionally beneficial, such a chelating agent must not only have an equal or stronger binding affinity than phytic acid for the element, but also be able to release the mineral at the mucosal cell surface or within the cell. However, as noted previously, solubility is a prerequisite for mineral release from phytic acid to other chelating agents.

The common food additive, EDTA, is one chelator that has been well studied. EDTA has been shown to reverse the deleterious effects of phytate on the bioavailability of zinc and increase zinc absorption in both chicks and rats (O'Dell et al., 1964; Oberleas et al., 1966b; Reddy et al., 1982). In a food system, Okubo et al., (1975) used a large molar excess of EDTA at pH 8.5 to facilitate dissociation of phytate complexes and subsequently removed phytic acid by ultrafiltration. O'Dell (1969) suggested that EDTA may form soluble complexes with zinc that compete with and inhibit the formation of zinc-phytate and calcium-zinc phytate complexes. Soluble zinc-EDTA complexes then may be absorbed intact or release zinc directly at the mucosal cell wall for rapid absorption.

Curiously, EDTA may either enhance iron absorption at low EDTA concentrations in the diet or inhibit iron absorption with EDTA:iron molar ratios of 1:1 or 2:1 (Cook & Monsen, 1976). NaFeEDTA is one of several EDTA complexes

Table IV. The effect of dietary calcium level upon growth and bone zinc in rats

Dietary calcium level (%)	Average wt gain in 21 days (g)	μg zinc in two tibias after 21 days
0.3	127.3 ± 5.1[a]	48.6 ± 2.5[a]
0.5	112.5 ± 4.8[a]	34.8 ± 1.1[b]
0.8	79.2 ± 16.4[b]	25.5 ± 3.7[c]
1.0	60.5 ± 8.0[c]	23.3 ± 3.1[c]

Source: Data (mean ± S.D.; n = 6) derived from Forbes et al., 1984. All diets contained 12 ppm zinc and 0.036% phytic acid and phytate:zinc molar ratios of 30. Values within a column not sharing a common superscript letter are statistically different (P < 0.05).

which has received interest as a mineral fortificant. Tea, but not wheat bran, is able to inhibit iron absorption from this complex (Mac Phail et al., 1981). This observation points to the complexity of mineral chelate interactions in the GI tract. Studies in rats (Forbes et al., 1984; Morris & Ellis, 1980b, for example) show that the presence of high levels of calcium and, to a lesser degree, magnesium (Forbes et al., 1984), in the diet can reduce the bioavailability of zinc when phytic acid is also present. Other divalent cations may also be deleterious as a number of interactions with phytic acid are possible. We believe that the negative effect of calcium is primarily exerted in the small intestine where highly insoluble calcium-zinc-phytate complexes form at neutral pH. Table IV shows how manipulation of dietary calcium levels from 0.3 to 1.0% at constant zinc and phytic acid levels (phytate:zinc ratio = 30) lowers growth and bone zinc deposition in rats.

In order to determine whether the negative effects of calcium occur during food processing or in the GI tract, our laboratory (Forbes et al., 1983) prepared soybean curd (tofu) with two different traditional coagulants, calcium sulfate or magnesium chloride. Diets (9 ppm zinc) were formulated from each of the freeze-dried tofu products and additional calcium and magnesium was added to result in final diet concentrations of 0.4, 0.7 or 1.2% dietary calcium and 0.1% magnesium. Although increasing total dietary calcium depressed weight gain and tibia zinc in rats, the tofu-making process (i.e., the type of coagulant) did not affect zinc bioavailability as judged by these parameters. It can be concluded from the tofu studies that, at least with these products, the negative impact of the higher dietary calcium most likely occurred in the gastrointestinal tract.

Yoshida & co-workers (1985) utilized germ-free and conventional rats to investigate the effect of gut flora on utilization of calcium, phosphorus and zinc from diets with and without phytate. Their results showed that gut flora increased fecal excretion of calcium and phosphorus and decreased bone zinc. Phytate also increased the percentages of fecal excretions of calcium, phosphorus and zinc.

The authors suggest the possibility that the "calcium-phytate formed in the digestive tract, which under practical dietary conditions may be predominantly insoluble metal-phytate complex at neutral pH, is actively hydrolyzed by the gut flora of rats and calcium is absorbed from the intestine."

Conclusions

Phytic acid, the hexaphosphate of myoinositol, is found in high concentrations in cereals and legumes and is a strong chelating agent. Chelation of phytic acid with divalent cations is implicated in reduced absorption of a number of mineral cations including zinc, calcium and iron. This paper has reviewed phytic acid-mineral interactions, particularly those with zinc and calcium, that occur within cereal grains and legume seeds, during various food processing procedures and during the digestive processes in the stomach and upper GI tract. In unprocessed dry cereals and legumes, phytic acid apparently is not heavily chelated to minerals or bound to proteins. However, during hydration of seeds with or without milling or grinding, phytate complexation can occur. Germination or fermentation of cereals and legumes after hydration causes marked reduction of phytic acid due to action of phytase(s). With other food processing techniques such as pH modification, the prescence of EDTA or mineral supplements can also affect phytic acid binding. Within the GI tract phytate complexes from foods may be maintained, destroyed or new complexes may be formed depending upon the type and solubility of phytate complexes present, levels and types of minerals present in the GI tract, levels of other chelators (or ligands), and protease and phytase enzyme activity. Prediction of the overall effects of phytic acid on mineral bioavailability is difficult at this time. Any accurate assessment of the nutritional implications of phytate must consider the chemistry of phytic acid in foods, during food processing and in the GI tract.

References

Beal, L., Finney, P. L., & Mehta, T. (1984) *J. Food Sci.* 49, 637-641.

Bindra, G. S., Gibson, R. S., & Thompson, L. U. (1986) *Nutr. Res.* 6, 475-483.

Cheryan, M. (1980) *CRC Crit. Rev. Food Sci. Nutr.* 13, 297-335.

Cook, J. D., & Monsen, E. R. (1976). *Am. J. Clin. Nutr.* 29, 614-620.

Cosgrove, D. J. (1966) *Rev. Pure. Appl. Chem.* 16, 209-224.

Crean, D. E. C, & Haisman, D. R. (1963) *J. Sci. Food Agric.* 14, 824-833.

de Boland, A. R., Garner, G. B., & O'Dell, B. L. (1976) *J. Agric. Food Chem.* 24, 804-808.

de Rham, O., & Jost, T. (1979) *J. Food Sci.* 44, 596-600.

Erdman, J. W., Jr. (1979) *J. Am. Oil Chem. Soc.* 56, 736-741.

Erdman, J. W., Jr., & Forbes, R. M. (1981) *J. Am. Oil Chem. Soc.* 58, 489-493.

Erdman, J. W., Jr., Garcia-Lopez, J. S., & Sherman, A. R. (1987) in *Nutrition 1987* (Levander, O. A., Ed.) pp 23-26, Bethesda, MD.

Erdman, J. W., Jr., Weingartner, K. E., Mustakas, G. C., Schmutz, R. D., Parker, H. M., & Forbes, R. M. (1980) *J. Food Sci.* 45, 1193-1199.

Fontaine, T. D., Pons, W. A., Jr., & Irving, G. W. (1946) *J. Biol. Chem.* 164, 487-507.

Forbes, R. M., Erdman, J. W., Jr., Parker, H. M., Kondo, H., & Ketelsen, S. M. (1983) *J. Nutr.* 113, 205-210.

Forbes, R. M., Parker, H. M., & Erdman, J. W., Jr. (1984) *J. Nutr.* 114, 1421-1425.

Fordyce, E. J., Forbes, R. M., Robbins, K. R., & Erdman, J. W., Jr. (1987) *J. Food Sci.* 52, 440-444.

Fulcher. R. G. & Wong, S. I. (1980) in *Cereals for Food and Beverages* (Inglett, G. & Munck, L., Eds.) Academic Press, New York.

Ketelsen, S. M., Stuart, M. A., Weaver, C. M., Forbes, R. M., & Erdman, J. W., Jr. (1984) *J. Nutr.* 114, 536-542.

Kivistö, B., Andersson, H., Cederblad, G., Sandberg, A. S., & Sandstrom, B. (1986) *Brit. J. Nutr.* 55, 255-260.

Lathia, D., Hoch, G., & Kievernagel, Y. (1987) *Plant Foods for Human Nutr.* 37, 229-235.

Lönnerdal, B., Belle, J. G. Hendricks, A. G., & Keen, C. L. (1986) *Am. J. Clin. Nutr.* 43, 674 (Abstract).

Lott, J. N. A., & Ockenden, I. (1986) in *Phytic Acid: Chemistry & Applications* (Graf, E., Ed.) pp 43-55, Pilatus Press, Minneapolis, MN.

Lui, N. S. T., & Altschul, A. M. (1967) *Arch. Biochem. Biophys.* 121, 678.

Mac Phail, A. P., Botwell, T. H., Torrance, J. D., Derman, D. P., Bezwoda, W. R., Charlton, R. W., & Mayet, F. (1981) *Br. J. Nutr.* 45, 215-227.

Maddariah, V. T., Kurnick, A. A., & Reid, B. L. (1964) *Proc. Soc. Exp. Biol. Med.* 115, 391-393.

Martinez, W. H. (1977) in *Evaluation of Protein for Humans* (Bodwell, C. E., Ed.) pp 304-317, AVI Publ. Co., Inc., Westport, CT.

Morris, E. R., & Ellis, R. (1980a) *J. Nutr.* 110, 1037-1045.

Morris, E. R., & Ellis, R. (1980b) *J. Nutr.* 110, 2000-2011.

Morris, E. R., & Ellis, R. *Biol. Trace. Element Res.* (in press).

Nayini, N. R., & Markakis, P. (1986) in *Phytic Acid: Chemistry and Applications* (Graf, E., Ed.) pp 101-118, Pilatus Press, Minneapolis, MN.

Oberleas, D. (1983) in *Nutritional Bioavailability of Zinc* (Inglett, G. E., Ed.) pp 145-158, Washington, DC.

Oberleas, D., & Harland, B. F. (1981) *J. Am. Diet. Assn.* 79, 433-436.

Oberleas, D., Muhrer, M. E., & O'Dell, B. L. (1966a) *J. Nutr.* 90, 56-62.

Oberleas, D., Muhrer, M. E., & O'Dell, B. L. (1966b) in *Zinc Metabolism* (Prasad, A. S. Ed.) pp 225-238, C. C. Thomas, Springfield, IL.

O'Dell, B. L. (1969) *Am. J. Clin. Nutr.* 22, 1315-1322.

O'Dell, B. L., de Boland, A. R., & Koirtyohann, S. R. (1972) *J. Agric. Food Chem.* 20, 718-721.

O'Dell, B. L., Yohe, J. M., & Savage, J. (1964) *Poult. Sci.* 43, 415-419.

Okubo, K., Waldrop, A. B., Iacobocci, G. A., & Myers, D. V. (1975) *Cereal Chem.* 52, 263-271.

Phillippy, B. Q., Johnston, M. R., Tao, S.-H., Fox, M. R. S., & White, K. D. (1988) *J. Food Sci.* 53, 496-499.

Pons, W. A., Jr., Stansbury, M. F., & Hoffpauir, C. L. (1953) *J. Assoc. Off. Agric. Chem.* 36, 492-504.

Ranhotra, G. S., Loewe, R. J, & Puyat, L. V. (1974) *J. Food Sci.* 39, 1023-1025.

Reddy, N. R., & Salunkhe, D. K. (1980) *J. Food Sci.* 45, 1708-1712.

Reddy, N. R., Sathe, S. K., and Salunkhe, D. K. (1982) *Adv. in Food Res.* 28, 1-92.

Rizk, S. W., & Clydesdale, F. M. (1985) *J. Food Prot.* 48, 35-38.

Sandberg, A. S., & Andersson, H. (1988) *J. Nutr.* 118, 469-473.

Sandberg, A. S., Andersson, H., Carlsson, N.-G., & Sandstrom, B. (1987) *J. Nutr.* 117, 2061-2065.

Sudarmadji, S., & Markakis, P. (1977) *J. Sci. Food Agric.* 28, 381-383.

Vohra, P., Gray, G. A., & Kratzer, F. H. (1965) *Proc. Soc. Exp. Biol. Med.* 120, 447-449.

Widdowson, E. M. (1941) *Nature* (London) 148, 219.

Yoshida, T., Shinoda, S., Kawaai, Y, Iwabuchi, A., & Mutai, M. (1985) *Agric. Biol. Chem.* 45, 2199-2202.

Yui, S. H. & Mongeau, R. (1987) *Food Microstructure* 6, 143-150.

12

Low Gastric Hydrochloric Acid Secretion and Mineral Bioavailability[1,2]

Elaine T. Champagne

Low secretion of hydrochloric acid by gastric parietal cells occurs in young infants (Mason, 1962; Ródbro et al., 1967a,b; Agunod et al., 1969;) and in approximately 30% of the elderly (Villako et al., 1976). In the infant, low acid secretion is due to immaturity of the gastric parietal cells (Agunod et al., 1969). The reduced acid secretion in older people is a result of both a loss in parietal cells as well as a decrease in the secretory capacity of existing cells (Meyers & Necheles, 1940; Fikry, 1965). The incidence and severity of the condition increases with advancing age (Bhanthumnavin & Shuster, 1977). The severity can range from mild atrophic gastritis with hypochlorhydria to total gastric atrophy with achlorhydria. Table I allows a comparison of average acid outputs following histamine stimulation in infants, children, and normal adults.

Hydrochloric acid performs several functions which assist digestion (Vander et al., 1975). High acidity in the stomach denatures food proteins and disrupts intermolecular bonds, thereby breaking up connective tissue and cells. Ionized species are released into solution. With high acidity, minerals dissociate from food complexes. Hydrochloric acid initiates the process by which inactive pepsinogen splits off peptides to form the proteolytic enzyme pepsin. Furthermore, hydrochloric acid activates pepsin by providing a high hydrogen ion concentration.

Low hydrochloric acid secretion leads to raised intraluminal gastric pH values, reduced pepsin formation from pepsinogen, and reduced pepsin activity. Besides affecting the dissociation of food complexes, low acidity could lead to the formation of insoluble mineral complexes in the stomach (e.g., hydroxides, phytates, fiber complexes). Low pepsin formation and activity could prevent the digestion of food proteins to polypeptides in the stomach and the subsequent complete

---

1 The mention of firm names or trade products does not imply that they are endorsed or recommended by the U.S. Department of Agriculture over other firms or similar products not mentioned.

2 This article is not copyrighted, therefore is in the public domain.

Table I. Gastric hydrochloric acid outputs of infants, children and adults following histamine stimulation

Mean Age	HCl output (meq/10 kg/h)
Birth	0.15[a]
1st month	0.31[a]
3 months	1.22[a]
20 months	2.18[b]
16 years	2.02[c]
Adult*	1.02-2.71[d]

[a] Agunod et al., 1969.
[b] Rodbro & Christiansen, 1966.
[c] Ghai et al., 1965.
[d] Ardeman et al., 1964; Yamaguchi & Glass, 1967.
* Adults with normal gastric biopsy specimens.

breakdown to amino acids and smaller peptides in the small intestine following digestion by pancreatin. Poor digestion of protein-mineral complexes could affect the release of the minerals for absorption at intestinal sites (Champagne & Phillippy, 1989).

These observations raise the concern that low gastric hydrochloric acid secretion may decrease the bioavailabilities of nutritionally important minerals, such as iron, zinc, and calcium. The purpose of this article is to review the possible effects of low gastric hydrochloric acid secretion on iron, zinc, and calcium absorption as studied by *in vivo* and *in vitro* methods.

Iron Absorption

Clinical studies have demonstrated that the absorption of ferric iron by achlorhydric subjects is lower than by normal subjects (Choudhury & Williams, 1959; Goldberg et al., 1963; Jacobs et al., 1964; Bezwoda et al., 1978). Achlorhydria, however, does not affect the absorption of ferrous and heme iron (Biggs et al., 1962; Jacobs et al., 1968). The differences in absorption of ferric iron by achlorhydric and normal individuals have been attributed to the differences in pH of their gastric juices (Jacobs et al., 1968; Bezwoda et al., 1978). In the normal individual, ligands (e.g. proteins, amino acids, ascorbic acid, sugars, components of gastric juice) combine with iron at low pH to form complexes that remain in solution after neutralization in the duodenum, thereby maintaining the iron in a form suitable for absorption. In the achlorhydric individual, ferrous iron will form soluble complexes with ligands in the less acidic stomach, but ferric iron will not (Conrad & Schade, 1968). The onset of precipitation of ferric hydroxide occurs at approximately pH 3 (Britton, 1925). Ferric ions precipitate irreversibly upon hydrolysis forming large macromolecules (Spiro & Saltman, 1974). Once precipitated these ferric ions cannot be resolubilized through binding with complexing agents. Ferrous iron can be complexed at either acid or slightly alkaline pH values. Reducing substances such as ascorbate, succinate, fructose, and cysteine serve in preventing ferrous iron from oxidizing to ferric iron (Pollack et al., 1964). The hydroxides of ferrous iron do not begin to precipitate until pH 8 (Britton, 1925), thus stomach pH is of no consequence to their absorption. Heme iron is absorbed independently of intraluminal factors (Turnbull et al., 1962).

The diets of many elderly contain little or no meat, and thus little heme iron. Since the iron obtained from plant foods is mainly in the ferric form (Jacobs & Owen, 1969), there is a likelihood of iron deficiency developing in those with high gastric pH values. The low bioavailability of iron in infant formulas (5-10%) is partly compensated by iron supplementation (Saarinen et al., 1977; McMillan et al., 1977; Lönnerdal et al., 1983). Maintaining iron in the reduced ferrous form in infant formulas could be of particular importance in the iron nutriture of the young infant.

Dietary fiber has been implicated in reducing the absorption of iron into the body from the gastrointestinal tract (reviewed in: Kelsay, 1982; Harland & Morris, 1985). The possible effects of high intraluminal gastric pH values on the absorption of iron from high fiber plant foods have not been ascertained. The extent of iron binding by dietary fiber depends on pH and on the presence of competing iron-binding ligands. Figure 1 shows the binding of iron by enzymatically isolated, dephytinized wheat bran fiber as a function of pH in the presence of various iron-binding ligands (Leigh & Miller, 1983). The iron binding by the dietary fiber source increased from pH 2.0 to a maximum in the pH 3.5-5.0 range and then decreased at higher pH values, except when EDTA was the ligand. Steric changes in the fiber structure and increased ionization of the fiber functional groups appear to lead to the increase in iron binding in the lower pH range. The decrease in iron binding by the dietary fiber in the higher pH range may be attributed to the fiber functional groups being unable to compete with the ligands used or with polymer formation at these pH values (Leigh & Miller, 1983). The presence of a reducing agent, such as ascorbate, maintains the iron in the ferrous form and thus suppresses polymer formation. This permits more extensive binding of the iron by the dietary fiber (Leigh & Miller, 1983).

Reilly (1979) and Thompson & Weber (1979) have shown that the effects of pH on endogenous iron binding by dietary fiber are reversible over the pH 1.0 to 7.0 range. It is then possible that the final amount of ferrous iron bound by dietary fiber during passage through the intestinal tract could depend only on the presence of iron-binding ligands and not on intraluminal gastric pH values. In the case of ferric iron, low intraluminal gastric pH values would permit the formation of soluble iron complexes with ligands which can compete with the fiber functional groups for the low molecular weight iron. With high intraluminal gastric pH values, insoluble ferric hydroxide polymers form. Iron-binding ligands would not resolubilize these precipitated ferric ions and it seems unlikely that soluble fiber sources would. Thus, less ferric iron would reach intestinal sites in soluble forms.

The results of studies (Kojima et al., 1981; Reinhold, 1982) have indicated that some types of dietary fiber or factors associated with the fiber source may promote the oxidation of ferrous iron to ferric iron at pH values in the 4.0-7.0 range. As discussed earlier, the conversion of ferrous iron to ferric iron in the stomach at higher pH values will lead to its polymerization and precipitation,

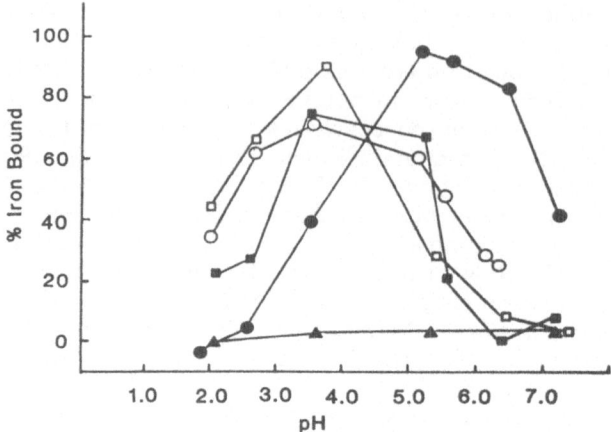

Figure 1. Binding of iron by enzymatically isolated, dephytinized wheat bran fiber as a function of pH and iron-binding ligand. Iron-binding ligands: 1:1 Fe:EDTA (▲), 1:1 Fe:NTA (○), 1:5 Fe:Ascorbate (●), 1:1 Fe:Citrate (□), 1:1 Fe:Lactobionate (■). Redrawn from Leigh & Miller (1983) with permission.

thereby lowering its availability for absorption from the intestine. Considering that the elderly are being encouraged to consume liberal intakes of fiber to help avoid or alleviate constipation, investigations are needed to assess the effects of dietary fiber on iron nutriture in those with high intraluminal gastric pH values.

Zinc Absorption

The effects of low hydrochloric acid secretion on zinc absorption have not been established clinically. The low bioavailability of zinc from plant foods has been attributed to their phytate content (reviewed in: Cheryan, 1980; Oberleas, 1983; Davies, 1982). If sufficient dietary calcium is present, zinc coprecipitates with the calcium phytates at intestinal pH values (Wise, 1983). The insolubility of these complexes prevents the absorption of zinc at intestinal sites. Raised intraluminal gastric pH values could cause the precipitation of calcium-zinc phytates in the stomach. There would then be a decrease in the zinc that would reach intestinal sites in soluble forms and be absorbed before precipitation with phytate occurs.

High intraluminal gastric pH values in young infants could possibly lead to lower absorption of zinc from soy protein isolate formulas. Recently, an *in vitro* study was undertaken to (1) evaluate possible effects of gastric pH values on the solubilities and complexes of zinc following pepsin treatments of soy protein isolate and to (2) determine whether gastric pH values would affect resultant zinc solubilities following subsequent digestion of the soy protein with pancreatin. The experimental details of this study are reported elsewhere (Champagne & Phillippy, 1989).

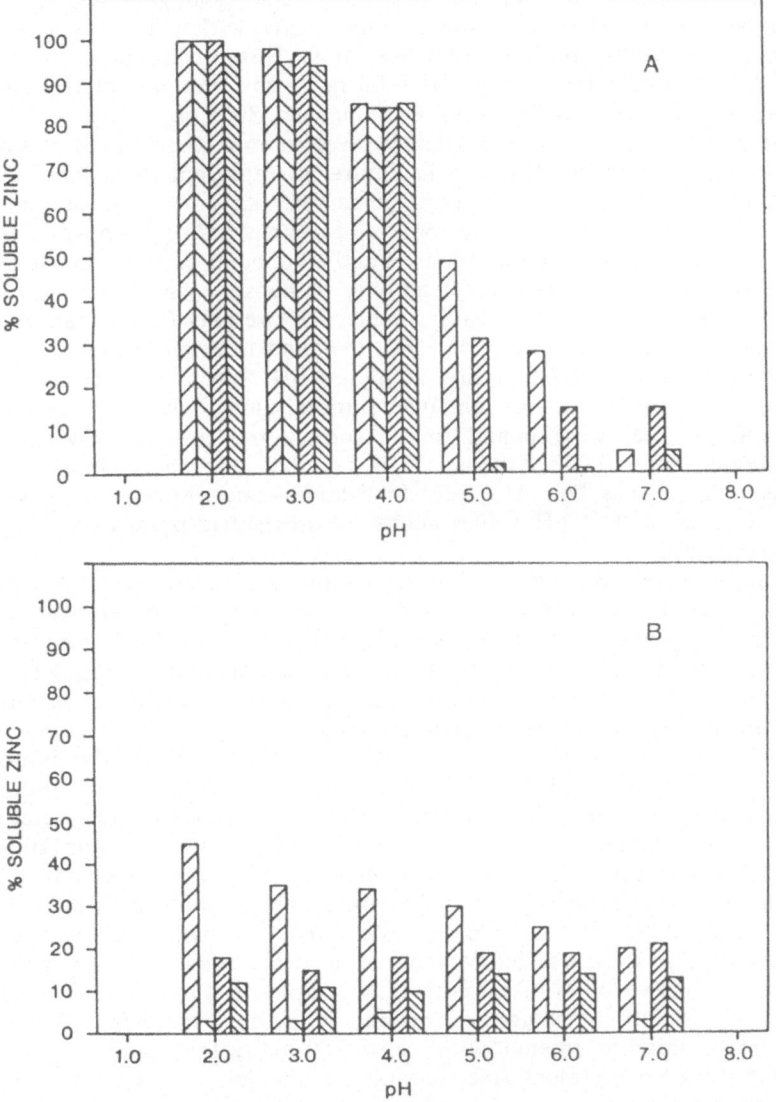

Figure 2. Solubility profiles of zinc as functions of pH in soy protein isolate treated with pepsin (A) and with subsequent pancreatin digestion at pH 7.0 (B). The isolate [Ralston Purina Protein 1711 (pH 6.9)] contained 2.0 mg calcium/g soy, 0.04 mg zinc/g soy, 1.3% phytic acid. Calcium chloride and zinc sulfate were used as exogenous sources. 0.04 mg Zn/g soy, 2.0 mg Ca/g soy ; 0.04 mg Zn/g soy, 30.0 mg Ca/g soy ⫟ ; 0.24 mg Zn/g soy, 2.0 mg Ca/g soy ⫟ ; 0.24 mg Zn/g soy, 30.0 mg Ca/g soy ⫟ .

Figure 2A depicts the solubility profiles of zinc (endogenous and exogenous) following *in vitro* treatments of soy protein isolate with pepsin as a function of pH. The zinc solubility profiles are those for soy protein isolate with endogenous levels of zinc and calcium (0.04 mg and 2.0 mg/g soy protein isolate, respectively) and with zinc and calcium levels of 0.24 mg and 30.0 mg/g soy protein isolate, respectively. The higher zinc and calcium levels mimic those found in soy protein isolate formulas. The solubility data in Figure 2A represent the solubilities of zinc in the stomach as a function of gastric juice pH. At normal intraluminal gastric pH values (2.0-3.0), all of the zinc (both endogenous and exogenous) was soluble. At these pH values, zinc solubility was found to depend entirely on the pH of the treatment and not on the presence or activity of pepsin. There was no binding of the soluble zinc to soy proteins having molecular weights larger than 10,000 daltons at these pH values (i.e., zinc was free or bound to small ligands).

Zinc solubilities declined rapidly at higher pH values. At pH values 6.0 and 7.0, over 50% of the zinc that remained soluble, along with some of the soluble calcium and phytate, were bound to the soluble soy proteins having molecular weights larger than 10,000 daltons. It is possible that this soluble zinc at pH values 6.0 and 7.0 was bound as protein-calcium-zinc-phytate complexes, which are postulated to exist at pH values above the isoelectric point of the soy protein (Prattley et al., 1982).

The addition of 28.0 mg calcium/g soy protein isolate did not significantly affect zinc solubilities at pH values in the 2.0-4.0 range. However, at higher pH values little if any zinc (endogenous or exogenous) was soluble in samples containing this amount of added calcium. At the higher pH values, zinc coprecipitated with calcium as calcium-zinc-phytates. The added calcium did not precipitate the zinc as protein-calcium-zinc-phytates, since the level of calcium did not significantly affect resultant protein solubilities. Furthermore, the insoluble soy zinc at pH values 5.0 and 6.0 in samples without exogenous calcium was not present as protein-calcium-zinc-phytate complexes, because phytate solubility was 100% in these samples. Therefore, insoluble soy protein-calcium-zinc-phytate complexes did not appear to be present in samples with or without added calcium. This observation could have nutritional significance for those with high intraluminal gastric pH values. It has been suggested that zinc associated with a protein-phytate complex is even less bioavailable than zinc associated solely with phytate due to the poor digestibility of these ternary complexes (Prattley et al., 1982).

Figure 2B depicts the solubilities of zinc following pancreatin digestion at pH 7.0 of samples initially treated with pepsin at pH values in the 2.0-7.0 range. These solubility data represent zinc solubility in the small intestine following pancreatin digestion of soy protein isolate as a function of gastric juice pH. A comparison of Figures 2A and 2B permits an evaluation of the changes in zinc solubilities following pancreatin digestion of pepsin treated samples. Zinc solubilities decreased following pancreatin digestion of samples initially treated with pepsin at pH values in the 2.0-6.0 range. In samples with added calcium or zinc, calcium-zinc-phytates precipitated at the higher pH value of the pancreatin digestion. However, in samples without added calcium or zinc, the amount of calcium and zinc available was insufficient to precipitate the phytates. All (98-100%) of the phytate was soluble. It is possible that the lowering of zinc solubilities following pancreatin digestion in these samples was due to the formation of insoluble hydroxides and insoluble bile salt complexes at pH 7.0. Pancreatin digestion of the pH 7.0 pepsin treated samples resulted in higher zinc solubilities, reflecting the release of zinc from insoluble protein complexes by the action of pancreatin.

Following pancreatin digestion, all of the soluble zinc and approximately 90% of the soluble phytate passed a 10,000 dalton molecular weight cut-off filter. Some of the zinc that passed the filter was possibly in the form of amino acid/low molecular weight peptide-zinc-calcium-phytate complexes. The bioavailability of zinc from such complexes (assuming that they exist) is unknown.

The pH of the initial pepsin treatment only affected resultant zinc solubilities following pancreatin digestion in the samples without added calcium or zinc, as shown in Figure 2B. In these samples, zinc solubility decreased from 45% to 20% as the pH values of the initial pepsin treatment increased from 2.0 to 7.0. Considering solubility as a criterion for bioavailability, it appears that intraluminal gastric pH values could have a noticeable effect on zinc availability from soy protein isolate not supplemented with calcium or zinc. Supplementation with calcium alone would not be beneficial in increasing the amount of zinc available to the person with high intraluminal gastric pH values, since less zinc was soluble in the pancreatin digests that contained added calcium. Since soy protein isolate formulas are supplemented with calcium and zinc, intraluminal gastric pH values possibly do not affect the amount of zinc absorbed by infants.

Thirty-two percent of men and 39% of women age 65 and above have serum zinc levels below 80 μg/100 ml (considered to be less than adequate) (Schlenker, 1984). Whether these low serum zinc levels reflect low dietary intake of zinc, a metabolic response of the aging process, or result from high intraluminal gastric pH values is not known. In view of the results of our *in vitro* study, clinical evaluations of the effects of intraluminal gastric pH values on zinc absorption from phytate-containing plant foods are warranted. Zinc supplementation would probably be of particular benefit to the elderly with high intraluminal gastric pH values.

Calcium Absorption

The popular use of calcium carbonate supplements in the prophylactic treatment of osteoporosis in the elderly has led to a need for evaluating the effects of low gastric hydrochloric acid secretion on calcium absorption. It has been postulated that ingested calcium carbonate dissolves in the acidic stomach to form the soluble chloride salt, which is absorbed in the small intestine (Clarkson et al., 1966). The solubility of calcium as the carbonate would be expected to decrease with high gastric pH values, and thus less calcium would be available for absorption.

Conflicting results have been obtained in clinical studies of the effects of intraluminal gastric pH values on calcium absorption from the carbonate salt. Bo-Linn et al. (1984) concluded that gastric acid secretion had no effect on calcium absorption after calcium carbonate ingestion, while Recker (1985) found calcium absorption from the carbonate salt to be markedly lower in achlorhydric subjects than in normal subjects. Russell (1986) has suggested that the lavage of the subjects in the Bo-Linn study may have dissolved some of the calcium carbonate permitting its absorption.

Fiber and phytic acid bind calcium, decreasing its bioavailability (reviewed in: Davies, 1982; Harland & Morris, 1985; Morris, 1986). The possible effects of high intraluminal gastric pH values on calcium absorption from plant foods which are high in fiber and phytate have not been determined. The binding of calcium by dietary fiber increases with increasing pH (Platt & Clydesdale, 1987). The onset of precipitation of calcium phytates occurs in the pH 4-6 range (Martin & Evans, 1986). At low gastric pH values (2-3), phytate does not bind calcium (Martin & Evans, 1986) and calcium binding by dietary fiber would be weak if at all (Platt & Clydesdale, 1987). Thus, in normal individuals calcium would reach intestinal sites as soluble species. Depending on the concentrations and binding strengths of various food ligands, some of the calcium will be absorbed at the intestinal sites while the remainder becomes bound as insoluble fiber and phytate complexes. In the individual with high intraluminal gastric pH values, insoluble calcium-fiber and calcium phytate complexes would form in the stomach. Based on the argument above, less calcium would be available for absorption at intestinal sites.

In a recent *in vitro* study (Champagne & Phillippy, 1989), all (97-100%) of the calcium in soy protein isolate samples that contained various amounts of calcium was soluble at pH values in the 2.0-4.0 range, as shown in Figure 3A. The percentages of calcium solubilized depended only on the pH of the pepsin treatment and not on the extent of proteolysis of the protein, as determined by the amount and activity of the pepsin present. The addition of calcium as the chloride or carbonate (Champagne, unpublished data) did not affect the percentages of calcium solubilized at pH values in the 2.0-5.0 range, with the exception of a small decrease in the percentages of soluble calcium with the addition of 28.0 mg calcium/g soy protein isolate at pH 5.0. At pH 6.0, the addition of 5.0 mg calcium (as the chloride)/g soy protein isolate led to a decline in overall calcium solubility to approximately 67%; at pH 7.0 the percentage of calcium solubilized remained unchanged (38%). Calcium solubility was lower when 5.0 mg of calcium was added as the carbonate: 38% at pH 6.0 and 11% at pH 7.0. These percentages decreased to 14% and 4% at pH values 6.0 and 7.0, respectively, when 28.0 mg calcium (as the carbonate)/g soy protein isolate was added. In contrast, higher percentages (78%) of calcium were soluble in the samples supplemented with 28.0 mg calcium/g soy protein isolate as the chloride salt than in samples with lower levels of calcium chloride at pH values 6.0 and 7.0. This observation can be explained by the insoluble calcium binding sites being full at the higher calcium chloride levels. Excess calcium was present and thus the percentages of soluble calcium increased. The lower solubility of calcium when it was added as the carbonate at pH values 6.0 and 7.0 reflects the insolubility of the carbonate salt at these pH values. More calcium precipitated with phytate in samples supplemented with calcium as the chloride than as the carbonate.

Figure 3B depicts the effects of pancreatin digestion at pH 7.0 on the calcium solubility profiles of samples initially treated with pepsin at pH values in the 2.0-7.0 range. Calcium solubility in the pancreatin digests without added calcium decreased from approximately 94% to 72% as the pH value of the initial pepsin treatment increased from 2.0-7.0. In digests containing added calcium chloride or calcium carbonate, the pH of the initial pepsin treatment had little effect on the percentages of calcium solubilized for values in the 2.0-7.0 and 2.0-5.0 ranges, respectively. Calcium solubilities were markedly lower in calcium carbonate supplemented digests which were initially treated with pepsin at pH 6.0 and 7.0.

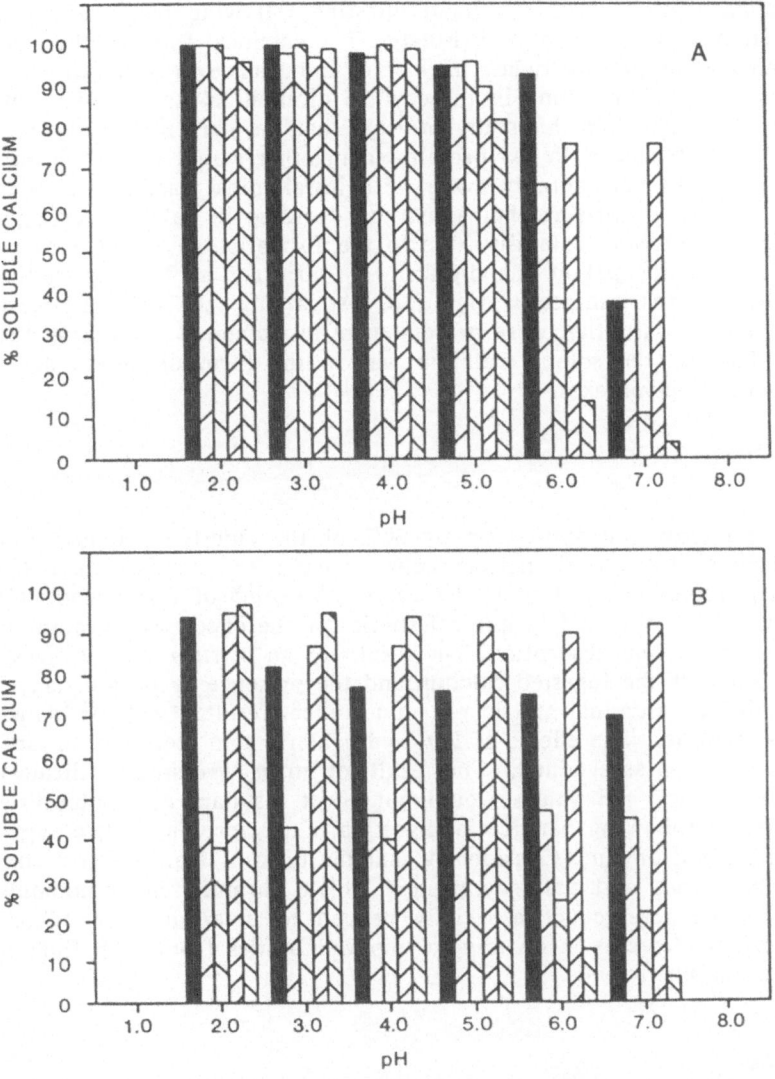

Figure 3. Solubility profiles of calcium as functions of pH in soy protein isolate (Ralston Purina Protein 1711) treated with pepsin (A) and with subsequent pancreatin digestion at pH 7.0 (B). 2.0 mg Endogenous Ca/g soy ▉ ; + 5.0 mg Ca (as chloride)/g soy ▨ ; + 5.0 mg Ca (as carbonate)/g soy ▧ ; + 28.0 mg Ca (as chloride)/g soy ▨ ; + 28.0 mg Ca (as carbonate)/g soy ▧ .

Keeping in mind the limitations of *in vitro* investigations, the results of this study suggest that intraluminal gastric pH values less than 6.0 will not affect resultant calcium solubilities in the small intestine following pancreatin digestion of calcium supplemented soy protein isolate. The chemical form of the calcium ingested with the soy protein isolate may be of importance in resultant calcium solubilities in the small intestine in those with intraluminal gastric pH values higher than 5.0. The results of this study indicate that the percentages of calcium, ingested as the carbonate with soy protein isolate, that would be soluble in the small intestine could be considerably lower with intraluminal gastric pH values higher than 5.0. It was surprising that a marked decrease in calcium (endogenous and that added as chloride) solubility due to the formation of calcium carbonate did not occur when the pH of the digests were adjusted to 7.0 with sodium bicarbonate prior to the pancreatin digestion. Apparently the protein digestion products or the bile salts that were present were instrumental in keeping the calcium soluble. Possibly the soluble calcium was in the form of amino acid/peptide-calcium-phytate complexes.

Summary

Young infants and approximately 30% of the elderly have low secretion of hydrochloric acid by gastric parietal cells. It has been established that low hydrochloric acid secretion can lead to decreased absorption of ferric iron. Conflicting results have been obtained in clinical studies of the effects of intraluminal gastric pH values on calcium absorption. The results of an *in vitro* study suggest that the chemical form of the ingested calcium and the presence of protein may influence whether high intraluminal gastric pH values affect resultant calcium solubilities in the small intestine. The effects of low hydrochloric acid secretion on zinc absorption have not been ascertained. The results of an *in vitro* study indicate that high intraluminal gastric pH values would not affect resultant zinc solubilities in the small intestine following pancreatin digestion of soy protein isolate supplemented with calcium and/or zinc. Considering that the diets of many elderly contain primarily plant foods and that soy protein isolate formulas are commonly fed to infants, further research is especially needed to determine the effects of low hydrochloric acid secretion on mineral bioavailabilities from high fiber and phytate containing plant foods.

References

Agunod, M., Yamaguchi, N., Lopez, R., Luhby, A. L., & Glass, G. B. J. (1969) *Am. J. Dig. Dis.* 14, 400-414.

Ardeman, S., Chanarin, I., & Doyle, J. C. (1964) *Brit. Med.* J. 2, 600-603.

Bezwoda, W., Charlton, R., Bothwell, T., Torrance, J., & Mayet, F. (1978) *J. Lab. Clin. Med.* 92, 108-116.

Bhanthumnavin, K., & Shuster, M. M. (1977) in *Handbook of the Biology of Aging* (Finch, C. E., & Hayflick, L., Eds.) Van Nostrand Reinhold Co.Inc., New York.

Biggs, J. C., Bannerman, R. M., & Callender, S. T. (1962) *Proc. 8th Congr. Europ. Soc. Haemat.*, 1961, pt1, no. 236.

Bo-Linn, G. W., Davis, G. R., Buddrus, D. J., Morawski, S. G., Santa Ana, C., & Fordtran, J. S. (1984) *Am. Soc. Clin. Invest.* 73, 640-647.

Britton, H. T. S. (1925) *J. Chem. Soc.* 127, 2110-2120.

Champagne, E. T., & Phillipy, B. Q. (1989) *J. Food Sci.* in press.

Cheryan, M. (1980) *Crit. Rev. Food Sci. Nutr.* 13, 297-335.

Choudhury, M. R., & Williams, J. (1959) *Clin. Sci.* 18, 527-532.

Clarkson, E. M., McDonald, S. J., & DeWardner, H. E. (1966) *Clin. Res.* 30, 425-438.

Conrad, M. E., & Schade, S. G. (1968) *Gastroenterology* 55, 35-45.

Davies, N. T. (1982) in *Dietary Fiber in Health and Disease* (Vahouny, G. V., & Kritchevsky D., Eds.) pp 105-116, Plenum Press, New York.

Fikry, M. E. (1965) *Gerontol. Clin.* 1, 216-226.

Ghai, P., Singh, M., Walia, B. N. S., & Gadekar, N. G. (1965) *Arch. Dis. Child* 40, 77-79.

Goldberg, A., Lockhead, A. C., & Dagg, J. H. (1963) *Lancet* 1, 848-850.

Harland, B. F., & Morris, E. R. (1985) in *Dietary Fibre Persceptives: Reviews and Bibliography* (Leeds, A. R. & Avenell A., Eds.) pp 72-82, John Libbey Co. Ltd., London.

Jacobs, A. M., & Owen, G. M. (1969) *J. Gerontol.* 24, 95-96.

Jacobs, P., Bothwell, T. H., & Charlton, R. W. (1964) *J. Appl. Physiol.* 19, 187-188.

Jacobs, P., Charlton, R. W., & Bothwell, T. H. (1968) *S. Afr. J. Med. Sci.* 33, 53-57.

Kelsay, J. L. (1982) in *Dietary Fiber in Health and Disease* (Vahouny, G. V., & Kritchevsky D., Eds.) pp 91-103, Plenum Press, New York.

Kojima, N., Wallace, O., & Bates, G. W. (1981) *Am. J. Clin. Nutr.* 34, 1392-1401.

Leigh, M. J., & Miller, D. D. (1983) *Am. J. Clin. Nutr.* 38, 202-213.

Lönnerdal, B., Keen, C. L., Ohtake, M., & Tamura, T. (1983) *Am. J. Dis. Child* 137, 433-437.

Martin, C. J., & Evans, W. J. (1986) *J. Inorg. Biochem.* 27, 17-30.

Mason, S. (1962) *Arch. Dis. Childhood* 37, 387-391.

McMillan, J. A., Oski, F. A., & Lourie, G. (1977) *Pediatrics* 60, 896-900.

Meyers, J., & Necheles, H. (1940) *J. Am. Med. Assoc.* 115, 2050.

Morris, E. R. (1986) in *Phytic Acid: Chemistry and Applications* (Graf E., Ed.) pp 57-76, Pilatus Press, Minneapolis.

Oberleas, D. (1983) in *Nutritional Bioavailability of Zinc*, ACS Symposium Series 210 (Inglett, G. E., Ed.) pp 145-158, American Chemical Society, Washington, D.C.

Platt, S. R., & Clydesdale, F. M. (1987) *Cereal Chem.* 64, 102-105.

Pollack, S., Kaufman, R. M., & Crosby, W. H. (1964) *Blood* 24, 577-581.

Prattley, C. A., Stanley, D. W., Smith, T. K., & Van de Voort, F. R. (1982) *J. Food Biochem.* 6, 273-282.

Recker, R. R. (1985) *N. Engl. J. Med.* 313, 70-73.

Reilly, C. (1979) *Biochem. Soc. Trans.* 9, 202-204.

Reinhold, J. G. (1982) in *Nutritional Bioavailability of Iron*, ACS Symposium Series 203 (Kies, C., Ed.) pp 143-162, American Chemical Society, Washington, D. C.

Rodbro, P., & Christiansen, P. M. (1966) *Scand. J. Gastroent.* 1, 292-298.

Rodbro, P., Krasilnikoff, P. A., & Bitsch, V. (1967a) *Scan. J. Gastrol.* 2, 257-260.

Rodbro, P. Krasilnikoff, P. A., & Christiansen, P. M. (1967b) *Scan. J. Gastrol.* 2, 209-213.

Russell, R. M. (1986) in *Nutrition and Aging* (Hutchinson, M. L., & Munro, H. N., Eds.) pp 56-69, Academic Press, New York.

Saarinen, U. M., Siemes, M. A., & Dallman, P. R. (1977) *J. Pediatr.* 91, 36-39.

Schlenker, E. D. (1984) in *Nutrition in Aging* pp 121-123, Times Mirror/Mosby College Publishing, St. Louis.

Spiro, T. G., & Saltman, P. (1974) in *Iron in Biochemistry and Medicine* (Jacobs, A., & Worwood, M., Eds.) pp 1-28, Academic Press, New York.

Thompson, S. A., & Weber, C. W. (1979) *J. Food Sci.* 44, 752-754.

Turnbull, A., Cleton, F., & Finch, C. A. (1962) *J. Clin. Invest.* 41, 1897-1907.

Vander, A. J., Sherman, J. H., & Luciano, D. S. (1975) in *Human Physiology: The Mechanisms of Body Function* (Adams, T. A. P., & First, C., Eds.) p 367, McGraw-Hill Inc., New York.

Villako, K., Tamm, A., Savisaar, E., & Ruttas, M. (1976) *Scand. J. Gastroenterol.* 11, 817-827.

Wise, A. (1983) *Nutr. Abs. Rev.* 53, 791-806.

Yamaguchi, N., & Glass, G. B. J. (1967) *Ann. NY Acad. Sci.* 140, 924-944.

13

Effect of Age and the Milk Sugar Lactose on Calcium Absorption by the Small Intestine

H. James Armbrecht

There is a marked decrease in the capacity of the small intestine to absorb Ca with age. Older adults also tend to consume diets with less than the recommended daily amount of Ca. This combination of decreased absorption of Ca and decreased intake of dietary Ca may contribute to the decrease in bone mass seen in the elderly. Therefore, it is important to understand the mechanisms responsible for the decrease in intestinal Ca absorption with age. Knowledge of the mechanisms involved may suggest ways of improving Ca absorption and utilization in the elderly.

We have used the Fischer 344 male rat as an animal model in which to study the age-related decline in intestinal Ca absorption. We have also investigated ways of enhancing Ca absorption in older animals. In particular, we have studied the response of older animals to 1,25-dihydroxyvitamin D, the hormonal form of vitamin D. In young animals, 1,25-dihydroxyvitamin D markedly stimulates Ca absorption by the small intestine. In addition to 1,25-dihydroxyvitamin D, we have studied the effect of certain dietary constituents, such as the milk sugar lactose, on Ca absorption throughout the lifespan. Dietary factors which enhance Ca absorption may be important in the elderly, who have altered vitamin D metabolism.

This chapter is divided into three sections. In the first section, we will discuss changes in Ca absorption by the small intestine with age. In the second section, the effect of 1,25-dihydroxyvitamin D on Ca absorption with age will be reviewed. Finally, the stimulation of Ca absorption by lactose and its relationship to 1,25-dihydroxyvitamin D stimulation will be addressed.

Changes in Intestinal Absorption of Ca with Age

Several human studies have demonstrated a decrease in the absorption of Ca with age (Alevizaki et al., 1973; Avioli et al., 1965; Bullamore et al., 1970). The time of greatest decrease is unclear from these clinical studies. One study reported an exponential decline (Alevizaki et al., 1973), another reported a linear decline (Avioli et al., 1965), and a third reported a decline after age 60 (Bullamore et al., 1970).

The effect of age on Ca absorption has also been studied in the rat. Everted duodenal sacs were used to measure active transport of Ca *in vitro* (Armbrecht et al., 1979; Armbrecht et al., 1980). Active transport is the energy-dependent movement of Ca against an electrochemical gradient, and it is greatest in the proximal duodenum. Active transport was measured by initially placing equal amounts of radiolabeled Ca on each side of the everted sac. After a 1.5 hour incubation, the amount of radioactivity on each side of the sac was assayed by scintillation counting. The ratio of the inside to the outside counts was calculated, and a ratio greater than 1.0 was considered indicative of active transport.

Active transport was found to decrease markedly between 1.5 and 12 months of age. At 1.5 months the ratio was 2.7 ± 0.4, and at 12 months the ratio was 0.7 ± 0.1 (Armbrecht et al., 1979). The effect of age on the passive uptake of Ca by the distal small intestine (jejunum and ileum) could not be studied in this way.

To study Ca uptake in both proximal and distal intestine, everted intestinal sacs with radiolabeled Ca on one side only were used (Armbrecht, 1986). Briefly, the small intestine was removed from the animal and everted. Two cm sacs were tied off with nylon thread. The sacs were then incubated in buffered salt solution containing 0.25 mM radiolabeled Ca for 15 min. Radiolabeled Ca in intestinal mucosa was quantitated and expressed per wet weight of tissue.

Using this technique, Ca uptake was found to decline markedly with age in certain regions of the intestine (Armbrecht, 1986). In young animals (2-3 months), there was a progressive decrease in Ca uptake as distance from the pylorus increased. In adult (12-14 months) and old animals (22-24 months), Ca uptake was relatively constant along the whole length of the intestine. In the duodenum, there was a greater than 50% decrease in Ca uptake in adult and old rats compared to young rats; there was no difference in Ca uptake between adult and old animals. No age-related changes in Ca uptake were seen in the jejunum and ileum of the three age groups. These studies are in agreement with the previous studies (Armbrecht et al., 1979; Armbrecht et al., 1980), which showed that the major changes in Ca absorption with age are in the duodenum and that the greatest decrease in Ca absorption takes place between 2-3 and 12 months.

Since intestinal absorption of Ca declines with age in both man and rats, we have used the rat to explore the biochemical mechanisms responsible for the decline.

Figure 1 shows a model for the absorption of Ca by the intestinal epithelial cell (Wasserman et al., 1984). Ca may be absorbed by either cellular or paracellular routes. In the cellular routing, luminal Ca enters the cell by crossing the brush border membrane. Movement across the brush border membrane is thought to involve a carrier-mediated process, but metabolic energy is not required, since the luminal Ca concentration is higher than the intracellular Ca concentration. Once inside the cell, there is a net movement of Ca through the cytoplasm from the brush border to the basal lateral membrane. A cytosolic protein which is thought to play a role in facilitating Ca movement is the vitamin D-dependent Ca-binding protein (CaBP). This soluble protein binds Ca with high affinity, is markedly stimulated by 1,25-dihydroxyvitamin D, and correlates well with Ca absorption (Wasserman & Fullmer, 1983). At the basal lateral surface of the cell, Ca is actively pumped out of the cell by an ATP-dependent pump (Figure 1-lower

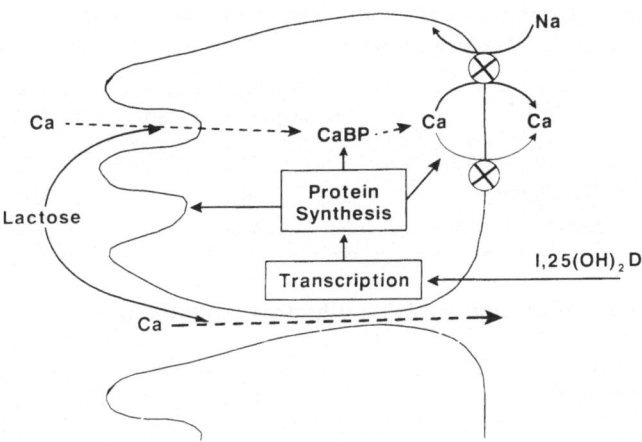

Figure 1. Possible model for the absorption of Ca by small intestinal epithelial cells. The brush border side of the cell (facing the lumen) is on the left, and the basal side of the cell is on the right. The actions of 1,25-dihydroxyvitamin D and lactose in enhancing Ca absorption are shown. See text for details. Note: intensities of arrows are not related to magnitude of Ca fluxes.

pump) and/or by a Na-Ca exchange mechanism (Figure 1-upper pump)(Ghijsen et al., 1982). Physiologically, the ATP-dependent pump is probably the most important. The paracellular route of Ca absorption does not require metabolic energy and involves the diffusion of Ca between cells from the lumen to the blood. The mechanisms involved in the possible regulation of this pathway are not well understood.

In the F344 rat, there are significant age-related changes in the CaBP and basal-lateral membrane components of the Ca transport system. Intestinal CaBP levels, as measured by a specific antibody, decline markedly between 2 and 12 months of age (Armbrecht et al., 1979). This decline parallels the decline in duodenal active transport of Ca. In the basal lateral membrane, the capacity to actively pump Ca also declines with age (Armbrecht & Doubek, 1987). This capacity was measured by isolating basal lateral membrane vesicles and measuring their capacity to pump Ca in the presence and absence of ATP. There was a 5-fold decrease in the active transport of Ca across vesicles isolated from adult rats as compared to young rats. This difference was seen only in the presence of ATP. No age differences were seen in the absence of ATP. The movement of Ca across the brush border membrane has not been reported to be age-dependent. However, age differences in glucose transport by brush border membranes have been described (Doubek & Armbrecht, 1987). The age-related changes in the components of the Ca transport system are summarized in Table I.

Table I. Changes in the components of the intestinal
Ca transport system with age

Site	Energy Required	Age Changes
Brush border membrane	No	No
Cytosolic CaBP	No	Yes
Basal lateral membrane	Yes	Yes

Stimulation of Ca Absorption by 1,25-dihydroxyvitamin D

In young animals, Ca transport is markedly stimulated by 1,25-dihydroxyvitamin D (DeLuca, 1979). 1,25-dihydroxyvitamin D is the metabolite of vitamin D with the most biological activity in the intestine. 1,25-dihydroxyvitamin D is produced in the kidney from 25-hydroxyvitamin D, which in turn is produced in the liver by the hydroxylation of vitamin D itself.

Possible actions of vitamin D in stimulating intestinal Ca absorption are shown in Figure 1 (Wasserman et al., 1984). At the brush border membrane (Figure 1-left side of cell), 1,25-dihydroxyvitamin D acts to enhance Ca entry into the cell. This may involve alteration in the lipid composition of the brush border membrane and/or the synthesis of new brush border proteins. In the cytoplasm, 1,25-dihydroxyvitamin D markedly increases the amount of CaBP. At the basal lateral membrane (Figure 1-right side of cell), 1,25-dihydroxyvitamin D increases the capacity of the basal lateral membrane to actively pump Ca (Ghijsen & Van Os, 1982). Possible effects of 1,25-dihydroxyvitamin D on paracellular Ca transport have not been well characterized.

Serum levels of 1,25-dihydroxyvitamin D decline with age in humans (Manolagas et al., 1983) and in rats (Armbrecht et al., 1984). In the F344 rat, the greatest decline in serum 1,25-dihydroxyvitamin D is between 2-3 and 12 months of age. In fact, the decline in serum 1,25-dihydroxyvitamin D closely parallels the age-related decline in CaBP and Ca active transport (Armbrecht et al., 1980). Thus, the age-related decline in serum 1,25-dihydroxyvitamin D could account for the decline in CaBP. The decline in CaBP, in turn, could account for the decline in Ca transport, assuming that the intestinal concentration of CaBP is rate-limiting for Ca absorption.

Since the age-related decline in Ca absorption may be related to the decline in serum 1,25-dihydroxyvitamin D, we have examined the possibility of enhancing Ca absorption in older animals by 1,25-dihydroxyvitamin D administration. In one series of experiments, rats were made deficient in 1,25-dihydroxyvitamin D by feeding dietary strontium, which blocks the renal production of 1,25-dihydroxyvitamin D (Armbrecht et al., 1980). Rats were then given a single maximal dose of 1,25-dihydroxyvitamin D, and intestinal Ca transport and CaBP levels were measured. 1,25-dihydroxyvitamin D significantly increased active Ca transport, as measured by everted intestinal sacs, in both young and adult animals. However, the increase was much less in the adult, and the adult never reached the levels of active transport seen in the young. In the same experiments, the induction of CaBP by 1,25-dihydroxyvitamin D was virtually identical in terms of time course and maximal induction.

In a second series of experiments, the effect of 1,25-dihydroxyvitamin D administration on intestinal uptake of Ca was studied in vitamin D replete animals (Armbrecht, 1986). A maximal dose of 1,25-dihydroxyvitamin D significantly stimulated Ca uptake by 52% and 64% in young and adult rats respectively (P < 0.05, t-test). Although the per cent stimulation was actually higher in the adult rats, the absolute Ca uptake was still much less in the adults compared to the young. In the jejunum and ileum, 1,25-dihydroxyvitamin D significantly stimulated Ca uptake in young animals, but it had no detectable effect in the adults.

In summary, 1,25-dihydroxyvitamin D significantly enhances both active Ca transport and Ca uptake in the rat duodenum. However, maximal levels of Ca transport are never achieved in the adult, suggesting that there is some defect in the Ca absorptive mechanism of adult rats. This defect does not appear to involve CaBP, since maximal amounts of CaBP are induced by 1,25-dihydroxyvitamin D regardless of age. The jejunum and ileum of adult rats appear to be unresponsive to 1,25-dihydroxyvitamin D, in contrast to the responsiveness seen in the young animal. In terms of human studies, older adults appear to respond to exogenous 1,25-dihydroxyvitamin D (Gallagher et al., 1979), but the responsiveness of a younger group was not determined for comparison.

Stimulation of Ca Absorption by Lactose

Studies in both humans and animals have shown that the milk sugar lactose influences Ca metabolism. In humans, lactose has been shown to improve Ca absorption (Kocian et al., 1973; Cochet et al., 1983) and Ca balance (Condon et al., 1970; Recker & Heaney, 1985) in lactose-tolerant individuals. In rats, dietary lactose significantly improves Ca retention and balance (Evans & Ali, 1967; Schaafsma & Visser, 1980).

The mechanism by which lactose improves Ca intestinal absorption has been extensively studied in rats. Using ligated intestinal loops, it has been shown that lactose acts rapidly to stimulate Ca absorption and that this stimulation is not dependent on vitamin D (Lengemann, 1959; Lengemann et al., 1959). In these studies, lactose caused the greatest stimulation in the ileum, although significant stimulation was also seen in the duodenum and jejunum. Using everted intestinal sacs, it was found that lactose enhances the initial influx of Ca into intestinal tissue (Armbrecht & Wasserman, 1976). This increased influx involved cellular pathways, since the increased influx could not be accounted for by an increase in extracellular space in the presence of lactose. In these studies, the effects of lactose were not blocked by metabolic inhibitors, and lactose did not need to be physically present with Ca to enhance Ca uptake.

Based on these experimental findings, a working model for the action of lactose can be proposed (Figure 1). The fact that lactose exerts its effect in the ileum and in the absence of metabolic energy suggests that it affects primarily the passive component of Ca transport. Both the cellular and paracellular passive component appear to be altered. The fact that lactose works in the absence of vitamin D suggests that the mechanism of lactose action is separate from that of vitamin D action. Lactose appears to act directly with the tissue to alter Ca permeability rather than to interact with Ca in solution.

Since lactose stimulates Ca absorption in young animals, we were interested in whether lactose also stimulates absorption in adult and old animals. We studied this question by measuring Ca uptake in everted intestinal segments from young, adult, and old F344 rats (Armbrecht, 1987). Segments were preincubated in the presence or absence of 160 mM lactose for 45 min., and then Ca uptake was measured. We found that lactose significantly (P < 0.05, t-test) increased Ca uptake by 20-54% in the duodenum and by 42-64% in the ileum, regardless of age. It was of interest that lactose had an effect in both the duodenum and ileum, even in old animals.

The effect of feeding lactose on intestinal CaBP levels also has been studied as a function of development (2-5 months) in the rat (Pansu et al., 1979). As reported previously, intestinal CaBP levels declined with age. However, feeding lactose decreased CaBP levels even further in all age groups. These studies point out the difference in the mechanism of action of lactose and 1,25-dihydroxyvitamin D. Both substances increase Ca absorption, but 1,25-dihydroxyvitamin D affects mainly the energy-dependent pathways while lactose acts on passive, diffusional pathways. In fact, the movement of Ca through the passive pathways tends to shut down the vitamin D-dependent active pathways, which include CaBP.

Since both lactose and 1,25-dihydroxyvitamin D stimulate Ca absorption in the duodenum, the question arises as to whether the action of lactose is additive to that of 1,25-dihydroxyvitamin D. To answer this question, serum 1,25-dihydroxyvitamin D levels were measured in the same animals in which the effect of lactose was measured (Armbrecht, 1987). When Ca uptake in the absence of lactose was plotted against serum 1,25-dihydroxyvitamin D, there was a significant positive correlation between serum 1,25-dihydroxyvitamin D and Ca uptake, as would be expected. Lactose, in turn, increased Ca uptake by about the same amount at each serum 1,25-dihydroxyvitamin D concentration. These results suggest that the stimulatory effect of lactose is additive to the effects of 1,25-dihydroxyvitamin D.

Finally, since lactose enhances intestinal Ca absorption and Ca balance, the effects of lactose on bone mineralization itself have been investigated. In animal studies, weanling rats were fed a vitamin D-deficient diet containing either 20% sucrose or lactose for four weeks (Miller et al., 1988). At that time, the lactose-fed rats were found to have greater bone weights, increased bone Ca content, and a greater endochondral (membraneous) bone growth rate than the sucrose-fed rats. In human studies, postmenopausal women fed milk supplements containing lactose had improved Ca balance but no detectable increase in bone mass (Recker & Heaney, 1985). However, bone remodeling was not suppressed as much in these women as in those given calcium carbonate only.

Conclusion

In conclusion, the capacity of the intestine to absorb Ca declines with age in both humans and rats. In rats, this decline parallels the age-related decline in serum 1,25-dihydroxyvitamin D. Decreased serum 1,25-dihydroxyvitamin D may account for the decreased amounts of intestinal CaBP and the decreased pumping capacity of the basal lateral membranes seen in older animals.

1,25-dihydroxyvitamin D stimulates intestinal Ca absorption in older animals, but not to the same levels seen in young animals and only in the duodenum. In a clinical situation, the administration of 1,25-dihydroxyvitamin D to increase Ca absorption must be carefully monitored, since it may also increase bone resorption (DeLuca, 1979). The use of vitamin D and 25-hydroxyvitamin D, the precursors of 1,25-dihydroxyvitamin D, to enhance Ca absorption in older mammals may be less effective, since the renal conversion of 25-hydroxyvitamin D to 1,25-dihydroxyvitamin D declines with age (Armbrecht et al., 1984).

Lactose stimulates intestinal Ca uptake in older animals by a largely unknown mechanism which is independent of and additive to that of 1,25-dihydroxyvitamin D stimulation. Lactose stimulates uptake in the ileum as well as the duodenum, and it does not act directly on bone. The disadvantage of lactose is that it is not well tolerated by some older individuals who have decreased levels of intestinal lactase activity. However, there is evidence that this relative lactose intolerance can be overcome by the feeding of smaller amount of lactose in conjunction with other foods (Newcomer & McGill, 1984).

In addition to lactose, other substances such as amino acids, phosphoproteins, and oligosaccharides have been reported to enhance Ca absorption. Along with lactose, these substances may be useful in enhancing Ca absorption, improving Ca balance, and decreasing bone loss in the elederly.

Acknowledgments

This research was supported by the Veterans Administration, the National Dairy Council, and the National Dairy Board.

References

Alevizaki, C. C., Ikkos, D. G., & Singhelakis, P. (1973) *J. Nucl. Med.* 14, 760-762.

Armbrecht, H. J. (1986) *Biochim. Biophys. Acta* 882, 281-286.

Armbrecht, H. J. (1987) *Nutrition Research* 7, 1169-1177.

Armbrecht, H. J. & Doubek, W. G. (1987) *Fed. Proc.* 46, 888.

Armbrecht, H. J., Forte, L. R., & Halloran, B. P. (1984) *Am. J. Physiol.* 246, E266-E270.

Armbrecht, H. J., & Wasserman, R. H. (1976) *J. Nutr.* 106, 1265-1271.

Armbrecht, H. J., Zenser, T. V., Bruns, M. E. H., & Davis, B. B. (1979) *Am. J. Physiol.* 236, E769-E774.

Armbrecht, H. J., Zenser, T. V., & Davis, B. B. (1980) *Endocrinology* 106, 469-475.

Armbrecht, H. J., Zenser, T. V., Gross, C. J., & Davis, B. B. (1980) *Am. J. Physiol.* 239, E322-E327.

Avioli, L. V., McDonald, J. E., & Lee, S. W. (1965) *J. Clin. Invest.* 44, 1960-1967.

DeLuca, H. F. (1979) *Nutr. Rev.* 37, 161-193.

Bullamore, J. R., Gallagher, J. C., Wilkinson, R., & Nordin, B. E. C. (1970) *Lancet* II, 535-537.

Cochet, B., Jung, A., Griessen, M., Bartholdi, P., Schaller, P., & Donath, A. (1983) *Gastroenterology* 84, 935-40.

Condon, J. R., Nassim, J. R., Millard, F. J. C., Hilbe, A., & Stainthorpe, E. M. (1970) *Lancet* I 7655, 1027-1029.

Doubek, W. G. & Armbrecht, H. J. (1987) *Mech. Aging and Develop.* 39, 91-102.

Evans, J. L., & Ali, R. (1967) *J. Nutr.* 92, 417-424.

Gallagher, J. C., Riggs, B. L., Eisman, J., Hamstra, A., Arnaud, S. B., & DeLuca, H. F. (1979) *J. Clin. Invest.* 64, 729-736.

Ghijsen, W. E. J. M., De Jong, M. D., & Van Os, C. H. (1982) *Biochim. Biophys. Acta* 689, 327-336.

Ghijsen, W. E. J. M. & Van Os, C. H. (1982) *Biochem. Biophys. Acta* 689, 170-172.

Kocian, J., Skala, I., & Bakos, K. (1973) *Digestion* 9, 317-324.

Lengemann, F. W. (1959) *J. Nutr.* 69, 23-27.

Lengemann, F. W., Wasserman, R. H., & Comar, C. L. (1959) *J. Nutr.* 68, 443-456.

Miller, S. C., Miller, M. A., & Omura, T. H. (1988) *J. Nutr.* 118, 72-77.

Manolagas, S. C., Culler, F. L., Howard, J. E., Brinckman, A. S., & Deftos, L. J. (1983) *J. Clin. Endocrinol. Metab.* 56, 751-759.

Newcomer, A. D., & McGill, D. B. (1984) *Clin. Nutr.* 3, 53.

Pansu, D., Bellaton, C., & Bronner, F. (1979) *J. Nutr.* 109, 508-512.

Recker, R. R., & Heaney, R. P. (1985) *Am. J. Clin. Nutr.* 41, 254-263.

Schaafsma, G., & Visser, R. (1980) *J. Nutr.* 110, 1101-1111.

Wasserman, R. H., Armbrecht, H. J., Shimura, F., Meyer, S. & Chandler, J. S. (1984) *Prog. Clin. Biol. Res.* 168, 307-312.

Wasserman, R. H. & Fullmer, C. S. (1983) *Annu. Rev. Physiol.* 45, 375-390.

14

Dietary Fiber or Bile-Sequestrant Ingestion and Divalent Cation Metabolism

Marie M. Cassidy and Don W. Watkins

The most rapidly developing area of nutritional science in the past fifteen years has been the study of physiological sequelae of enhanced dietary fiber intake. Original ethnographic observations by Burkitt & Trowell (1975) led to substantive epidemiologic studies relating decreased consumption of fiber to a variety of disease patterns. A major medical advance of the 19th century was the recognition that infectious disease was related to environmental factors. The recognition that chronic noninfective diseases characteristic of modern Western culture and lifestyle are linked to environmental aspects may prove to be the most significant medical advance of the 20th century. There has been considerable growth in knowledge of the effects of fiber on gastrointestinal physiology and function and the utilization of fiber regimens in the treatment of specific human disorders. These include such diseases as those of the cardiovascular system, colon cancer, diabetes and lesser metabolic disorders including obesity, ulcers, and gall-stones. For a comprehensive overview of the development and current research activity in this field the reader is referred to the proceedings of three international conferences on the subject held in 1981 (Vahouny & Kritchevsky, 1982), 1984 (Vahouny & Kritchevsky, 1986), and 1988 (Kritchevsky & Anderson, 1988). In the context of the effects of diet fiber or fiber components on mineral balance, a brief summary of accepted definitions of such materials, their analytical determination and the relationship of fiber chemistry to function and the putative mechanisms of action is presented.

What is dietary fiber?

A classical definition of these substances describes them as endogenous components of plant material in the diet which are resistant to digestion by enzymes present in man. They are predominantly nonstarch polysaccharides and lignin and may include, in addition, associated substances. The physical and chemical characteristics of isolated or semi-purified materials, as well as the physiological effects they induce, differ from those present in the original complex matrix of the

193

Table I. Dietary fiber constituents

Mixture in diet	Terminology in metabolic studies on diet supplements	Analytic definition
Proteins Lipids Inorganics		Non-dietary fiber constituents
Resistant starch Lignin Cellulose Other non-starch polysaccharides	Cellulose Pectic substances	Dietary fiber constituents
	Pectins Gums Mucilages Algal polysaccharides Modified cellulose	Polysaccharide food additives

plant. Table I shows the major dietary fiber constituents from plant cell walls, together with other substances which are either integral to the plant wall structure or are associated with it.

Modern concepts of the physiological functions of fiber classifies fiber sources as soluble or insoluble. This is an operational definition and, in general, soluble fibers include the gums, pectins, mucilages and some hemicelluloses. Insoluble fibers include cellulose, lignin and other hemicelluloses. Health positive effects consequent to enhanced fiber intake may vary, depending on whether the source is fiber-rich foods such as whole grains, legumes, beans, fruits and vegetables, or fiber supplements such as wheat, oat or corn brans or purified materials such as cellulose, pectins or gums. The portion and maturity of the plant consumed and food processing techniques also affect the relative fiber composition.

Analytical Methodology for the Measurement of Dietary Fiber

The chemical complexity of dietary fiber materials does not permit a single agreed upon technique which is satisfactory for the determination of dietary fiber from all sources. Available methods can be used to render a single value for total dietary fiber or values for the individual constituents. Gravimetric methods yield a weight measurement of the residue remaining after chemical or enzymatic solubilization of other components. The measurements are corrected for nitrogen content, which is considered to represent protein. Recent refinements permit the estimation of soluble and insoluble fractions, the sum of which is considered to be total dietary fiber. Chemical methods involve the assay of neutral sugar constituents of fiber polysaccharides by high-pressure liquid chromatography, or by gas chromatography following acid hydrolysis and derivatization. Gravimetric techniques are used for human and animal foodstuffs and were approved by the Association of Official Analytical Chemists in 1984 (Prosky, 1986). The neutral detergent fiber (NDF) method of Van Soest & Wine (1967), and the Southgate fractionation procedure (1988) to measure unavailable carbohydrate are also in current use. Comparative available data strongly suggest that there are significant differences in the assessment of fiber from several foods by chemical versus gravimetric methods. Further detailed study is warranted before a consensus is reached concerning the utility and validity of these techniques. It is also true that precise analytical measurements of fiber properties, *in vitro*, of such factors as absorption, water holding capacity, and osmolality, may not correlate with properties under physiological conditions, because alterations may occur during passage through the gastrointestinal tract. The principal physicochemical properties of fiber as they relate to physiological effects are shown in Table II.

Mechanisms of Action of Dietary Fiber

A variety of mechanisms have been proposed by which dietary fiber may influence the digestion and absorption of nutrients. These include alterations in:

[1]   Gastric filling and emptying, with subsequent perceptions of satiety levels.

[2]   Gastric acidity and the pH profile in the gastrointestinal tract.

[3]   Small intestinal mixing and transit times.

[4]   Intraluminal digestion, including pancreatic and biliary secretion and digestive enzyme activities.

[5]   Interactions with the intestinal surface, and effects on surface interactions.

[6]   Bile salt metabolism including interference with micelle formation, lipid absorption and bile acid resorption.

[7]   Bulk interference with nutrient diffusion and absorption and modifications of mucin synthesis and secretion.

[8]   Gastrointestinal hormone and peptide release.

[9]   Sites of absorption and sites of maximal transport of sugars, lipids, minerals and vitamins.

[10] Changes in intestinal morphology and altered rates of mucosal cell proliferation and repair.

Considerable evidence now exists in the literature documenting the existence of many of these mechanisms. Two principles are emerging: 1) Since dietary fiber does not cross the gastrointestinal barrier whole-body effects or those apparent in other organ systems probably originate in neuronal or hormonal signals that are perceived by the gut mucosal lining and relayed elsewhere. 2) Acute short-term effects are likely to be elicited when the fiber is co-administered with the particular nutrient being studied. Other effects can be shown to occur following chronic ingestion of dietary fiber constituents; an adaptational response of the

Table II. Physiochemical properties of dietary fibers and predicted physiological responses*

Property	Fiber Physiochemical Characteristics	Predicted Responses
Bulk		Increased mastication; slower intake; satiation
Water-holding capacity	Particle size; ionic properties	Altered stool bulk, laxation and transit time
	Gel formation	Delayed gastric emptying; satiation; delayed or impaired nutrient availability; unaltered or increased transit time; altered bile acid metabolism
Cation-exchange capacity	Polyuronic acids; associated oxalate and phytate	Modified mineral and cation metabolism
Bile acid binding	Pectins; gums; lignins	Laxation; altered enterohepatic circulation; modified lipid digestion and absorption
Bacterial metabolism	Polysaccharides	Altered hydratability, microfloral growth; production of short-chain fatty acids by fermentation; osmotic catharsis

* Adapted from Vahouny (1982).

rapidly renewed cells of the gastrointestinal tract to increased fiber ingestion is one such effect. Most of these mechanisms have been originally probed in animal models and are being partially substantiated in normal human volunteers and selected clinical populations.

Dietary Intake of Fiber in the US Population

Data on this point is somewhat lacking. A recent study in which information derived from twenty-four hour recall data from adults interviewed for the Second National Health and Nutrition Examination Survey (NHANE bII) is shown in Table III (Lanza et al., 1987). The mean dietary fiber intake in the US population (19 years of age) is 11.1 g/d, using food fiber values compiled from the literature by the National Cancer Institute and 13.3 g/d based on the Southgate methodology. On a per 1000 kcal basis women consume more dietary fiber (6.5 g/1000 kcal) than men (5.5 g/1000 kcal) in every age group. This study (Lanza et al., 1987) indicates that dietary fiber intake in the USA is considerably lower than that pre-

Table III. Mean dietary fiber intake by urban versus rural residence, race, and sex

	Mean Fiber (g) (SEM)		Mean Fiber (g/1000 kcal) (SEM)	
	Urban	Rural	Urban	Rural
Black females	8.0 ± 0.3	8.4 ± 0.6	5.7 ± 0.2	6.0 ± 0.4
White females	9.6 ± 0.2	9.6 ± 0.2	6.6 ± 0.1	6.6 ± 0.1
Black males	11.4 ± 0.4	8.4 ± 0.6	5.3 ± 0.2	4.6 ± 0.3
White males	12.9 ± 0.2	13.5 ± 0.4	5.5 ± 0.1	5.5 ± 0.1
Total	10.9 ± 0.1	11.5 ± 0.2	6.0 ± 0.1	6.0 ± 0.1

Data of Lanza et al. (1987).

viously reported and is 50-70% less than that consumed in other developed countries.

Dietary Fiber and Gastrointestinal Function

The physical and chemical characteristics of fibers are, to some degree, predictive of the *in vivo* response to these food components and these responses occur throughout the entire alimentary tract. The increased consumption of fiber-rich foods has been shown to cause increases in fecal volume, dry weight and fecal energy content. There is also evidence that specific dietary fibers affect the digestion and absorption of other nutrients, including minerals. These studies also suggest that, in addition to the acute effects caused by viscous fibers, there are chronic adaptive responses in the intestine to fiber-containing diets. Nutrient absorption is depressed by binding of fiber to luminal constituents and by modification of the mucosal surface barrier to transport. This barrier has been described as an unstirred water layer associated with the apical brush border membranes. However, there is an extensive mucin coat which is dynamic in nature and arises from the goblet cells, which constitute about one of every eight cells on the villous column. Fiber interacts with mucin (Vahouny et al., 1986) and increased turnover of intestinal mucins in response to prolonged ingestion of several different types of fiber has been reported (Vahouny et al., 1985; Cassidy et al., 1981). The acute effects of fiber derivatives on nutrient absorption *in vitro* are not observed when intestinal tissues are well rinsed prior to transport studies.

Effects of Fiber on Mineral Bioavailability and Metabolism

A number of reports have indicated that fiber in the diet may result in diminished or negative mineral balances in human subjects and in some animal models. The literature reflects considerable disagreement and the evidence is less than clear-cut except in the case of special sub-populations e.g., geriatric subjects. In reviewing the effects of fiber on mineral balances several factors need to be taken into consideration: these include the kind and level of fiber, level of mineral intake, the study design and length of test period, the presence of other mineral complexing agents such as phytic and oxalic acids and the levels of protein intake.

Many studies have been performed on vegetarians who have higher fiber intakes than those of omnivores. The mineral status of both groups appear to be equivalent. There is little evidence of mineral deficiences in Third World populations where fiber is a significant component of the diet (Walker, 1985). Blood serum values for minerals are not likely to be altered by fiber unless a deficiency is well advanced because homeostatic mechanisms contribute to maintain serum levels. Anderson et al. (1981) determined that serum values for calcium, iron and magnesium and total iron-binding capacity and hemoglobin levels were normal in 15 diabetic patients fed high-fiber diets for a period of 21 months. Serum levels of iron, calcium, phosphorus, zinc and magnesium were within the normal range for 68 adults consuming 2 tablespoons of bran for 6 months. Nine adolescents (Rattan et al., 1981; Godara et al., 1981) fed 21 g cellulose for 21 days, were compared to a control low-fiber group. Serum calcium, inorganic phosphate and iron levels were significantly decreased with this supplement. The use of test meals makes it possible to assess the effects of fiber from a particular meal, but does not necessarily predict the bioavailability of minerals in the whole diet. If minerals are bound by fiber, increased fecal mineral excretion should be observed. Dintzis et al. (1985) showed significant alterations in copper, iron, zinc and calcium in fiber sources during their passage through the gastrointestinal tract. More complete information can be obtained from *in vivo* studies if both urinary and fecal losses are determined. Unrefined cereals are high in phytate, which accounts for negative mineral balances reported with brown bread consumption. The removal of the phytate led to an improvement in mineral balance. In addition, the high levels of oxalic acid in foods such as spinach appears to be partially responsible for negative effects originally attributed to fiber. Almost all of the negative balances reported resulted from intakes of more than 25 g/day of insoluble fiber. Most of the study periods were from 2-4 weeks in length. Longer experimental time-frames generally indicate an adaptation to the decreased mineral availability. Moderate levels of fiber intake of 20-25 g/day would not appear to be problematic except in cases of marginal deficiency for other reasons, or generalized malabsorptive states.

In a series of studies aimed at defining the mechanism of action of dietary fibers relating to morpho-functional aspects of the gastrointestinal tract, we investigated calcium, magnesium, iron and zinc status and balance. In the first study the effects of the bile acid sequestrant, cholestyramine, which is a very effective medication for hyperlipidemia, were studied. Several reports of chemical abnormalities arising from this medication, including alterations in the handling of calcium, magnesium and iron, have been published. Runeberg & coworkers (1972) demonstrated modification of acid-base balance in patients with impaired renal function and this was accompanied by moderate increases in urinary magnesium excretion. Cholestyramine has also been shown to decrease the absorption of iron in normal iron-loaded and hemorrhaged animals.

Because of the intestinal mucosal injury in the rat induced by feeding cholestyramine, in conjunction with its role as co-carcinogen in the development of chemically induced colonic tumors, we investigated the influence of cholestyramine on dietary balance of the four major mineral elements (Watkins et al., 1985).

Two paired groups of animals housed in individual metabolic cages were fed either a control diet or one containing 2% cholestyramine for four weeks. The results indicate that chronic administration of this agent, which possesses some similar physicochemical properties to certain dietary fiber components, disturbed the metabolism of all four cations to varying degrees and with different time courses. After a 10-day period of accommodation to their environment, rat food consumption was monitored thrice weekly and fecal and urine samples were collected. Net balances for the four cations are shown in Table IV. Urinary pH and urinary excretion for the four elements are depicted in Table V. Both groups of rats gained equivalent amounts of weight during that study and the balance data was derived from three 3-day balance periods at the end of weeks 2, 3 and 4 of the study.

Calcium

Cholestyramine-fed rats had a negative net calcium balance in weeks 2 and 3 in contrast to the positive net balances achieved by the control rats. This was a consequence of a larger fecal and urinary calcium excretion by the cholestyramine group (Figure 1). However, there was no significant difference between the two groups in week 4 in terms of the net calcium balance, fecal excretion, or urinary excretion. This was due to a reduction in both the fecal and urinary calcium excretion by the cholestyramine group in week 4 compared to the previous weeks (Table V).

Magnesium

Animals from the cholestyramine-fed group had a near-zero magnesium balance in week 2 compared to the positive balance of those in the control group (Figure 2). Net magnesium balances for the two groups were not different for weeks 3 and 4. However, the urinary magnesium excretion was significantly higher in the cholestyramine-fed than the control animals In all three balance periods.

Iron

Rats fed cholestyramine had a smaller positive net balance for iron than did the control rats in all three balance periods (Table IV). This resulted from a greater fecal iron excretion with resin feeding throughout the study (Figure 3). Urinary iron concentrations were too low to be detected by the atomic absorption methodology used in this study.

Zinc

A smaller positive net balance for zinc was observed in the cholestyramine-fed rats than in the control rats in all balance periods. This resulted from a

Table IV. Net balances for four cations*

Balance period at end of week	Control (N = 4)	Cholestyramine (N = 5)
Calcium (meq/100 g/day)		
2	0.862 ± 0.550	-1.20 ± 0.590[a]**
3	0.990 ± 0.523	-2.42 ± 0.350[c]
4	0.200 ± 0.372	-0.358 ± 0.168
Magnesium (meq/100 g/day)		
2	0.179 ± 0.043	-0.006 ± 0.044[a]
3	0.180 ± 0.035	-0.120 ± 0.019
4	0.129 ± 0.019	-0.108 ± 0.018
Iron (meq/100 g/day)		
2	0.086 ± 0.013	0.027 ± 0.015[b]
3	0.073 ± 0.016	0.013 ± 0.004[b]
4	0.053 ± 0.010	-0.012 ± 0.009[b]
Zinc (μeq/100 g/day)		
2	10.8 ± 2.21	-1.29 ± 2.94[c]
3	11.0 ± 2.31	-1.30 ± 1.50[d]
4	7.74 ± 1.65	1.43 ± 1.16[c]

* Data of Watkins et al. (1985). Net balances are positive except for those preceded by a minus sign which indicates a net loss of the cation in question. The figures represent the net balance ± SE, that is, food intake minus the urine and fecal excretion, for each element at the time periods shown.
** Statistically significant differences between the control and cholestyramine-treated rats are indicated by lower-case letters. Control values for a given element are not different between weeks.
a, $P < 0.05$; b, $P < 0.02$; c, $P < 0.01$; d, $P < 0.005$.

higher fecal zinc excretion with the cholestyramine diet (Figure 4). In contrast, animals fed the resin additive had a lower urinary zinc excretion than the control animals in weeks 3 and 4, although the urinary zinc excretion comprised only a very small portion of total zinc excretion.

Tissue Cation Composition and Urine pH

The mineral content of intestinal scrapings and blood obtained at the end of the study is shown in Table VI. There was no difference between the two groups in gut tissue levels of any of these ions. However, the serum magnesium

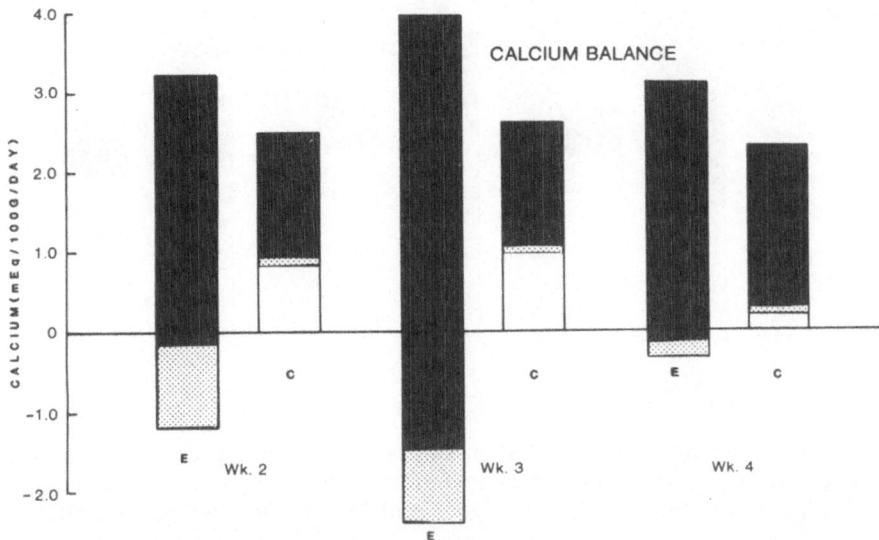

Figure 1. Average balances and calcium excretion rates are shown for control (C) and cholestyramine (E) animals for balance periods of three days at weekly intervals. The total bar height from the baseline upward represents the dietary intake of Ca, and excretion is plotted downward from the top of the bar. Fecal Ca is in black, urine in grey and positive net Ca balance in white, if present. Extension of the bar below the baseline indicates a net negative balance. Cholestyramine fed rats had larger fecal and urinary Ca excretion.

concentration of the cholestyramine animals was significantly lower than in controls. Urine pH of the cholestyramine-fed rats was significantly more alkaline than that of controls during the balance periods of weeks 3 and 4 (Table V).

The effect of cholestyramine was most pronounced on the calcium balance. This resin has been shown to decrease the absorption of Vitamin D, probably through interference with bile salt metabolism (Thompson & Thompson 1969). Inadequate Vitamin D could also account for the lesser effects on magnesium. While inadequate Vitamin D absorption may underlie the observations concerning high fecal excretion of Ca^{2+}, Mg^{2+} and Zn^{2+}, it does not adequately explain the elevations of urinary Ca^{2+} and Mg^{2+}. As shown in Table VII urinary phosphate excretion at 2 and 3 weeks following cholestyramine administration was only 1/6 to 1/15 the excretion rate in control rats. Such extremely low levels of urinary phosphate with cholestyramine is suggestive of a state of phosphate depletion which would explain the failure of the kidney to reabsorb filtered calcium and magnesium. Phosphate depletion has been reported to evoke hypercalciuria, magnesuria and an alkaline urine pH (Sutton, 1983; Dirks, 1983). Excretion of an alkaline urine by the rats fed the bile sequestrant may be an important clue to a significant metabolic disturbance. Our control rats achieved a consistently larger net iron balance than did the cholestyramine animals throughout the experiment.

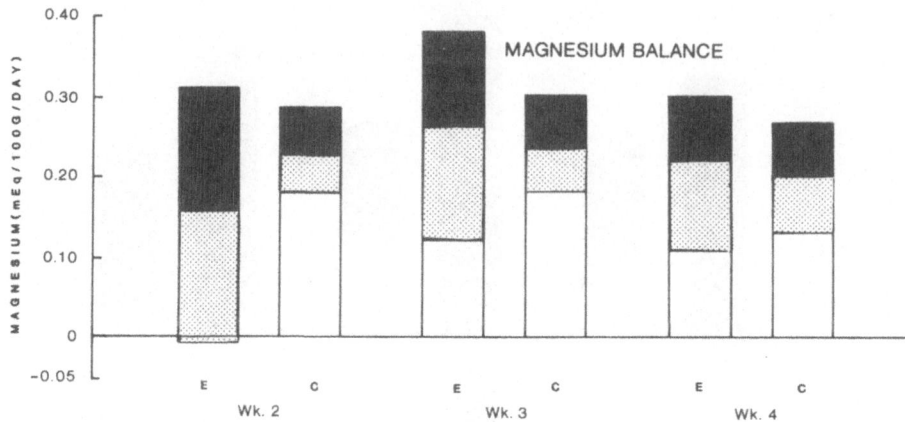

Figure 2. Balances are plotted in the same way as Figure 1. Urinary Mg was larger for cholestyramine-fed animals in all periods. In week 2, cholestyramine rats had a larger fecal but smaller net balance than controls.

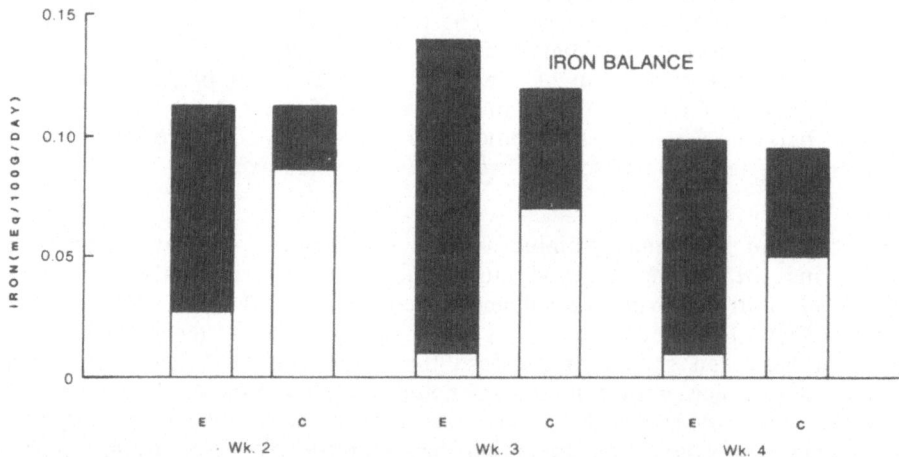

Figure 3. Cholestyramine-fed animals had a larger fecal Fe and smaller net Fe balance than controls during all balance periods. See Figure 1 for the plotting methods.

The apparent effect of cholestyramine in increasing the fecal iron could be due to the erosion of the intestinal mucosa with a resulting loss of epithelial iron (Cassidy et al., 1980) or to bleeding into the lumen from reported lesions. In addition, cholestyramine has been reported to bind iron (Thomas et al., 1971) thereby inhibiting iron and hemoglobin iron absorption in acute experiments in rats.

Thus, cholestyramine feeding induced variable alterations in the metabolism of the four divalent cations. The observed changes in calcium, magnesium, and zinc

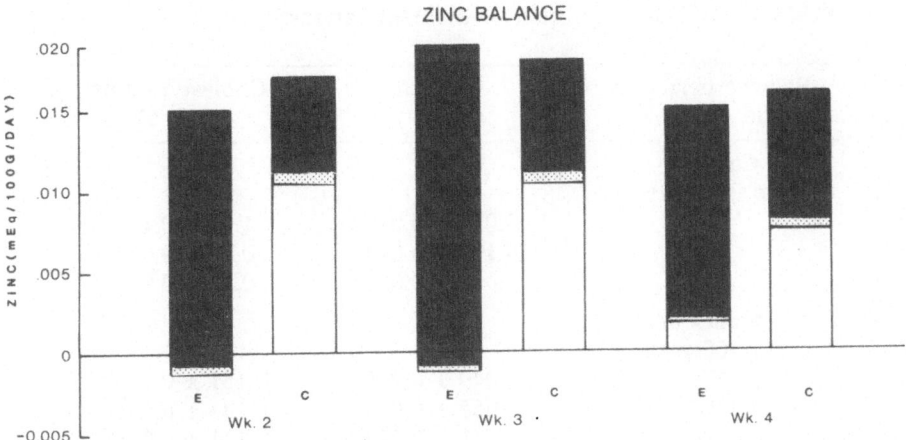

Figure 4. Fecal Zn excretion of cholestyramine-fed rats was larger, but urinary Zn was smaller than controls during all periods. Statistics are given in Tables 4 and 5.

excretion might be explained by inadequate vitamin D absorption and a resultant increase in parathyroid hormone secretion. The increased excretion of iron may be due to intestinal lesions or the binding of the metal or other factors, to the resin itself. However these effects may also have been caused by a failure of these young rats to stabilize their mineral metabolism when fed cholestyramine and housed individually. The multiple disturbances in mineral balances of cholestyramine fed animals appear to diminish with time, suggesting an ability of the intestine to adapt to this relatively harsh dietary additive.

In another study a wide spectrum of fiber types and derivatives were fed to rats, maintained in normal housing, for a period of 4 weeks. The basal diet consisted of the following components (g/100 g): dextrose, 55; casein, 25; corn oil, 14; salt min, 5; vitamin mix, 1. Additions to this diet included 10% soft white wheat bran (Archer Daniels Midland, Decatur, IL); 10% mixed fiber (Fibyrax) (Farma Foods, McLean, VA); 10% alfalfa (North Hampton County Farm Bureau, Nazareth, PA); 5% guar gum (Freeman Industries, Tuckahoe, NY); 5% methoxylated (7%) citrus pectin (Freeman Industries); 10% psyllium preparation (Metamucil) (50% sugar; Searle, Skokie, IL); 2% cholestyramine (Questran; Mead-Johnson, Evansville, IN). All diets were mixed, pelleted and analyzed by Bio-Serv, Frenchtown, NJ.

Fecal excretion of calcium, magnesium, iron and zinc was measured in samples obtained over a 3-day period (day 26-28) at the end of the dietary regimen. Apparent balances of Ca^{2+}, Mg^{2+}, Fe^{2+} and Zn^{2+}, based only on measured dietary intakes and fecal outputs, were positive after 4 weeks for animals fed any of the defined diets. Measurements of urinary mineral excretion indicated that such losses would not significantly influence retention. Thus, data on divalent cation balances obtained for rats in a more "normal" housing environment gave no indication of imbalances induced by relatively high levels of insoluble or soluble dietary fiber supplements. These data are entirely consistent with studies on mineral

Table V. Urinary excretion of divalent cations*

Balance period at end of week	Control (N = 4)	Cholestyramine (N = 5)
Calcium (meq/100 g/day)		
2	0.061 ± 0.017	1.02 ± 0.19[c]**
3	0.160 ± 0.005	0.90 ± 0.05[d]
4	0.063 ± 0.033	0.20 ± 0.07
Magnesium (meq/100 g/day)		
2	0.049 ± 0.028	0.151 ± 0.019[b]
3	0.055 ± 0.015	0.143 ± 0.014[c]
4	0.071 ± 0.017	0.111 ± 0.008[a]
Zinc (μeq/100 g/day)		
2	0.014 ± 0.010	0.073 ± 0.019
3	0.153 ± 0.031	0.047 ± 0.007[c]
4	0.123 ± 0.028	0.043 ± 0.008[b]
Urine pH		
2	6.22 ± 0.25	7.30 ± 0.37[a]
3	6.20 ± 0.12	7.68 ± 0.39[b]
4	6.35 ± 0.29	7.98 ± 0.15[c]

* Data of Watkins et al. (1985). The figures represent the urinary output of the individual cations ± SE, or the urine pH, at the time periods shown.
** Statistically significant differences between the control and cholestyramine-treated groups are indicated by lower-case letters: a, $P < 0.05$; b, $P < 0.02$; c, $P < 0.005$; d, $P < 0.001$.

availability in rats fed "fiber-filler" (a mixed fiber source) using radioactive cations to assess absorption (Fairweather-Tait et al., 1985).

Early information from feeding studies had suggested that high fiber intakes might be a factor in the potentially negative mineral balances, specifically, balances of calcium. More recent reports on studies in humans (Rattan et al., 1981) and various literature surveys (Walker, 1985; Kelsay, 1985; Harland et al., 1985) suggest that when such imbalances appear in subjects shifting to a higher fiber diet, the response tends to be transient and is often followed by changes which indicate adaptation to the diet (Walker, 1985).

Fears that the proliferation of advice to the US population recommending higher intake of dietary fiber could result in negative physiological responses are being allayed by preview reports from a study of the Chinese population. A massive multinational and multidimensional study on the relationship between diet and disease is being carried out in China by Cornell University, the University of Oxford, and the Chinese Academies of Preventive Medicine and Medical Sciences.

Table VI. Tissue cation concentrations*

	Control (N = 4)	Cholestyramine (N = 5)
Calcium		
Duodenum (meq/g)	0.063 ± 0.0013	0.071 ± 0.002
Jejunum (meq/g)	0.019 ± 0.009	0.024 ± 0.009
Serum (meq/L)	4.70 ± 0.21	4.88 ± 0.05
Magnesium		
Duodenum (meq/g)	0.089 ± 0.017	0.084 ± 0.003
Jejunum (meq/g)	0.065 ± 0.002	0.068 ± 0.002
Serum (meq/L)	1.46 ± 0.07	1.25 ± 0.07[a]
Iron		
Duodenum (meq/g)	0.020 ± 0.003	0.025 ± 0.004
Jejunum (meq/g)	0.016 ± 0.001	0.016 ± 0.002
RBC (meq/L)	42.0 ± 2.9	41.0 ± 2.0
Zinc		
Duodenum (meq/g)	0.0023 ± 0.0003	0.0030 ± 0.005
Jejunum (meq/g)	0.0028 ± 0.0001	0.0028 ± 0.0002
RBC (meq/L)	0.36 ± 0.07	0.28 ± 0.02

* Data from Watkins et al. (1985). The figures shown represent the mean ± SE of the concentration indicated. Significant differences between the control and cholestyramine groups are indicated by a superscript a ($P < 0.05$).

Table VII. Urinary excretion of phosphate*

Week	Control (N = 4)	Cholestyramine (N = 5)
2	3.36 ± 0.62	0.23 ± 0.07[b]
3	1.49 ± 0.38	0.26 ± 0.07[b]
4	0.88 ± 0.18	0.30 ± 0.06[a]

* The figures shown represent the mean ± SE of the daily phophate excretion (mg/day). Significant differences determined by the t-test are indicated by: a, $P < 0.02$; b, $P < 0.01$.

Samples from large cohorts of people are being analyzed in laboratories around the world. Data assembled thus far include information on hormone, mineral and fat levels among some 350 variables being recorded. Access to the primary data will be available late in 1988. Some of the preliminary findings (Table VIII) show that despite the consumption of more than 3 times the level of fiber than is usual in the US, mineral uptake is not hampered, and plasma iron, zinc and magnesium are all at healthy levels.

Table VIII. China study on the relationship between diet and disease*

Study Design

1. 6,500 people from 130 villages studied 5 yrs.
2. Data collected from blood and urine, and on lifestyle. Food samples and diaries analyzed multinationally.

Preliminary Findings

1. Chinese consume ~20% more calories than Americans, but there is little obesity.
2. Fats comprise only 15% of caloric intake, less than half of American intake.
3. Serum cholesterol levels are at very bottom of the scale for US population.
4. Fiber intake is 34 g/day, almost 3 times US average.
5. Plasma Fe, Zn, Mg, hemoglobin and hematocrit levels are moderately high.

---

* From Anderson (1988). Principal investigators are:
T. C. Campbell, Cornell U., R. Petro, U. of Oxford, and
the Chinese Academies of Preventive Medicine and Medical Sciences.

In conclusion, the present state of knowledge concerning the effect of dietary fiber on mineral balance suggests that imbalances observed in short term or acute studies are transient in nature and that intestinal adaptation to an altered diet restores mineral homeostasis within a period of a few weeks in both animals and man.

Acknowledgements

We wish to gratefully record our thanks to several of our collaborators in these studies: D. Kritchevsky, S. Satchithanandam, R. Khalafi, J. Story and others. The untimely death of a major colleague in 1986, George V. Vahouny, who initiated these studies, leaves a void in the dietary fiber nutritional research field.

References

Anderson, A. (1988) *Nature* 332, 100.

Anderson, B. M., Gibson, R. S., & Sabry, J. H. (1981) *Am. J. Clin. Nutr.* 34, 1042-1048.

Anderson, J. W., Ferguson, S. K., Karounos, D., O'Malley, L., Sieling, B., & Chen, W. (1980) *Diabetics Care* 3, 38-40.

Asano, T., Pollard, M., & Madsen, D. (1975) *Proc. Soc. Exp. Biol. Med.* 150, 780-785.

Burkitt, D., & Trowell, H. L. (Eds.) (1975) in *Refined Carbohydrate Foods and Disease. Some Implications of Dietary Fiber*, Academic Press, London.

Cassidy, M. M., Lightfoot, F. G., Grau, L., Roy, T., Kritchevsky, D., & Vahouny, G. (1980) *Dig. Dis. Sci.* 25, 504-512.

Cassidy, M. M., Lightfoot, F. G., & Vahouny, G. V. (1982) *Adv. Lipid Res.* 19, 203-229.

Cassidy, M. M., & Vahouny, G. V. (1987) in *Cardiovascular Disease* (Gallo, L., Ed.) Plenum Press, New York.

Cassidy, M. M., Lightfoot, F. G., & Vahouny, G. V. (1981) in *Structure and Function in Epithelia* (Dinno, M., Ed.) pp 97-127, Liss, New York.

Dintzis, F. R., Watson, P. R., & Sandstead, H. H. (1985) *Am. J. Clin. Nutr.* 41, 901-908.

Dirks, F. H. (1983) *Kidney Int.* 23, 771-777.

Fairweather-tait, S. J., & Wright, A. J. A. (1985) *Br. J. Nutr.* 54, 585-592.

Godara, R., Kaur, A. P., & Bhat, C. M. (1981) *Am. J. Clin. Nutr.* 34, 1083-1086.

Harland, B. F., & Morris, E. R. (1985) in *Dietary Fiber Perspectives. Reviews and Bibliography* (Leeds, A. R., Ed.) pp 72-82, John Libbey, London.

Kelsay, J. L. (1986) in *Dietary Fiber: Basic and Clinical Aspects* (Vahouny, G. V., & Kritchevsky, D., Ed.) pp 361-372, Plenum, New York.

Kritchevsky, D., & Anderson, J. (Eds.) (1988) in *The Vahouny Fiber Symposium: Dietary Fiber in Health and Disease* Plenum, New York.

Lanza, E., Jones, Y., Block, G., & Kessler, L. (1987) *Am. J. Clin. Nutr.* 46, 790-797.

Prosky, L., Asp, N. G., Furda, I., DeVries, J. W., Schweizer, T. F., & Harland, B. F. (1985) *J. Assoc. Off. Anal. Chem.* 68, 677-679.

Rattan, J., Levin, N., Graff, E., Weizer, N., & Gilat, T. (1981) *J. Clin. Gastroenterology* 3, 389-393.

Runeberg, L., Miettinen, T. A., & Nikela, E. A. (1972) *Acta. Med. Scand.* 192, 71-76.

Southgate, D. & Englyst, H. (1985) in *Dietary Fiber, Fiber Depleted Foods and Disease* (Trowell, H., Burkitt, D., Heaton, K., Eds.) pp 31-35, Academic Press, New York.

Sutton, R. A. L. (1983) *Kidney Int.* 23, 665-673.

Thompson, W. G., & Thompson, G. R. (1969) *Gut* 10, 717-722.

Vahouny, G. V. (1982) *Fed. Proc.* 41, 2801-2806.

Vahouny, G. V., & Kritchevsky, D. (Eds.) (1982) in *Dietary Fiber in Health and Disease* Plenum, New York.

Vahouny, G. V., Le, T., Ifrem, I., Satchithanandam, S., & Cassidy, M. M. (1985) *Am. J. Clin. Nutr.* 41, 895-900.

Vahouny, G. V., & Kritchevsky, D., (Eds.) (1986) in *Dietary Fibre: Basic and Clinical Aspects* Plenum, New York.

Vahouny, G. V., Khalafi, R., Satchithandam, S., Watkins, D. W., Story, J. A., Cassidy, M. M., & Kritchevsky, D. (1987) *J. Nutr.* 117, 2009-2015.

Van Soest, P. J., & Wine, R. H. (1967) *J. Assoc. Agric. Chem.* 50, 50-55.

Walker, A. (1985) in *Dietary Fibre, Fibre Depleted Foods and Disease* (Trowell, H., Burkitt, D, Heaton, K., Eds.) pp 361-375, Academic Press, New York.

Watkins, D. W., Khalafi, R., Cassidy, M. M., & Vahouny, G. V. (1985) *Dig. Dis. Sci.* 30, 477-482.

Index

Absorption,
    calcium ... 9, 21, 36, 45-61, 96-99, 122-124, 126, 135, 147, 149-152, 156,
        168-169, 174, 176, 179-180, 182, 185-191, 198, 201, 203
    copper ... 7, 106-107
    iron ... 27-42, 96, 101-102, 117-120, 122-129, 135, 147, 167-169, 174-176,
        182, 198-199, 201-203
    minerals ... 11, 41, 95-97, 101, 108, 133-135, 143, 147, 151, 156, 158, 165,
        167-169, 174, 182, 195, 197, 203
    nonheme iron ... 101-102, 118-120, 122-128
    radioiron ... 118-120, 122, 127
    substrates ... 95, 147
    zinc ... 3-11, 13-14, 16, 18-22, 24, 35-42, 102-108, 135, 147, 165-169, 174,
        176, 179, 182, 198, 201, 203
Achlorhydria ... 124, 128, 173, 175
Acrodermatitis enteropathica ... 103-104
Active transport (*see* Transport)
Anemia ... 37, 102
Anorexia ... 110
Antinutritional factors ... 163
Ascorbic acid (ascorbate) ... 28-29, 33, 36, 102, 120, 123, 127, 129, 135, 143,
    167, 175
ATPase ... 8, 46, 50, 60
ATP-dependent ... 8, 46, 48-49, 56, 61, 187
Availability (*see* Bioavailability)
Balance ... 70, 118-119, 156, 189-191
    calcium ... 97, 99-100, 107, 190, 198-199, 201, 203-204
    copper ... 7, 198
    zinc ... 3, 7, 21, 107, 198-199, 201, 203
Basolateral membrane ... 8-9, 46, 48-49, 52, 56-57, 60-61, 88, 103
Bicarbonate ... 67-78, 83, 87-91, 182
Binding sites ... 4, 20, 40, 67-70, 72-74, 76, 78-81, 83, 85, 87-89, 138,
    140-142, 157, 165, 175, 180
Bioavailability,
    copper ... 106, 198
    iron ... 96, 101-102, 117-120, 122-129, 143, 164, 168-169, 175, 198
    mineral ... 96, 103, 133-134, 143, 147, 156-157, 164-165, 168-169, 173, 198
    zinc ... 3-4, 11, 24, 102-103, 106, 135, 147, 164-169, 176, 179, 198

Brush border membrane ... 4-6, 28, 31, 33, 46, 49-50, 56, 59-60, 103, 186-188, 197

Brush border vesicles ... 5-6, 28-29, 31, 33, 46, 187

Ca-binding protein (CaBP) ... 50, 52, 55-60, 97, 187-190

Cadmium ... 37, 39-42, 81, 83

Calbindin-D ... 46, 50, 52-54, 56-58, 60

Calcium ... 6, 8-9 18, 21, 30-31, 36, 45-46, 48-58, 60-61, 96-97, 99-100, 122-124, 126, 135-138, 140-141, 143, 149, 151-158, 163-164, 166, 168-169, 174, 176, 178-180, 182, 185-191, 198-199, 201, 203-204

Calcium phytate ... 123-124, 126, 163, 166, 168-169, 176, 178-180, 182, 198

Calcium pump ... 46, 48, 56-57, 61, 187-188

Calciuria ... 100

Calmodulin ... 46, 52, 59-60

Cardiomyopathies ... 110

Cereals ... 117, 120, 125-126, 129, 161-163, 166, 169, 198

Chelating agents ... 5, 29-31, 70, 81, 97, 101, 106, 161, 163, 165-169

Chromium ... 38-39

Colon ... 21, 105, 148, 151-153, 193
    distal ... 148, 151-153
    proximal ... 105, 148, 151-153

Corn bran ... 134-138, 140-141, 143, 147, 151, 154, 157-158, 161-162, 194, 203

Crohn's disease ... 100

Cytosolic facilitator, of Ca ... 60

Deficiency,
    iron ... 101, 120, 127, 175, 198
    vitamin D ... 49
    zinc ... 5-6, 13, 103, 105-106, 109-110, 198

Diet,
    American ... 101, 122
    legume-based ... 120
    self-selected ... 100
    semi-synthetic ... 53
    standard ... 122
    vegetable (plant) ... 97, 101, 109, 128, 163-164, 175-176, 179-182, 194
    Western ... 101, 117-118, 128-129, 193

Dietary
    components ... 3-5, 10, 96, 103, 106, 143, 193-195, 197, 199
    factors ... 5, 7, 11, 103, 111, 117, 120, 124, 176, 185, 193, 195, 203

Dietary fiber ... 3-4, 123, 133-133-143, 147, 167, 174-176, 180, 182, 193-199, 203, 205-206

Diffusion ... 5, 10, 46, 48, 56-58, 60, 187, 195

Diffusional translocator ... 46

Digesta ... 4, 105-106, 125, 136, 148-149, 151-155, 157-158, 166, 179-180, 182

Digestion, products of ... 95-96, 102, 125-126, 156, 165-166, 182

Duodenum ... 21, 28, 30, 33, 41, 106, 155, 167, 175, 186, 189-191

Dysfunction, taste and smell ... 13-14, 19

EDX analysis ... 147-148, 157-158

Electron microprobe ... 49, 149

Electropotential gradient ... 46, 61

Endocytosis ... 49

Energy-dispersive X-ray (*see* EDX analysis)

Enzymes, digestive ... 3, 169, 195

Epithelial cells ... 4-5, 46, 57, 186

Equilibrium ... 4, 67-69, 77, 79, 81-82, 87, 135-136

Equilibration time ... 87

Exchange mechanism, Na-Ca ... 187

Excretion, calcium ... 99-100, 168-169, 198-199, 201, 203

Exocytosis ... 46, 49

FeEDTA ... 29

Fermentation ... 163-164, 169

Ferritin ... 37, 101, 119-120, 127-128, 133

Fiber (*see* Dietary fiber)

Foods (*see* Diet)

Fortification ... 118-119, 127

Gastrointestinal conditions ... 125, 127, 133-135, 143, 195

Gastrointestinal conditions, simulated ... 125, 134

GI tract ... 147-148, 151-158, 166-169

Hemoglobin repletion method ... 118

Hemosiderin ... 119, 127

Homeostasis, calcium ... 45-46, 50

Homeostatic ... 6, 10, 198

Hormonal ... 49, 96, 100, 185, 195

Hormone ... 45, 50, 60, 97, 100, 195, 203, 205

Hypochlorhydria ... 173

Hypoxia ... 28-31

Hypozincemia ... 105

Ileum ... 21, 105, 107, 147-148, 151-156, 166, 186, 189-191

Insufficiency ... 106, 108, 110

Insufficiency, manganese ... 108

Intestinal mucosa ... 6, 10, 28, 40, 53, 55-56, 95-96, 101, 104, 107, 166, 186, 195, 197, 199, 202

Intestinal segments ... 3, 39, 53, 190

Iron ... 27-29, 33, 35, 42, 67-71, 76, 79, 81, 89, 117-129, 135-138, 142-143, 163-164, 167-169, 198-199, 201-203, 205

    ferric ... 67, 101, 122, 124, 128, 175-176, 182

    ferrous ... 70, 87, 101-102, 124, 142, 175-176

    heme ... 96, 101, 110, 119-120, 127-128, 175

    nonheme ... 101-102, 118-120, 122-128

Iron status ... 120, 127, 129, 198

Jejunum ... 21, 97, 105-108, 128, 186, 189

Kinetics(s) ... 5, 7-8, 10, 13-14, 16-19, 22, 24, 27-28, 41, 85, 105

Lactoferrin ... 67-68, 128

Lactose ... 97, 185-186, 189-191

Lignin ... 133, 142-143, 194

Linear free energy relationships (LFER) ... 81-87

Lumen ... 4-6, 9-10, 46, 48, 58, 95-97, 107-108, 147, 186-187

Magnesium ... 36, 96-97, 99-100, 135-138, 141, 147, 163, 166, 168, 198-201, 203, 205

Magnesuria ... 100, 201
Malabsorption ... 4, 11, 100
Manganese ... 36, 39, 41-42, 108, 163, 166
Meal(s) (*see* Diet)
Mechanism,
    active transport ... 46, 48, 189
    endocytotic-exocytotic ... 46, 60
    Fe-absorbing ... 41
    Fe-transport ... 40
    of mucosal iron uptake ... 27-28
Metabolism ... 35-37, 69, 91, 96, 101, 106, 156, 185, 189, 193, 195, 199, 201
    zinc ... 3, 7, 13-14, 16, 18-19, 21-22, 24, 170, 203
Metallothioneins ... 6-7, 9, 11, 39-40, 103
Milk ... 97, 102-104, 106-108, 122, 124, 127-129, 166, 185, 189-190
    breast ... 102-104, 106-108
    cow's ... 103, 106-108, 128
Milk products ... 97, 108, 122, 124, 127, 166
Model(ing) ... 3, 5-6, 9-10, 13-14, 16, 18-22, 24, 28, 61, 89, 118, 133-135,
        142-143, 147, 185-186, 189, 196-197
Mucosa(l) ... 6, 8, 10-11, 27-31, 39-41, 53, 55-56, 95-97, 101, 104, 107, 110,
        119, 133, 166-167, 186, 195-197, 199, 202
Myoglobin ... 101, 119
Nonheme iron (*see* Iron)
Nonsaturable ... 5-6, 8, 10, 29, 46, 48, 53
NTA ... 28-31, 33, 70, 175
Oat hulls ... 147-149, 151-158, 161
Oligopeptides ... 97, 102, 105-108
Osteoporosis ... 61, 100, 179
Pancreatic juices ... 104, 155
Pancreatin ... 124-125, 174, 176, 179-180, 182
Paracellular (*see* Transport)
Parietal cells, gastric ... 173, 182
Passive transport (*see* Transport)
Pectin(s) ... 133-134, 141, 143, 194, 203
pH, gastric ... 136, 142-143, 174-176, 178-180, 182, 195
Phosphoprotein ... 102, 106, 191
Phosphorus ... 97, 99-100, 152-153, 156, 161, 166, 168-169, 198
Phytase ... 163-164, 166, 169
Phytic acid (phytate) ... 106, 123-126, 133, 142-143, 161-169, 174-180, 197-198
Picolinic acid ... 104
Pig ... 109, 143, 147-148, 151-152, 154-158
Potassium ... 122, 135-136, 149, 151-152, 154-155, 157-158, 163
Proteases ... 46, 95, 167, 169
Pump activity ... 46, 52
Pump, ATP-dependent ... 46, 48, 56, 61, 187
Rat ... 5-6, 8, 10, 21, 36-37, 39, 49, 52-53, 56, 58, 97, 100-101, 103-108,
        118, 164, 166-169, 185-190, 199-203
Rectum ... 147-148, 151-154, 158
Rickets ... 49

Saturable ... 5-6, 8, 10, 27, 48, 53
Selenium ... 109-110
Skin lesions ... 13, 103
Small intestine ... 21, 36, 41, 97, 101, 105, 126, 136-138, 155, 158, 166-168, 174, 179, 182, 185-186
Sodium ... 8, 28, 46, 70, 124, 152, 154-156, 158, 182
Soybean
    curd ... 168
    flour ... 123, 125, 127-128, 164
    formula ... 108, 127, 164, 176, 178-179, 182
    hull ... 134-138, 140-143, 148
    protein ... 102, 106, 108, 122-125, 127-128, 163-165, 176, 178-180, 182
Status, zinc ... 7, 22, 24, 105, 108, 166, 198
Stomach ... 21, 101, 106, 136-138, 142-143, 147-148, 151-155, 157-158, 166-167, 169, 173-176, 178-180
Sufficiency,
    copper ... 106
    iron ... 101, 129
Sulfur ... 109-110, 152-153, 156
Supplementation,
    ascorbic acid ... 129
    iron ... 129, 175
    zinc ... 40, 203
Tannin ... 126, 133, 143
Theophylline, effects of ... 58
Toxicity, of manganese ... 108
Transferrin ... 37, 67-73, 75-79, 81-85, 87-91, 101, 128
Transport,
    active ... 46, 48, 53, 57, 106, 161, 167, 186-189
    calcium ... 6, 8, 31, 36, 45-60, 97, 186-189
    carrier-mediated ... 41, 187
    cellular ... 3-5, 7, 10-11, 33, 46, 189
    copper ... 7, 36, 39-41, 106-107
    facilitated ... 46, 58, 97, 126, 137, 167, 187
    iron ... 27-28, 31, 33, 35-36, 40-42, 67, 69, 101, 205
    kinetics ... 5, 7-8, 10, 13, 41, 105
    mechanism ... 5-6, 8, 10, 13, 19-20, 27-28, 31, 33, 36, 40-41, 45-46, 48, 58-59, 97, 101, 108, 110, 133, 189
    membrane ... 3-6, 8-9, 28, 31, 33, 39, 46, 58-60, 88, 103, 187-188, 197
    non-facilitated ... 46
    paracellular ... 28-29, 33, 3-6, 10, 46, 48, 61, 104, 186-189
    passive ... 5, 33, 186, 189
    transcellular ... 3, 5, 8-9, 46, 61
    water ... 97, 107, 197
    zinc ... 3-11, 13-14, 18, 20, 35-36, 39-41, 88, 103, 105, 107-108
Trypsin inhibitors ... 163
Uptake, iron ... 27-33, 101, 205
Vitamin D ... 9, 45-46, 49-50, 52-55, 58-60, 96-97, 185, 187-191, 201, 203
Vitamin E ... 109

Wheat bran ... 161-162, 164, 166, 168, 175, 194, 203
Wilson's Disease ... 7, 40
Zinc ... 3-11, 16-22, 24, 74-78, 81, 83, 88-90, 102-110, 135-138, 141-142,
       163-169, 174, 176, 178-179, 182, 198-201, 203, 205
Zinc deficiency ... 5-6, 13, 40, 103, 105-106, 109-110, 198